Human Epidemiology
and Animal Laboratory Correlations
in Chemical Carcinogenesis

CURRENT TOPICS IN BIOMEDICAL RESEARCH

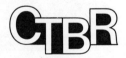

Coulston and Dunne, (Eds.) • The Potential Carcinogenicity of Nitrosatable Drugs: WHO Symposium, Geneva, June 1978, *1980*

Coulston and Shubik, (Eds.) • Human Epidemiology and Animal Laboratory Correlations in Chemical Carcinogenesis, *1980*

Human Epidemiology and Animal Laboratory Correlations in Chemical Carcinogenesis

Frederick Coulston
Philippe Shubik

editors

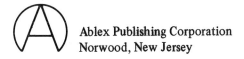

Ablex Publishing Corporation
Norwood, New Jersey

Printed in the United States of America.

Library of Congress Cataloging in Publication Data
Main entry under title:

Human epidemiology and animal laboratory
    correlations in chemical carcinogensis.

    (Current topics in biomedical research)
    Includes bibliographies and index.
    1. Carcinogenesis–Congresses.   2. Oncology,
Experimental–Congresses.   3. Epidemiology–
Congresses.   4. Cancer–Animal models–Congresses.
5. Pharmacology, Experimental–Congresses.
I. Coulston, Frederick.   II. Shubik, Philippe.
III. Series.
RC268.5.H85   616.9'94071   79-25466
ISBN 0-89391-026-0

ABLEX Publishing Corporation
355 Chestnut Street
Norwood, New Jersey 07648

Contents

Participants

Dr. C.A. Anderson
Mobay Chemical Corp.
Kansas City, Missouri

Mr. Walter Appleby
Shell Chemical Company
San Ramon, California

Mr. Marvin C. Bachman
IMC Chemical Group
Terre Haute, Indiana

Dr. Del Barth
U.S. Environmental
    Protection Agency
Washington, D.C.

Dr. Samuel Battista
Arthur D. Little
Cambridge, Massachusetts

Dr. Etcyl Blair
Dow Chemical Co.
Midland, Michigan

Dr. Charles C. Brown
National Cancer Institute
Bethesda, Maryland

Prof. Dr. K.H. Buechel
Bayer AG
Central Research
Leverkusen, GERMANY

Dr. Orhan Bulay
Eppley Institute for
    Research in Cancer
Omaha, Nebraska

Dr. John J. Burns
Hoffman-La Roche
Nutley, New Jersey

Dr. William H. Butler
St. George's Hospital Medical School
London, ENGLAND

Dr. John J. Clary
E.I. duPont de Nemours & Co.
Wilmington, Delaware

Dr. David Clayson
Eppley Institute for Research in Cancer
Omaha, Nebraska

Dr. J. Clemmesen
Institute for Cancer Epidemiology
Copenhagen, DENMARK

Dr. Allan H. Conney
Hoffman-La Roche
Nutley, New Jersey

Dr. Peter Conradt
Albany Medical College
Holloman AFB, New Mexico

Dr. Frederick Coulston
Albany Medical College
Albany, New York

Dr. Morris F. Cranmer
National Center for Toxicological
  Research
Jefferson, Arkansas

Dr. Bruce I. Doerr
Hoechst-Roussel Pharmaceuticals
Somerville, New Jersey

Dr. Alfred Farah
Sterling-Winthrop Research Institute
Rensselaer, New York

Dr. John Farmer
National Center for Toxicological
  Research
Jefferson, Arkansas

Dr. Robert Felt
Albany Medical College
Holloman AFB, New Mexico

Dr. Robert Fisher
University of Arkansas
Little Rock, Arkansas

Dr. Lawrence Fishbein
National Center for Toxicological
  Research
Jefferson, Arkansas

Dr. James Flanders
Hercules Incorporated
Wilmington, Delaware

Dr. Edgar M. Flint
Ciba-Geigy Corporation
Ardsley, New York

Dr. Ralph Gingell
Eppley Institute for Research in Cancer
Omaha, Nebraska

Prof. Dr. Miki Goto
Gakushuin University
Tokyo, JAPAN

Dr. Peter Greenwald
New York State Department of
  Health
Albany, New York

Dr. Travis B. Griffin
Albany Medical College
Holloman AFB, New Mexico

Dr. Walter H. Grimes
Mobay Chemical Corporation
Kansas City, Missouri

Dr. E. Cuyler Hammond
American Cancer Society
New York, New York

Dr. Manfred Herbst
C.H. Boehringer Sohn
Ingelheim am Rhein, GERMANY

Dr. Donald Hill
University of Arkansas
Little Rock, Arkansas

Dr. Benjamin Holder
Dow Chemical Company
Midland, Michigan

Ms. Rose Houle
Albany Medical College
Albany, New York

Dr. Jerry Hutton
Foremost Foods Company
San Francisco, California

Dr. Klaus W. Jager
Shell Internationale Research
The Hague, Netherlands

Dr. Charles J. Kensler
Arthur D. Little, Inc.
Cambridge, Massachusetts

Dr. A. Fred Kerst
Velsicol Chemical Corporation
Chicago, Illinois

Dr. Werner Klein
Gesellschaft fur Strahlen-und
  Umweltf.m.b.h.
Neurherberg, GERMANY

Dr. Albert C. Kolbye, Jr.
Food and Drug Administration
Washington, D.C.

Dr. Herman F. Kraybill
National Cncer Institute
Bethesda, Maryland

Ms. Joanna Lowry
National Center for Toxicological
   Research
Jefferson, Arkansas

Dr. Frank C. Lu
University of Miami
Coral Cables, Florida

Dr. Joseph Lyon
University of Utah
Salt Lake City, Utah

Dr. Peter Magee
Fels Research Institute
Philadelphia, Pennsylvania

Ms. Ruth S. Magee
National Center for Toxicological
   Research
Jefferson, Arkansas

Dr. Ezzat Mahboubi
Eppley Institute for Research in Cancer
Omaha, Nebraska

Dr. E. Truman Mays
University of Kentucky
Lexington, Kentucky

Dr. James A. Miller
McArdle Laboratory for Cancer
   Research
Madison, Wisconsin

Dr. Carol Mitchell
University of Arkansas
Little Rock, Arkansas

Dr. Ch. Mofidi
University of Tehran
Tehran, IRAN

Prof. Dr. Ulrich Mohr
Med. Hochschule Hannover
Hannover, GERMANY

Dr. Roscoe M. Moore, Jr.
National Institute for
   Occupational Safety and Health
Rockville, Maryland

Dr. Emil Mrak
University of California
Davis, California

Dr. Robert E. Mrak
Vanderbilt University
Nashville, Tennessee

Dr. Wolfgang Mueller
Albany Medical College
Holloman AFB, New Mexico

Dr. Vaun A. Newill
Exxon Corporation
Linden, New Jersey

Dr. Maureen T. O'Berg
E.I. duPont deNemours & Company
Wilmington, Delaware

Dr. Lawrence Plumlee
U.S. Environmental Protection Agency
Washington, D.C.

Prof. Dr. R. Preussmann
Deutsches Krebsforschungszentrum
Heidelberg, GERMANY

Dr. Parviz Pour
Eppley Institute for Research in Cancer
Omaha, Nebraska

Ms. Sandra Rankin
National Center for Toxicological
   Research
Jefferson, Arkansas

Dr. Ira Rosenblum
Albany Medical College
Albany, New York

Dr. Herbert C. Rosenkilde
Hoechst-Roussel Pharmaceuticals
Somerville, New Jersey

Dr. Karoly Rozman
Albany Medical College
Holloman AFB, New Mexico

Dr. Theodore Sandberg
Mobay Chemical Corporation
Kansas City, Missouri

Dr. Irving J. Selikoff
Mount Sinai School of Meicine
New York, New York

Dr. Thomas Shellenberger
National Center for Toxicological
   Research
Jefferson, Arkansas

Dr. Charles J. Krister
E.I. duPont deNemours & Company
Wilmington, Delaware

Dr. Donald Lamb
Mobay Chemical Corporation
Kansas City, Missouri

Dr. Dale Lindsay
Tucson, Arizona

Dr. Philippe Shubik
Eppley Institute for Research in Cancer
Omaha, Nebraska

Dr. M.J. Sloan
Shell Chemical Company
Washington, D.C.

Dr. M.B. Slomka
Shell Chemical Company
San Ramon, California

Dr. James T. Stevens
Ciba-Geigy Corporation
Greensboro, North Carolina

Dr. D.E. Stevenson
Shell Toxicology Laboratory
   (Tunstall)
Sittingbourne, Kent, U.K.

Dr. E. Thorpe
Shell Toxicology Laboratory
   (Tunstall)
Sittingbourne, Kent, U.K.

Prof. Dr. Rene Truhaut
Universite Rene Descartes
Paris, FRANCE

Dr. William M. Upholt
U.S. Environmental Protection Agency
Washington, D.C.

Dr. H.G.S. van Raalte
Shell Internationale Research
The Hague, NETHERLANDS

Dr. J. Henry Wills
National Institute for
   Occupational Safety and Health
Rockville, Maryland

Dr. Ernst L. Wynder
American Health Foundation
New York, New York

Dr. John A. Zapp, Jr.
E.I. duPont deNemours & Company
Wilmington, Delaware

Human Epidemiology
and Animal Laboratory Correlations
in Chemical Carcinogenesis

DR. COULSTON: It's a great pleasure for me on behalf of Drs. Shubik, Mrak, and Cranmer to welcome you to the Inn of the Mountain Gods. Last night, it looked as if the Gods were saying something to us, but today the sky is clear and, hopefully, we can proceed on a good note and have our meeting.

I wish to make a few opening remarks that I think are important. You are probably all wondering what the International Academy of Environmental Safety is, and I'd like to mention that this is a group which was organized some five years ago in Munich, Germany, and limited to 100 members worldwide. There are many members of this academy in the audience, and we are fortunate to have the president of the academy with us today, Dr. Mrak, who will say a few words later.

This group was formed simply to provide a forum to discuss certain pertinent and important problems in the field of drugs, food additives, health effects, and environmental quality and safety.

We are here this morning primarily through the good offices of the supporting group, which is the National Center of Toxicological Research. We are all indebted to them for their good offices in providing much of the support for this meeting, but even more than that for their good sense in recognizing the importance of this meeting.

The cochairman of this meeting, Dr. Shubik, must be mentioned, with many thanks from all of us for his good wishes and help in organizing the meeting. I hope in his opening remarks he will set the tone for the entire meeting.

A key issue today, at least in the United States, is the prediction of chemical carcinogenesis from animal data to man. We've all struggled with this problem over the years and there is as yet no real answer, it seems to me. The real answer in the final analysis will be human experience, since we cannot do studies on man with so-called chemical carcinogens, except in cases where the subjects already have cancer. Some of you might be interested to know that we can use true, absolute, chemical carcinogens for the treatment of cancer. This is a paradox, of course, but it is a fact. Several chemicals have been designated as human carcinogens based on this kind of therapy for the treatment of cancer. The issue to be still resolved is, How to predict from animals to man?

Obviously, human epidemiology is a good answer, if we could do proper epidemiological studies at least on compounds that have been around for a long time. With this information, we certainly should be able to guess, if not know, whether a particular chemical is a hazard to man or not. In the case of new chemicals, this, of course, is very difficult to do, if possible at all; but, we can also rely on experience within the factory itself where exposure may or may not take place, depending on the good practices in the factory and the protection of the workers.

The issue then really comes back to the animal. What is the animal model that really predicts correctly to man, and can we arrive at some kind of a solution to the problem? If we find a mouse on a very high dose with cancer in a lifespan study, but at lower doses we find absolutely nothing, should we ignore this? If the high dose is at the maximum tolerated level, it is really an LD_5 in the final analysis.

1

Then, indeed, we have to ask ourselves, is there a dose-response effect for a chemical carcinogen? Can you have a no-effect level based on lifespan studies in animals? Are there quicker ways to tell? All of these ramifications should be the substance of our program.

The key feature of our program is the bringing together of epidemiologists and animal research toxicologists to discuss—around a table, so to speak—the nature of the basic problem. It is very difficult to get toxicologists and epidemiologists to sit down together. I have tried before and others have also. We have been able to bring to this meeting a proper balance between good epidemiology and good animal laboratory practice. Hopefully, this will lead to the kind of understanding that will benefit us when we leave a few days from now.

It gives me great pleasure at this time to introduce the current president of the International Academy of Environmental Safety, a man I really don't need to introduce to you, you all know him, Dr. Emil Mrak.

DR. MRAK: Thank you, Fred. My comments will be very brief. The International Academy has been a fairly active organization in bringing groups of this type together. I'm very enthusiastic about this because it brings together people from around the world. We've had meetings not only in the U.S., but in Germany, France, Japan, and I've forgotten where else. But in the international community and in international thinking there's strength, and I find that there is less emotional thinking outside the United States than inside. At times it's very important to divorce emotional thinking from what I call realistic thinking.

Now our decisions are often made frankly on the basis of emotions, but if you talk to the decision-makers—do I see any here?—they will probably deny this. I have had several talks with administrators of EPA and FDA, among others, and they have said at times there may be overriding factors such as social, economic, political, and aesthetic; they don't admit that emotional aspects are taken into account.

I've always argued that it's okay; if you want to do it on that basis be sure that you have scientific input, tell the world about the scientific input, and then be honest in telling them what the basis for the real decision was.

So it's my hope that a meeting of this type will influence the decision-making one way or another, will produce world thinking divorced of emotion, and get sound and reasonable thinking into the picture. I think this will happen here and I really am very happy about the group that Dr. Coulston has brought together; I compliment him, Dr. Shubik, and Dr. Cranmer very much. Thank you all for coming.

DR. COULSTON: I would like now to turn over the meeting to Morris Cranmer for a few remarks. I'm sure he will have something important to say.

DR. CRANMER: I think it is absolutely appropriate that NCTR be able to join with the International Academy of Environmental Safety to put on this particular meeting. The mission of the National Center is to develop methods and protocols, to produce capabilities of extrapolating from high doses to low doses, and develop better information on the ability to extrapolate from experimental animal to man.

Of course, our particular activities are centered around the use of experimental animals and the prediction of risk to man, rather than in epidemiological studies. But the meeting of the two methods for safety evaluation is absolutely essential. I think in all of our opinions we're able to glean from both areas in better estimating human risk.

There will be times when it will be convenient and appropriate to be able to use animal studies in such a way that a potential chemical carcinogen is excluded from the environment. In other words, the societal need for a particular compound, once it's determined that it has a carcinogenic risk associated with it, will not be great enough for that compound to be manufactured. There will be other times when the manufacturer of these compounds, even knowing that there is some associated risk, will find it necessary to market them. The case of lifesaving drugs may be an example. There will be still other examples where there are compounds in the environment not likely to be removed in the near future, and which we know carry a carcinogenic risk. If we're to allocate our limited resources for public health appropriately, it will be necessary to estimate those risks more accurately than we are doing today.

So, it seems to me that the epidemiologists, working with human populations and collecting information, are able to produce part of the data to answer the problem. Since these studies are complicated by many uncontrollable variables, the animal toxicologist enters the scene. When we are better able to understand mechanistically the relationships between selected animal models and man, we will be able to estimate those risks with greater accuracy.

Therefore, it's with great enthusiasm that NCTR joins with the International Academy in putting on this meeting. I think I would be remiss if I didn't tell you a short story about how the discussions of such a meeting originally started. Fred Coulston, Bob Pfizer, Don Hill, and myself, and several of our colleagues in the Department of Pediatrics at the University of Arkansas Medical Sciences campus, were visiting Fred's laboratory, which I hope you will take advantage of visiting, because it is absolutely a unique facility and some great work is going on there. At any rate, we were there one evening discussing great scientific issues, as you might imagine. Bob Pfizer suggested that Mescalero would be an absolutely perfect place for a meeting, and various topics were suggested. I think Bob's final and best offer was "Pediatrics for the Aged," but Dr. Coulston thought the particular problem that we are addressing today might be the best even though past efforts had been, in several people's opinion, not very successful in bringing these groups together.

I must really compliment Dr. Shubik and Dr. Coulston for the fine work they've done in putting the program together, and thank you for the opportunity of speaking to you.

DR. COULSTON: Before I proceed, there is one man at this end of the room that I think we would like to hear from, and I'm sure he'd like to say something. There are in this room some of the real pioneers in the field of toxicology, such as Phil Shubik, John Zapp, Charles Kristor, Herman Kraybill, Dale Lindsay, and Charles Kensler. I'm not going to put Peter Magee in that group because he's too young, but as I look around the room I can pick out some first-class people, who made modern toxicology possible.

But one from abroad that has been a pioneer from the start has been Dr. René Truhaut. I would like him to say a few words about whatever he wants to talk about, related to the subject of the meeting. Dr. Truhaut, please.

DR. TRUHAUT: May I say how pleased I am to be here attending a meeting where famous scientists are present, and supplement those who have already taken the floor. I am pleased for several reasons. First, I think personally that a risk of carcinogenicity to man is one of the most important problems to look at for a number of years; I have strongly favored the safe evaluation of chemical carcinogenicity risks.

But on the other hand, I have been impressed in recent years to see how people have been exaggerating this risk, and I say now that sometimes—in international meetings I have said to some of my old friends—they were too emotional. One of them turned as if to strangle me, because he said, "You told me I am emotional," and I said "I don't know, because I am emotional myself." This man said "emotional" in English, which at least means unscientific, without science at all. Please forgive me.

But by the way, the man I told you was emotional was very scientific in the strict sense of the term. When I explained to him—French science is emotional—he said, "Instead of strangling you, I will kiss you." My answer was, "If you would have been a pretty girl I would have said yes, but now I say no."

Now, being serious, I think that this meeting is very important, to put into the right perspective the problem of predicting carcinogenicity to man. Some day we will restrict or ban light because solar light is a carcinogen, too, and this means really we have to be at the same time competent to be rigid, to be cautious, but also reasonable. It is all I will say at the moment, Professor Coulston, but I wanted to say this because we have to be in the middle. To be rigid, to protect the health of the people; on the other hand, not to be stupid. I am crazy about carcinogenicity, but I am not stupid as a consequence. Thank you very much.

DR. COULSTON: I hope we will have extensive discussion and that this discussion will be the keynote of this meeting.

1. Statement of the Problem

Philippe Shubik
Eppley Institute for Research in Cancer
University of Nebraska Medical Center
Omaha, Nebraska

DR. SHUBIK: Thank you very much, Fred, for the wonderful introduction. This is a sort of "Alice in Wonderland" approach where you congratulate people in advance. I think we should delete all the congratulations and wait until after the talk and see how things come along. This is a hackneyed subject by now; it is extraordinarily difficult to really add much new.

Let me at the outset congratulate people on finding this wonderful place in which to have the meeting. I would like to say that I was unable to find it yesterday when I started out from El Paso. I certainly cannot take any of the credit at all for the one established fact I think will emerge, and that is that we are in a very beautiful place. Perhaps we can do something about the schedule, Professor Coulston, to allow these nice people to have an hour or two, perhaps in the afternoon, in which to appreciate this scenery, take a walk, and perhaps even float out onto the lake or do something else equally dangerous.

I would also like to say that the responsibility for a great part of this program fell upon the very broad shoulders of Dr. Mahboubi, who is the epidemiologist at the Eppley Institute. Perhaps Dr. Mahboubi could stand so we could thank him because, frankly, Dr. Mahboubi and also Dr. Clayson did an enormous amount of work in getting this program put together. I can take relatively little credit except for some initial discussions and laying out the program and, I think, having a lot of enthusiasm for the sorts of things we are trying to achieve.

We have on numerous occasions tried to get epidemiologists and lab people together, and up to this point I do not believe we can claim to have had any singular success. Perhaps we will change the picture; time will tell. But my thanks to everybody for getting us all together in this very fine place.

The meeting as far as I'm concerned has the prime requirement for success in this day and age. Every time I started to write my introductory remarks I discovered I was out of date because so much had happened this week or the week before. This is reflected in the basic approach that we've had to develop during our short stay with the Mountain Gods, who one hopes will be of more assistance to us than, for example, our friends in Congress, who seem to know more and more about the management and objectives of scientists as every day passes.

It hardly seems possible that this meeting was actually conceived before everything started to remind one of saccharin. We—and I speak for many people but not all—have been so proud of the fact that at long last someone had been imaginative enough to devise a study of a food additive in man and seemingly to demonstrate a lack of carcinogenic activity. This all happened a very, very long time ago and appears to have been relegated to the type of publication, I believe, is often called a fairy story, not all of which I think have happy endings.

There have been a series of meetings dealing with saccharin along with numerous congressional hearings, and now our friends at the Office of Technology Assessment have done a rapid evaluation of the story of which I have yet to hear the results. For some strange reason that I'm entirely unable to fathom, those epidemiologists who are most involved with the studies of the possible carcinogenicity of saccharin in man have chosen essentially to remain silent and have not appeared at various meetings, nor have their names been prominently mentioned in the discussion of the issues.

Indeed, ever since the Canadian Health Protection Branch drew attention to the fact that, whether we like it or not, there is a problem with saccharin, the most vociferous and I think the most cogent epidemiologists and biometrists have been those who have pointed to the not inconsiderable problems of undertaking studies with diabetic populations and standardizing for their peculiarities, the taking of large quantities of saccharin being only one.

Dr. Schneiderman's testimony before a Senate committee recently, for example, cannot be dismissed. Dr. Muir of the International Agency for Research on Cancer at a recent meeting of the World Health Organization held in conjunction with the Toxicology Forum took note of the studies of Doll and his coworkers and concluded that, although it would be justifiable to feel that a high incidence of cancer as a result of taking saccharin had probably been excluded, by no means had low incidences in normal populations been shown surely not to be a potential hazard.

However, to put the matter into a practical context, Dr. Muir also said, in response to a question, that he would not rate highly the potential carcinogenicity of saccharin to man, any more than I would. In fact, he said he wouldn't really like to put that on his agenda as the sort of problem he felt worth tackling. It still leaves us with the problem, and I hope somehow we will thrash out some of this during the course of this meeting.

This meeting represents one of several attempts on my part to get epidemiologists and lab workers together. This objective I now rate as No. 1 priority to our society in dealing reasonably with the problems in toxicology that beset us. It is not enough to take the relaxed attitude recently expounded to me by a reasonable and able toxicologist (not present in this room) who still found it possible to work with the U.S. federal government.

This toxicologist felt that in the not too distant future the severity of our toxicological regulations may well have caused such obvious economic havoc that our attitude will have to be changed. I hope that we will not get to that stage and that science will prevail and retain its credibility. I think that before us today our first problem is the retention of the credibility of scientists and medical men in the area of toxicology.

In the course of the meeting, we hope to outline a series of situations amenable to additional study, either by the epidemiologist or by the animal experimentalist, that will provide us with complete packages and a basis for placing more reliance on individual components of the evaluation of hazards.

Let me say here in this introductory talk that I'm going to be quite selective; I'm not going to deal with problems and mechanisms in biochemistry which will be dealt with by others but to which I do give an enormously high priority.

We have before us examples of chemical carcinogenesis studies in which there are pointers from either epidemiological investigations or from animal studies, but the total picture is not amenable to complete understanding. Even the most complete cases still provide a lot of leeway for additional study.

Let me illustrate the point in a boring and old-fashioned way by starting with a discussion of the first chemical carcinogen to be discovered. The demonstration that coal tar was carcinogenic was made by Yamagiwa and Ichikawa in 1915 as a result of their familiarity with the observations of Percival Pott in 1776. We would like to shorten this latent period between the reaction of the laboratory worker and the observations of the clinical man. I think 150 years is a little too long. The studies of Yamagawa and Ichikawa were carried out in the rabbit. Tar was applied to the skin and, incidentally, a meticulous account provided the pathology and life history of the tumors induced.

Indeed, the paper bears rereading from time to time since much of it has been repeated. Much of the work of Peyton Rous and myself and others, in fact, had partly been done by these people.

A few years later another Japanese investigator, Dr. Tsutsui, induced skin tumors in the mouse. Within a few years Murphy and Sturm at the Rockefeller Institute observed that not only did the painted mice develop skin tumors but they also developed lung tumors, the first report of lung adenomas in mice.

My mentor, Dr. Berenblum, noted that there was a considerable discrepancy between the effects of coal tar on the mouse and on the rabbit, the rabbit being much more sensitive. This sensitivity was measured by the rapidity with which skin tumors appeared. Berenblum had become intrigued by the fact that the carcinogen benzo(a)pyrene, isolated from coal tar by Kennaway and Cook and assumed to be the active principle of coal tar, was, in point of fact, more potent in the mouse than in the rabbit. The opposite was true of coal tar. In fact it was found to be quite difficult to induce tumors in the rabbit with benzo(a)pyrene by injection, and induction in the skin was much, much slower than with coal tar.

My first study (in which, as a result of strange British legislation, I was not allowed to touch an animal until, after some months, I'd managed to find two members of the Royal Society to sign my application for a license) consisted of fractionating a barrel of coal tar provided by Dr. Berenblum from the Leeds gas works where the coal tar is carcinogenic. I was asked to follow up the observations of Berenblum and Schoental, that fractions of coal tar containing no benzo(a)pyrene were singularly carcinogenic to the skin of the rabbit but not to the mouse.

The active principle in this fraction of coal tar (that has no benzo(a)pyrene in it and happens to be the material that produces the tumors Yamagawa and Ichikawa were looking at) has not yet been isolated and identified in mice.

Dr. Wallcave and I are still toying with the idea of finishing the study, which is much more amenable to solution now than it was 30 years ago, when we didn't have mass spectrometers, and so forth.

The fact remains that we still do not know the nature of the active principle of the first carcinogenic mixture to be identified. Is this important? Well, I think so and will point out why for those to whom the answer is not apparent.

If we know that benzo(a)pyrene is not the active principle in rabbit skin carcinogenesis, we certainly do not know whether it, or the unknown factor, gives rise to rapid carcinogenesis. There is, as you know, a widespread assumption that benzo(a)pyrene is unequivocally a carcinogen to man. Indeed, documents produced by our learned organization, the National Academy of Sciences, have used benzo(a)pyrene as a standard from which detailed calculations of the level of human hazard are deduced. There are many prolonged and painstaking mathematical deductions made on this basis. In some countries automobile exhaust emissions are gauged for level of hazard using benzo(a)pyrene studies. I think these assumptions are all totally and absolutely unwarranted.

Another area of ignorance concerns the possible systemic effects of exposure to coal tars and related products. Although there is good skin cancer data from British registries, there is little good information on the systemic effect of these compounds. Perhaps the new emphasis on occupational cancer will change all that; and I'm sure Dr. Selikoff, who I understand is coming tomorrow, will know much more about recent advances than I do.

In any event, our animal studies tell us that these compounds, when applied to the skin, not only have a local effect but also cause lung tumors, lymphomas, mammary tumors, etc. They seem to have a local inducing effect, giving rise to neoplastic lesions seen only rarely or not at all in the test animal, and in addition do enhance the incidence of tumors usually seen in that species.

Does this happen in man? Do carcinogens have this double effect in man, or not? Here is an example, then, that has not really been followed through. Perhaps someone at the meeting might be able to answer the question, or at least decide how an answer may be obtained.

So much for coal tar, except to say that problems applicable to it are quite the same for a range of petroleum products. The catalytically cracked residues of petroleum have both animal and human data similar to those for the tars, except that there is somewhat more chemical analytical data. However, once again there is no pinning down of the exact nature of the active principle. Dr. Saffiotti and I studied the rabbit-mouse difference and found that it also occurred with fractions of catalytically cracked petroleum. In this instance we managed to find a carcinogenic fraction that was active alone in the rabbit, but only served as a potent promoting agent in the mouse.

Again, there's a lack of full knowledge of the systemic effects of these agents. As a matter of fact, we tried to isolate the promoting factor in this fraction way back when but didn't have the chemical know-how.

In the instance of the petroleum carcinogens, it's vitally important to know the nature of the active factors so the materials from the petroleum industry (and there are many of them) can be assessed for potential carcinogenic hazard by chemical analysis rather than by long-term bioassay in animals.

I think it's quite apparent that the cigarette problem inherently has many of the problems that I've described for the coal tars and petroleum products. Clearly, we still do not have a good animal model for the most important and well-established hazard to man. We have a national program for designing a safe cigarette based on the assay of tobacco tars on the skin of the mouse. I suppose if one had to choose between a tobacco tar that caused many tumors and one that caused none, one would be on reasonable ground suggesting the latter would likely be safer.

I have considerable doubt, however, that meaningful conclusions can be drawn from minimal quantitative differences observed in such a system. As with coal tar, we haven't the slightest idea of the active principle, if indeed there is one and not several.

Here we have a picture of a mixture containing polycyclic hydrocarbons, heterocyclic hydrocarbons, aromatic amines, nitrosamines, hydrazines, radioactive polonium, and as I have just recently learned, saccharin in the cigarette filters. In fact, I understand that one-third of all saccharin production goes into cigarette filters.

And, of course, some active promoters and without a doubt more new carcinogens will be discovered, if not by the end of this meeting, at least by next week.

In the hamster lung, it seems as though dibenzo(cg)carbazole, as well as one of the dibenzopyrenes, is a much more potent lung carcinogen than are other compounds. We don't know why this is, but it's certainly interesting.

Obviously, we need years and years of work on this problem. It might well be the wrong one to pick. It might turn out to be much too complicated for detailed analysis.

On the other hand, it is a situation for which the most human evidence is at hand. We do have the best quantitative data for man, and we're now about to compare the safe cigarettes with the old kind. I'm sure Dr. Wynder will be able to say something about this very thrilling development.

I think we should be thinking hard about how we can use these comparisons. We have evidence that cigarettes are not only associated with lung cancer but also with bladder cancer in man. Can we design studies to elucidate some of the questions here? It is possible that there is a problem of different carcinogens acting.

I think that by now all of you will have thought of enough experiments with this one model to enable us to start another industry.

The matter of what happens to smokers is a fundamental issue to students of carcinogenesis. Some early studies into the stages of carcinogenesis that I was privileged to undertake demonstrated that a single application of a subeffective dose of a carcinogen resulted in an irreversible change on the skin that persisted for the lifetime of the mouse.

When mice started to live longer in a more opulent society, it was found that this wasn't exactly so. Recent examination of the matter leaves it fractionally up in the air. The effect persists for at least 43 weeks.

You apply a carcinogen on the mouse in a subeffective dose and do nothing for 43 weeks; then you apply a promoting agent, such as phorbol ester, and you get the same number of tumors as if you put it on the day after you applied the carcinogen.

However, after a time some of the effects perhaps disappear, but not in a way that's really convincing. Intervening factors occur that make the study on mice difficult to interpret as if it were being done in man.

It would seem likely, however, that carcinogenesis is a similar, basic biological phenomenon in mouse and in human lung, and the effect is essentially an irreversible one. The exposure, even though stopped, carries a risk, although it is apparently reduced little by little. I think more comparative studies of this sort are absolutely essential.

When it was first shown that isoniazid was capable of inducing lung adenomas in mice, it seemed more than reasonable to suggest that the significance of this animal study could be translated to man. There were at that time many, many people who had been treated with isoniazid, so meetings were arranged with the National Cancer Institute. In fact, this was one of my earlier efforts to get things along these lines done. The Veterans Administration was consulted since they had records on perhaps half a million people treated with isoniazid. The sad conclusion of our discussions was that there was no profit in trying to use these data since (a) they were complicated by the presence of tuberculosis, (b) no normals treated with isoniazid could be found, (c) the tubercular scars were said in the old pathological literature to be associated with cancer of the lung, (d) the tuberculosis patients had been X-rayed with much greater frequency than the general population, and (e) the patients had usually been given additional drugs, such as streptomycin. For none of these situations could controls be found.

It was concluded that the retrospective study of the material would be unlikely to yield results. As a matter of fact, I believe somebody came up with a figure of 3 million cases needed to provide us with some sort of reasonable levels.

I'd like to hear that discussed and perhaps have different views expressed during the meeting. It was concluded that a retrospective study was not a good idea. A prospective study of children given prophylactic isoniazid was then recommended. Such a study was begun. I really don't know what's happened to it; perhaps someone can tell us some more about it now.

There are a series of drugs known to be carcinogenic in animals which have not been studied in man which will be discussed tomorrow.

In addition to those on the program, there are many others of considerable interest which I shall mention in passing, and I'm sure Dr. Clayson will deal with them in much more detail. I include griseofulvin, apparently carcinogenic in rats as well as in mice. It has been administered not only to many patients in this country and others, but also prophylactically to a large proportion of the U.S. army in Vietnam.

The antischistosomal drug, niridazole, a matter of considerable concern to Dr. Clayson and myself, as well as to Dr. Bulay who is here with us, represents a situation in which I believe animal data should be taken into epidemiology straight away. Niridazole is an antischistosomal drug; it is unequivocally carcinogenic to many tissues in three species.

A matter for consideration for the remainder of today is persistent chlorinated hydrocarbon pesticides. Isn't it reasonable to believe that the carcinogenic effects of DDT, if they applied to man, would have been manifested by now? We know of occupational groups exposed to very large doses of DDT, of geographical differences of exposure of several-fold. Not only do we know of these differences, but they can be confirmed by knowledge of levels of the compound in body fat.

These data do not seem to have been assembled for detailed evaluation of human risk. I wonder about this quite often, and I'm sure I'm going to find out why this hasn't been done in the course of this meeting, or perhaps that is has, and that I just don't know about it.

We're discussing the incredible state of affairs that exists in the instance of estrogenic hormones. When the birth control pill was first tested in rodents on any scale, induction of hepatomas was reported. This finding was not considered applicable to humans and indeed was officially said to be of no consequence in a report from Britain.

Somehow, the subject was not mentioned in this country at all. Recent reports demonstrate to the satisfaction of all those epidemiologists whom I know that there *is* an association between the occurrence of benign hepatomas in young women and the taking of the birth control pill.

At last we seem to be confronted with a complete package and must only elucidate the level of risk we are to encounter. For the moment we seem to have succeeded in being exceptionally nonchalant about the whole subject, when one considers the level of hysteria that can be engendered by something like TRIS.

On my wanderings from El Paso to this beautiful place yesterday I turned on the radio, and the first announcement was from some gentleman at Georgetown University, I believe, who was quoted as saying there was now unequivocal evidence that there was no carcinogenic potential whatsoever from the contraceptive pill and any such suggestion should be totally discounted. He had finally put together all the data in one big package, and he told everyone all was fine. What are these benign tumors that occur? I don't think that this man felt that one should be terribly worried about them.

Now I really don't know why one has to face this kind of curious dichotomy and schizophrenia in our population. There are problems here, there are problems in other places, and why we can't sit down and treat them in a proper and scientific way is beyond anyone's understanding.

Aflatoxins are among the few carcinogenic chemicals discovered in laboratory animals for which there is starting to be corresponding human data that might even eventuate in practical knowledge of safe levels for man. It would seem more than reasonable to believe that more and more carcinogens of natural origin will be found and will be shown to be of great importance in the origin of human cancer.

Recently, my colleague, Dr. Bela Toth, in a series of experiments pursued with enormous determination, demonstrated that there are potent carcinogens of the hydrazine group, particularly N-methylformylhydrazine, found in certain edible mushrooms.

Clearly, these observations open the way to various correlated studies in animals and man and provide for many conjectures on possible causes of well-established geographical differences. There are enormous differences in the eating of mushrooms around the world; and since the mushroom eaters and mushroom collectors are a group of people who get together quite a bit, they seem to know an awful lot about the sorts of things that are eaten and the things they poison themselves with from time to time, and how to avoid being poisoned, and so forth.

So there are some interesting studies to be done and, for certain, reasons for having meetings in even more amusing places as time goes on. I, in fact, have been faced recently with various requests for attending mushroom-hunting expeditions as part of cancer research. It seems to have come quite a long way.

We obviously will not have time to delve into each and every carcinogen discovered. The well-established occupational carcinogens, particularly the aromatic amines, have singularly interesting species specificities and dose requirements.

Although some of the more potent of these carcinogens, β-naphthylamine for example, seem to require only minute levels to induce cancer in man, it seems very large doses are required to induce bladder cancers in dogs and hamsters.

I have my personal doubts about some of the conclusions drawn from human studies in this instance and believe that here is a really fruitful area for additional research. I go to meetings from time to time and hear people chatter about β-naphthylamine and, way back when, Dr. Michael Williams used to tell us about his observations and the amount of β-naphthylamine he felt man had been exposed to, and the number of years it required to cause cancer. There is a vast compendium of evidence in this case about possible contamination of β-naphthylamine with other materials, for example with α-naphthylamine, making exact understanding difficult.

It seems to me that this area is one that needs to be focused on, that we really need to know in great detail exactly what these figures are because everything that one sees in the animal seems to indicate that β-naphthylamine, as far as I'm concerned, is a weak carcinogen. It's a weak carcinogen in the hamster; it needs at least 1% to produce tumors. In most of the dog studies, a very large amount was needed. Dr. Clayson and I have somewhat divergent views on this. We want to hear about it and discuss it and the other aromatic amines, because I think it's with examples like that—it's with real persistence—really going into the details, that we are going to find the crucial answers to the crucial questions of how much of these carcinogens are required, and learn something about the exact conditions of exposure, and so forth.

Indeed, it leads one straight into the question of what sorts of carcinogens are there, and are we going to be able to classify carcinogens in a meaningful manner into the various subgroups in which they belong, since they are not all the same? They obviously need different levels, different conditions of exposure, different cofactors and heaven knows what else, and at our present stage we must find out how to subclassify them. Perhaps the biochemists will be able to help us, since certainly we have situations in which biochemical mechanisms do not seem to be applicable across the board to some of those compounds which are being called carcinogens for regulatory purposes.

The data and the experimental evidence about vinyl chloride seem to me to provide a wonderful basic model system for the determination of the levels of exposure that correlate with human hazard.

Here again, it seems to me, we have a discrepancy between animal data and human data. There are these extremely low levels that Dr. Maltoni has reported as producing tumors in animals, and from anything that one sees of the human data it would appear that only men exposed to very large doses have, so far, developed cancer. It is always possible that later on there will be more men with cancer, possibly associated with lower levels of exposure to vinyl chloride, but it is the kind of thing that I think one needs to study very, very closely and look at the two systems together. The vinylidene chloride story coming along now, I think, again must be looked at very closely, and the two situations, the animal and the human situation, again meticulously compared.

The area that I think holds the most potential terror and should be at the top of the list is the subject that was to have been discussed by the man who was to have been the next speaker, Dr. Selikoff, and tomorrow he will get to that, namely, the question of asbestos.

There is absolutely no question that there is more and more asbestos around all the time—in the air, in water in food. It is absolutely essential that we have a proper scientific basis for the calculation of safe levels. Obviously, there have to be levels of safety. From everything we know, there must be.

Clearly, right now our animal models are totally and absolutely inadequate to answer all the obvious questions before us. We do not know clearly whether or not asbestos is indeed carcinogenic by mouth, in spite of the recent pronouncement in the IARC monograph which I hope will not be taken too seriously. I find it extremely bothersome that a group would have, in my view, misinterpreted some animal studies to say that they, in fact, feel that asbestos can be found to be carcinogenic by mouth.

I'm extraordinarily unhappy that Dr. Selikoff is not here so that we can set the stage for discussion of the real story with oral ingestion of asbestos. Dr. Selikoff, I think, now does not believe in his initial data on ingestion. I hope I'm not misquoting him, but this is what he's told me. The data in man apparently does not substantiate his original view that cancer in the gastrointestinal tract is associated with asbestos in occupational exposure.

I don't really believe there's any evidence to tell us that asbestos is, in fact, a hazard when taken by mouth, and neither is there animal work, I think, that says anything about that. Insofar as the levels of asbestos are concerned in lung carcinogenesis, there again we obviously have a series of terribly difficult problems—especially with the association of cigarette smoking in the instance of bronchogenic carcinoma. It seems to be an enormously important concomitant factor. Is it really necessary all the time? Probably not, but one doesn't really have the figures. There, again, is a sort of priority item which we really must know about. With asbestos accumulating in our general environment every day of our lives, obviously we need to know whether or not we are dealing with something real.

It is, I think, quite obvious that there are going to be a series of situations in which we will have toxicological data from the laboratory as a basis for regulatory decision-making. However, our model systems will have to be much more thoroughly evaluated before they can continue to be expanded, and perhaps one of the most important tasks that faces us now is the validation of these systems in general terms.

Recent studies with saccharin that have employed two-generation studies in rodents at high dose levels have posed a series of serious questions that cannot just be dismissed. One does not know the precise meaning of these studies. There is, of course, the hepatoma story which is now being joined by the bladder carcinogenesis story. What is the mechanism in these cases?

Here is a situation in which one has to underwrite a large amount of really good, basic research—biochemical, experimental, pathological, and so forth. I was really shaken, and am still shaken, by the fact that no one knows whether or not saccharin can get into cells. With 15 million dollars worth of toxicology done in the laboratory on a single substance for carcinogenicity, no one has bothered to take saccharin and find out whether or not saccharin crosses the cell membrane and goes into the cell.

At two meetings in which almost everybody concerned with saccharin was present, no one could answer that question. Someone forgot to look for it.

The question of the two-generation study is one that's going to prove particularly complicating when we find that everything that's been tested before is going to be retested by a method that will increase our sensitivity. Maximal tolerated dose levels may be effectively increased, possibly by several hundred-fold, by the use of this method as one example.

Opposing that, of course, we have a situation in which there are many, many substances that could be toxic to the fetus that have never been tested transplacentally, so there is a great need for transplacental studies.

But I think these methods have to be thought about with immense care, and the kind of method used contemplated and tailored to the conditions of use; the toxicologists should have the leeway to do this in the proper way and not just plunge straight into the kind of mindless two-generation study used in the saccharin situation.

The rapid test methods again are a major issue to the toxicologists, and with this as with transplacental studies, in the long run only a real knowledge of the mechanism or mechanisms of carcinogenesis is going to enable us to prognosticate what these things really mean.

For the moment we're stuck with more and more empiricism, and perhaps the only real debate, in fact, is on the basis of who wants to be more cautious. It's a sad state of affairs, but it's a question of the level of caution we're willing to impose upon our society; caution, of course, from many points of view—from the point of view of the future of the toxicologist involved, as well as society.

In summary, then, let me say that there appears at least superficially to be a range of examples in which there is knowledge about the action of a variety of carcinogens in the laboratory, and corresponding human studies would lead to much more knowledge, and vice versa.

There are a series of human investigations in which we note certain characteristics of carcinogens, and those characteristics have not been validated in animal studies or apparently are contradicted in some of them. In all cases the details of the knowledge gained from animals and humans must be examined carefully for missing links that can be provided by one group or another; details not only of the things I've mentioned but details of anything one knows about metabolism, about the excretion, the handling, and so forth, of the compound.

There are wide, wide gaps between the various groups in these fields, and continuous efforts such as those at this meeting have to be encouraged. I think that really what one needs is not just one meeting like this, but that this meeting hopefully should be the basis for the establishment of individual groups where people really have detailed knowledge of one compound or another. It's only by a study of every little detail that doesn't seem to be particularly important and contemplation of it in both systems, that I think we're going to finally elucidate some of the practical problems that we have before us.

And that I think is all I have to say, probably lots too much. Thank you.

Discussion

DR. COULSTON: Dr. Shubik, we all thank you very much for stating the problem, not only of this meeting but of future days. This is the issue, and hopefully in the next few days we can try to elucidate a little bit further. But I reiterate a plea he made when he said this should be the beginning of a whole series of meetings of this kind, particularly selecting, as we have tried to do, a few topics and to go in some depth to get a scientific basis for this problem.

You know, he questioned whether the toxicologist is in danger. Of course he's in danger. The toxicologist is becoming a "cookbook" type of technician, and I have said many times that this is the trend. In many instances, industry has promoted this situation.

The regulatory agencies demand certain tests to be done, they have a guide, and the management of big companies often says, "For heaven's sake, just do what they ask, and let it be so." But this is a far cry from even ten years ago when the problem of chemical safety was brought to a toxicologist in any organization, academic, industry, government, and the toxicologist devised, innovated, did all kinds of old and new tests that were perhaps never even thought of before. He thereby developed new concepts of safety evaluation.

Today, the idea of developing new concepts under a guide system set by regulatory agencies is almost impossible. What is the future of toxicology? How is it going to develop? This loss of research initiative in toxicology is a tragedy in my view.

I think that everything that Dr. Shubik said I can attest and agree to, and I think we all feel very much the same way.

I assure you that there is no press in this room and there is no press release to be made from this meeting, so you're free to say almost anything you wish with the understanding that you can delete anything you've said later, if you so desire.

This year the International Academy of Environmental Safety founded under its auspices a Society of Ecotoxicology and Environmental Safety. We would like to invite everyone in this group who is interested to join with us and become a charter member.

It gives me great pleasure to introduce Dr. Kraybill to you. Most of you know him very well; certainly he is one of the real pioneers on the subject of toxicology, and particularly the question of chemical carcinogenesis. He will speak of mice and men, the predictability of observations and experimental systems, and their significance in man.

2. From Mice to Men: Predictability of Observations in Experimental Systems and Their Significance in Man

H. F. Kraybill
National Cancer Institute
Bethesda, Maryland

I. INTRODUCTION

Animal models have been used traditionally in experimental toxicology to elucidate chronic effects from various chemical, biological, and physical agents. In this biomedical assessment of a probable adverse effect, one of the major concerns is that of the agent's capability to induce cancer. The armamentarium for testing and evaluating toxic effects has been extended by the more recent application of *in vitro* procedures, using bacterial systems and cell cultures, to delineate mutagenic effects or cell transformations. Direct observations on humans from systematic epidemiological studies (retrospective and prospective), including the fortuitous observations from occupational exposures, provide, of course, in almost all cases an irrefutable basis on carcinogenic risk.

In the past, carcinogenicity testing, a rapidly expanding branch of toxicology, had been based upon approaches and concepts that eventually came under intense scrutiny by biochemists, pharmacologists, toxicologists, and nutritionists. Scientists in these disciplines could not reconcile certain protocols and/or experimental designs with their previous experiences in these areas of toxicological research. Extrapolation of data and application of findings for interpretative statements on toxicologic and carcinogenic hazard on the basis of inapplicable or inappropriate protocols led to much debate with the hope that more sensitive, reliable and, perhaps, less expensive and more rapid methods for carcinogenicity testing could be developed. Roe and Tucker (1974), reflecting on the testing of the 1950-60 era, feel that even current procedures are based on completely outdated concepts of cancer and mechanisms in carcinogenesis. They are extremely critical of the investigative efforts when they state that "there was an increase in sophistication in that era to the extent that no tissue or body orifice of any laboratory species was spared the possibility that an ingenious and eager experimentalist would introduce a prospective carcinogen into it." Some data thus reported in the literature, viewed within the framework of current requirements and perspectives, are frequently irrelevant and inadequate to provide a meaningful basis in decision-making processes.

Direct observations and evidence from human studies are, as indicated earlier, the ideal for evaluation of carcinogenic hazard. Currently, many restrictive measures prevail for human testing which were not operable two or three decades ago. Man receives inadvertent and inescapable exposures to carcinogens in his environment or through the higher levels of carcinogenic stress in the workplace. Where such events prevail, epidemiological pursuits are of great value. However, for the wide spectrum of toxic chemicals that may be carcinogenic, reliance must be placed on experimental animal systems and other models for development of data which can be extrapolated to man in arriving at some decision on carcinogenic risk and the assessment of the risk.

It is this area which poses major problems and engages the attention of scientists, consumer activists, regulatory officials, industrial representatives, and legislators. It is an area of science and trans-science that reflects much emotionalism; it abounds with opinions conditioned by prior experiences and scientific indoctrination and opinions reflecting parochial interests and influence, that evolve into controversy until some resolutions can be achieved. In essence, in these developments it is invariably a situation where frequently more "heat is generated than light" and some issues, although apparently resolved by one means or another, are debated, scientifically, for years.

It is appropriate to delineate some of the problem areas inherent in making extrapolations to probable human risk and/or hazard utilizing animal resource data and findings. There are examples that demonstrate the need for restraints and limitations in making such extrapolations. Some of these principles will be discussed in the guidelines that may be used in data evaluation and the decision-making process.

II. GUIDELINES IN THE PREDICTION AND EVALUATION PROCESS

Prudent public health policy requires that remedial and protective measures be taken to regulate carcinogens when the experimental data is most convincing. The dominant approach is the Delaney Amendment to the Food, Drug, and Cosmetic Act, which dictates, for example, removal of a food additive from the marketplace on the basis of animal response data implicating that chemical food additive as a carcinogen. This decision, based on a judgment on a yes-or-no basis that it is a presumed human carcinogen, is not an easy one. Chemicals implied as carcinogens cannot all be removed from the environment. Therefore, the weight of the evidence must be evaluated by those in the regulatory or decision-making process. If available scientific data is inadequate to derive some estimate of the risk (for example at extremely low levels of exposure), mathematically derived extrapolation models are used to provide some rough estimate of the risk factor or numbers of excess cancers that may prevail. At this point, a societal decision must be made as to a permissive finite level of risk. These derivations are, of course, hypothetically based on some inherent mathematical assumptions. At best, they are extremely conservative and perhaps overstate the degree of human risk. This approach fills a void in the absence of sound biological data. Thus, it is at the outset generally recognized that a firmer scientific basis for achieving quantitative and qualitative extrapolations from either *in vivo* (animal) or *in vitro* bioassay data and procedures to the human situation is urgently required. In the following discussion of principles and guidelines, these discrepancies in our data bases and the fallacies in interpretations from extrapolations will be emphasized with illustrations, wherever possible, to clarify these issues.

A. Some General Criteria in Evaluation of Carcinogenicity in Experimental Animal Model Systems

A few general points will be emphasized. First of all, the typical bioassay with an assessment of positive findings on carcinogenicity implies a statistical relationship, that is to say, that the tumor incidence in the test chemical group is significantly in excess over that of the control group. That relationship and requirement would appear to be simple and straightforward. However, sometimes these relationships and the ultimate interpretative statements are based on inadequate numbers of control animals, reduction in size of animal groups because of premature mortalities (moribund animals due to intercurrent infections), and high incidence of mortalities prior to tumor development because of the overlay of overt toxicity at high dosage regimens. Carcinogenicity evaluations and conclusions derived from such inadequate experiments are suspect and open to criticism.

Data derived from several laboratories and findings that are duplicated and reproducible within a species and strains of species, insofar as a carcinogenic response is concerned, are invariably widely accepted and not challenged. Furthermore, if the response is duplicated in other species, and involves different target organ(s) over a wide range of doses, it usually provides a high index of credibility. Too often, such is not the case, which results in disagreement and debate. For example, response data from one laboratory sometimes cannot be duplicated elsewhere because of a different strain of the same species, variance in environmental conditions such as type and composition of diet, biorefractories (contaminants) in the water, pollutants in the air, animal care and/or husbandry, and others. The question then arises: Which experimental findings and which reports are authentic and recognized as a basis for an informed decision?

The pathological diagnosis is one of the most troublesome areas in the identification of lesions whether they are hyperplastic, or benign or malignant tumors in the various organs of the experimental animal. When one detects a variance in diagnosis, this divergence in professional opinion opens up the opportunity for debate. Thus, diagnosis should be confirmed by several pathologists as a basis for uniform agreement.

Another aspect in the acceptance of the conclusions in a final assessment of carcinogenicity is the observation that a dose-response relationship prevails. That is, if there is a dose-related increase in the incidence of tumors, then it would appear that the test chemical is evoking a response with an increased insult that is not overshadowed by the factor of overt toxicity. But this is not always the case. The question may then arise, are lower doses incapable of inciting a cellular transformation, or, if not observable, does it require a much larger population of animals to establish a finite tumor incidence? If the tumor incidence at the higher dose plateaus or decreases, then the question arises, is there a metabolic overload, or does the exposure produce an overt toxicity beyond which frank neoplasia may not be observed? Numerous examples could be cited here, but the work by Maltoni and Lefemine (1974) on vinyl chloride, and Cuthbertson et al (1976) and Adamson et al (1976) on the administration of aflatoxin to monkeys, are illustrative. In the first example, the liver angiosarcomas were not observable at extremely high doses; at low doses, the primary organ site was not the liver but other sites. In the second example, lethalities developed in monkeys at high exposure to aflatoxin while liver and biliary carcinomas developed only after a marked reduction or tolerance of the dose administered. For aflatoxin, Tulpule, Madhavan, and Gopolan (1964) found that daily doses of 500 μg/kg of body weight to monkeys were fatal whereas lower doses, 25-250 μg/kg of body weight, were tolerated.

Another factor of importance, to be discussed later, is the time-to-tumor incidence data which is dependent upon the design of the study. Here, the expectations are that increasing dose levels will result in a decrease in latency period, especially if the chemical is ultimately classified as a strong carcinogen. Conversely, if the agent is classified as one of low potency, then the latency period may be extended, perhaps beyond the lifespan of the animal. Excessive doses may bring the time-to-tumor formation within the animals lifespan but the experimental dose could be far beyond and not equated to the exposure situations for a human population, even at the high exposures in the workplace.

If the cancer incidence in animal studies is extremely low; that is, of the order of 10 or 15% for the test group, then the incidence could approach the one observed in a control group. Thus, a redesign of the study with the possible inclusion of larger numbers of animals, and various strains, may be requisite.

TABLE 1

PREDICTIVE FACTORS DEVELOPED IN ANIMAL MODEL ASSESSMENTS OF
CARCINOGENICITY WHICH REINFORCE POSSIBLE SIGNIFICANCE TO HUMANS

1. CONFIRMATION IN VARIOUS OR MULTIPLE SPECIES AND STRAINS

2. CONFIRMATION IN VARIOUS LABORATORIES

3. CONFIRMATION IN PATHOLOGICAL DIAGNOSES

4. ACCEPTANCE OF DESIGN OF EXPERIMENTS ON A PHARMACOLOGICAL
   AND BIOCHEMICAL BASIS

5. INCREASE OF TUMOR INCIDENCE ON DOSE-RESPONSE RELATIONSHIP

6. STATISTICAL SIGNIFICANT INCREASE OF TUMORS IN TEST GROUP
   VERSUS CONTROLS

7. EXPERIMENTAL DOSE RANGE USED IN TESTING WITHIN PROBABLE
   EXPOSURE RANGE FOR MAN.

Some of the essential factors in the acceptance of experimental data and extrapolation of such data and findings toward assessment of its probable significance to human exposure situations are summarized and presented in Table 1.

B. Some Specific Factors That May Confound Interpretations of Data in Carcinogenicity Studies

Inappropriate route of administration. Investigators, in their zealous endeavors to achieve a positive response in the experimental animal with a test agent, may resort to nonspecific or nonrelevant procedures. For example, it would be inappropriate to test food additives for carcinogenicity by injecting them subcutaneously or intramuscularly into rodents to ascertain whether (and how many) injection-site sarcomas develop. Hueper and Ruchhoft (1954), failing to demonstrate any marked response in rodents by administration by the oral route of adsorbates of industrially-polluted raw and finished water supplies, resorted to subcutaneous injection of these toxic fractions. Throughout the literature there are many examples of such inappropriate procedures, and interpretation should be made with caution.

Enhancement of risk by immunosuppression and hormonal action. Studies on laboratory animals (Allison & Law, 1968; Grant et al., 1966) and man (Penn, 1970) contain considerable evidence that immunosuppression, especially cell-mediated immunity using thymectomy and antilymphocyte serum, will enhance the chances of developing "spontaneous" neoplasms and increase the risk of

23

development of carcinomas in response to challenge by known carcinogens. Tumors thus appearing may not be induced by the immunosuppressant procedure or agent *per se* but may arise from transformed cells which are free to multiply under suppressed cell-mediated immunity. The problem arises that a positive response in a test animal might be construed, under such conditions, as that of cancer induced by the chemical under test. Similarly, under artificial laboratory conditions, an alteration in hormonal status could also reveal a positive response when the test chemical is administered. The result here involves a definition of carcinogenicity, which really embraces the feature of cocarcinogenicity.

Improper test species and strains. In various strains of animals the spontaneous tumor incidence (that is, for mammary, pituitary, and other tumors) has been ascertained through experience and surveys over the years. Thus, whatever the baseline tumor incidence may be, it can be anticipated that a test agent, for example in the rat, may increase, or in some cases appear to decrease, the risk of development of such tumors. Thus, any excess of tumors beyond the spontaneous incidence is assumed to be the result of induction by the test agent. For this purpose, the history of an animal model, insofar as sensitivity to induced cancers by known carcinogens is concerned, should be known. This background knowledge is particularly important when investigators attempt to use strains of animals with high spontaneous tumor incidence, especially where the test agent induces tumors in the same category as that for the control group. While some investigators recommend such purebred strains with high tumor incidence of a certain type, Roe and Tucker (1974) regard such advice as tantamount to recommending to an analytical chemist that he use a dirty test tube.

Therefore, the use of bioassay systems employing inbred strains with high incidence of particular tumors in the control group may be equivocal; basing interpretations on findings of this type may require caution unless further extensive evaluation is considered. In some instances, however, such well-controlled systems may have validity. Related to such procedures is the practice of adding a known carcinogen or cocarcinogen into the bioassay on an animal population (spontaneous tumor indicence known) where the tumor incidence for a test agent is to be quantified. This is another procedure that may be equivocal in interpretations unless adequate convincing evidence or additional studies are at hand.

Failures to consider the role of diet, state of nutrition, and diet contaminants. It is most distressing that so little attention is given to the role of micronutrients and macronutrients and dietary contaminants in the reporting of experimental findings where these factors are dependent variables. Tannenbaum and Silverstone (1949) and others (Kraybill, 1953; Tannenbaum, 1959) in their comprehensive treatment of this subject have shown how calorie intake and composition of the

TABLE 2

EFFECTS OF CALORIC RESTRICTIONS DURING

THE TWO STAGES OF CARCINOGENESIS*

GROUP	DIET IN PERIOD OF CARCINOGEN APPLICATION (10 WKS)	DIET IN PERIOD OF TUMOR FORMATION (52 WKS)	TUMOR INCIDENCE
HH	HIGH CALORIE	HIGH CALORIE	69
HL	HIGH CALORIE	LOW CALORIE	34
LH	LOW CALORIE	HIGH CALORIE	55
LL	LOW CALORIE	LOW CALORIE	24

TANNENBAUM, A. CANCER RES. 4: 673-677 (1974)

* BENZO(A)PYRENE IN SKIN CARCINOGENESIS IN MICE.

diet relevant to proportion of macronutrients (protein, fat, and carbohydrate) can influence the absence or existence of excess tumors from test chemicals compared to controls. In Table 2 the effects of caloric restriction on carcinogenesis are shown.

White et al. (1974) have shown the effect of low cystine in diet on the inhibition of leukemia induced by methylcholanthrene in DBA mice. Kline and co-workers (1943) noted the inhibition of skin tumors in pyridoxine deficient diets of mice, and Kensler et al. (1941) have shown the effect of riboflavin and casein in partial protection against liver cancer in rats administered dimethylaminoazobenzene. One might inquire why these factors, apparently well-recognized, are stressed. In spite of the fact that diets are presumably correctly formulated and properly stored, the processing of diets, storage, and addition of vitamin-mineral mixtures in correct amounts cannot be taken for granted. The question then arises as to whether proper attention is given to analysis to ascertain whether the diet and its composition is as it is intended to be for the study planned.

Roe and Tucker (1974) have shown convincingly the effect of diet intake in mice and the influence on tumor incidence (shown in Table 3). In addition, the test chemical may influence the palatability of the diet and, accordingly, influence intake; thus, a difference in tumor incidence from one group where caloric intake is higher, hence a built-in variation. Isocaloric intakes should be achieved for valid comparisons.

The aspect of diet contamination is one of the features in experimental

TABLE 3

CANCERS IN AFFLUENT MICE

| FEEDING PROCEDURE | TOTAL TUMORS (18 MOS) | TUMORS BY SITE | | | OTHER NEOPLASMS |
		LIVER	LUNG	LYMPHO-RETICULAR	
4 GMS DIET/DAY 1 MOUSE/CAGE	4	1	1	2	0
5 GMS DIET/DAY 1 MOUSE/CAGE	4	2	0	1	1-TESTIS
DIET AD LIBITUM 1 MOUSE/CAGE	32	15	2	11	2-TESTIS 1-KIDNEY 1-THYROID
DIET AD LIBITUM 5 MICE/CAGE	23	8	6	9	0

ROE AND TUCKER (1974) PROC. EUROP. SOC. FOR STUDY OF DRUG TOXICITY, 15: 171-177.

studies that is grossly neglected and its significance really never fully appreciated. For many years, prior to the wide utilization of laboratory animal chows which are formulated incorporating all essential macronutrients in proper proportion, the semisynthetic diets for laboratory animals were used. While the latter may have had trace contaminants and may be more costly, the problem of contaminants was a minor one in comparison to typical formulated animal laboratory chow. Ingredients such as fish meal and plant products such as wheat and soybean are ideal carriers for all the environmental contaminants and are one of the components in the food chain. To name but a few, one must expect pesticide contaminants, industrial chemicals (PBB, PCB, PCP, dioxins, etc.), heavy metals, estrogens or steroids, polycyclic aromatic hydrocarbons and, perhaps, mycotoxins.

In the design of experiments, careful investigators provide for the systematic or continuous analysis of the laboratory animal ration. At least this effort provides a profile on the extent and type of contamination that the laboratory must consider and evaluate. This information can be invaluable in interpretation of findings or results, especially where comparisons within test results are needed. In essence, a bioassay of a chemical for carcinogenic activity really reflects the response from an integrated insult of the test chemical, the diet contaminants, the biorefractories in the water supply, the contaminants in the air, plus other variants in the care and handling of the animals. Quite frequently, the removal or marked reduction in the level of the contaminant in the diet will completely alter the degree of tumor response or reverse the end result of the study.

One of the most illustrative cases wherein an elucidation of the effect of a diet contaminant not only altered the end result of a previous experiment but essentially negated a previous hypothesis is a 1954 study by Salmon and Copeland. These investigators reported that hepatomas occurred in rats that developed cirrhosis on a choline-deficient diet. In retrospect, it has been interesting to note that these hepatomas developed when commercial peanut meal was used as the protein source in the diet (Kraybill & Shimkin, 1964). However, in 1963 Salmon et al. found a decrease in the frequency of hepatomas when peanut meal in the diet was previously extracted with hot methanol. Supplementation of the diet with choline or methionine did not decrease the original frequency of hepatomas reported. It was soon discovered that solvent extraction of the peanut meal, chloroform being even more efficient than methanol, removed the contaminant aflatoxin, a potent hepatocarcinogen. Thus, the original concept of cirrhosis and hepatoma production being associated with choline deficiency was shattered by the discovery of the role of the contaminant. Thus, the question arises as to how many other bioassay results are really false positives. In Table 4 the results of these studies are shown.

Strain specific tumor incidence, genetic drift and understanding mechanisms for species variation. Many routine bioassays have been conducted without repeated surveillance of the animal model for definition and the true and current spontaneous tumor incidence. Throughout colonies of animals, over the years, genetic drift and other factors may escalate the overall tumor incidence. That is, for example, at one time the tumor incidence for a large population of a strain of mouse could be as low as 10%, but 10 or 15 years later could be escalated by

TABLE 4

HEPATOMAS IN RATS ON DIETS WITH AND WITHOUT EXTRACTED PEANUT MEAL

		PROTEIN SOURCES				
			PEANUT MEAL		AVE. TIME	
			NOT	FAT SOURCE	ON	
BEEF %	CASEIN %	EXTRACTED %	EXTRACTED %	IN DIET AND PERCENT	EXPERIMENT DAYS	HEPATOMA FREQUENCY
-	7.9	-	33.3	TALLOW 18.5	334	4/10
7.9	-	-	33.3	TALLOW 18.5	424	8/10
-	7.9	-	33.3	TALLOW 18.5	470	15/15
6.0	-	25.0	-	TALLOW 20.0	574	2/10
7.9	-	33.3	-	TALLOW 18.5	283	0/10
7.9	-	33.3	-	LARD 18.5	488	0/10
7.9	-	33.3	-	CRISCO 18.5	574	0/10

SALMON ET AL. FED PROC. 22: 262, ABSTRACT 609.

a factor of 5, 6, or 8 (Roe & Tucker, 1974). The important feature here is to know the standard to which the investigator can make his comparisons. The increased spontaneous tumor incidence could be decreased by appropriate procedures, one of which is dietary restriction.

One of the most puzzling problems in the reporting of bioassay results is the variability among strains within species and among species insofar as tumor response to the test of a chemical agent. These variations in response, needless to state, perplex the investigator. In the nonprofessional's mind, reading about these variations must conjure up some doubts as to the authenticity of the work or the significance of the findings. In essence, until one discovers or attempts to learn more about why tumors occur in the mouse liver and not the rat liver, or the lungs of the rat and not the mouse when the animal is challenged with a test chemical, we shall never advance the science of toxicology; neither shall we ever ascertain which indeed is the most appropriate species, the appropriate strain, perhaps which more nearly represents the animal model which may have good predictability for a human response.

Contaminants in test agent (chemical). Previous mention was made of the significance of dietary and water contaminants, but contaminants in the test chemical are not always recognized or identified. There are numerous reports in the toxicological literature that call attention to the fact that the biological response was frequently altered when impurities or contaminants in the chemical to be tested were removed by purification or a different synthesis. Many of the organic chemicals bioassayed for carcinogenicity would fall in the category where a systematic examination of the chemical for contaminants would be required. The so-called "technical grade" chemical, while perhaps representing the typical human exposure, can, in many instances, be purified and the response in animal systems determined. Assuming that the purified chemical does not evoke the carcinogenic response elicited by the contaminated chemical, then the effort to achieve purity and yield a negative response for carcinogenicity seems obvious and extremely worthwhile.

Body retention, body burden. Chemicals which are lipophilic and accumulate in adipose tissue or those that bind to other organs and tissues are usually assumed to be of greater hazard than those rapidly metabolized or excreted, although this may not always be the case. Conversely, the existence of a high excretion rate may not necessarily imply the existence of a no-effect level. The latter could prevail if the excretion of the chemical occurred independent of the concentration.

Chemicals retained in the organs or tissues and referred to as the body burden can be the result of naturally occurring exposures or exposures to environmental toxicants. Many of these chemicals can interact with other chemical moieties in the tissues and conjugate with some for longterm retention. Others may be slowly metabolized by the enzymes in the liver or detoxified in the kidney and, over a span of years, lead to a reduction in the body burden. Such a process may be slow as, for instance, the migration from the adipose tissue to the lean body mass. An example is the longterm retention of some of the organochlorine insecticides such as DDT and its metabolite DDE.

Some organic chemicals easily penetrate the body barrier and enter compartments such as the fat and lean body mass. They may not be deactivated and, as indicated earlier, reside as a burden and slowly dissipate across the barrier. Others, upon challenge to the mammalian system, pass across the placenta, such as did diethylstilbestrol used clinically as an abortifacient, only to have an effect on the progeny. With the slow release from adiposity to the lean body mass, and ultimately carried by the circulatory system to various organs and tissues, some are released during lactation through the breast milk.

It is interesting that DDT/DDE has represented an exposure to the population since the early forties. For all practical purposes it has now been banned for some time, yet both DDT and DDE appear in mothers' milk. Obviously, this is an observed phenomena of the so-called "sink effect" where the lipophilic organochlorine pesticide is spilling over, so to speak, from depot fat to muscle mass to venous system to mammary tissues and is excreted in milk. Perhaps this is a way for females to reduce the body burden, lowering their cellular insult to DDT/DDE, if the steady state is not enhanced by reintroduction of the environmental chemical. Table 5 shows some of the current levels of DDT/DDE, PCB, and PBB in human milk (U.S. EPA, 1976; Michigan State Dept. of Health, 1976).

TABLE 5

PCB AND DDE IN HUMAN MILK MONITORED IN ELEVEN STATES

	PCB	DDE
NUMBER OF SAMPLES	80	80
RANGE IN CONCENTRATION (PPM)	0 - 10.6	0.31 - 6.43
MEAN CONCENTRATION (PPM)	1.80	2.31
HIGHEST CONCENTRATION (PPM)	10.6	6.43

EPA PESTICIDE PROGRAM DATA FROM COLORADO STATE
UNIVERSITY PROJECT - AUGUST 1976

PCB AND PBB IN HUMAN MILK IN MICHIGAN

	PBB (FAT BASIS)	TOTAL PCB (FAT BASIS) AROCLOR 1254 & 1260
NUMBER OF SAMPLES	92	92?
RANGE IN VALUES (PPM)	0 - 0.30	0.08 - 0.810

MICHIGAN STATE DEPT OF HEALTH, OCTOBER 14, 1976 REPORT
COUNTIES OF CHIPPEWA, HOUGHTON AND INGHAM.

DDT/DDE has been characterized as a hepatocarcinogen by oral administration in several strains of mice (Innes et al., 1969; Tomatis et al. 1962). It is of interest that in the mouse (at least in the male), there was a significant increase in tumors at a dose level as low as 2 ppm; for a similar increase in the female a higher dose level was required. No convincing evidence of liver cell tumor induction has been noted in other species (rat, hamster, trout, dogs, and monkeys). As to man, no conclusive evidence is available. This subject will be discussed later under epidemiology.

PCB's (polychlorinated biphenyls) have also been identified, at least Kanechlor 500 by Ito et al. (1973) and Aroclor 1254 by Kimbrough and Linder (1974), as inducers of benign and malignant liver cell tumors in mice. No induction of malignant cells has been noted in rats, although multiple hyperplastic liver nodules were observed following oral exposure. No data is available thus far for humans.

The polybrominated biphenyls (PBB) are currently under test in the isomeric form of hexabromobiphenyl. The question arises as to the human significance of, perhaps, not just one of these lipophilic agents alone, but the effect of a carcinogenic integrated stress of two of these, DDT/DDE and PCB, and perhaps a promotion effect of PBB. Will these chemicals have a significant hazard from the body burden, and what impact will they have on infants who are breast-fed milk containing such exposures? In addition, these brominated and chlorinated compounds become a body burden through ingestion of foods other than human milk, that is, through the food chain, especially in fish. Nursing mothers should probably reduce considerably their intake of fish.

Animal exposure v. human exposure. In animal experimentation, we usually refer to the challenge from a test agent in terms of dose, and to the response as a dose-response relationship. In the human population laboratory, we have exposure with the corresponding exposure-response relationship. In these instances, we will refer to the response as a neoplastic disease. In the environment, man receives exposures from air pollutants, water biorefractories, diet contaminants, and, if drugs are taken, an added exposure from this source. If the individual is exposed to chemicals in the workplace and they are identified as carcinogens, then this may be the greatest added exposure. As to intensity of exposure, one could arbitrarily list the above in the following order: Workplace Exposure → Drugs → Food Contaminants → Air Pollutants → Water Biorefractories. The workplace exposures are usually by the dermal or inhalation route, while drugs and water biorefractories are by the oral route, with some drugs by oral, dermal, or inhalation route. The air pollutant exposures are, in general, by the inhalation route.

We have previously mentioned that diet, diet contaminants, and nutrition can have an impact on induction of cancer with the effect being in either a positive of negative direction. Many reviews have been written on the role of diet, and diet contaminants and cancer incidence in animals and man (Berg, 1975; Kraybill, 1963 1969; Kraybill & Shimkin, 1964; McLean, 1973; Tannenbaum, 1959; Tannenbaum & Silverstone, 1949). In this area each component may influence a response conditioned by nutritional and toxicological effects and each effect should be delineated.

In experimental studies, the effective dose for induction of a carcinogenic response may be dependent upon the concentration, the degree of absorption, activation by liver enzymes, potentiation, and other factors. Some potent carcinogens may require a low dose for short periods of time for induction (latency period). However, those of lower potency (so-called weak carcinogens) may require a high dose for a long latency period.

One of the most controversial areas in assessment of animal tumorigenic response and its probable predictive value to human hazard is the matter of large test doses that cannot be correlated to actual human exposures, sometimes exceeding comparable environmental exposures in man a hundred- or thousand-fold. For various chemicals the correlation of experimental doses in animals to calculated equivalent experimental exposures in man is shown in Table 4. The rationale for using small sample-size numbers of test animals at relatively high doses is an obvious compromise on a statistical basis. Some years ago, it was felt that the possibility of getting a negative response or not detecting a positive one, could be avoided by administering large doses which would bring into focus a response even if only 20, 50, or 100 animals were used per test group. However,

TABLE 6

CORRELATION OF EXPERIMENTAL DOSES IN
ANIMALS TO CALCULATED EQUIVALENT EXPERIMENTAL EXPOSURE IN MAN

CHEMICALS	EXPERIMENTAL DOSE	EQUIVALENCY CALCULATED HUMAN INTAKE LEVELS
CYCLAMATES	5% IN DIET (2.18 GMS/DAY)	552 BOTTLES OF SOFT DRINK (MAX)
OIL OF CALAMUS	5000 PPM IN DIET	250 QTS. OF VERMOUTH/DRY
SACCHARIN	5% IN DIET	800 12 OUNCE BOTTLES OF SOFT DRINK
DES (DIETHYLSTILBESTROL)	1 CLINICAL TREATMENT	5×10^6 LBS OF LIVER FOR 50 YEARS
SAFROLE	5000 PPM	613 BOTTLES OF ROOT BEER PER DAY
TCE (TRICHLOROETHYLENE) (IN DECAFFEINATED COFFEE)	900 MG/KG B.WT - FEMALE 1200 MG/KG B.WT - MALE	5×10^7 CUPS PER DAY* 10×10^7 CUPS PER DAY
DDT (DDE) - MOUSE DIET	316 MG/LIFETIME	853 TIMES GENERAL POPULATION EXPOSURE 3 TIMES WORK EXPOSURE

DATA FROM VARIOUS SOURCES
* CUP OF COFFEE = 9×10^{-4} MG OF TCE FOR 150 ML CUP.

we cannot generally state that any chemical given in sufficiently high doses will cause cancer, because there are many examples where the opposite is true.

The carcinogenesis process is a complex mechanism. This does not mean that one should not look for target organs at high dose, although the picture may be clouded by overt toxicity associated with cell injury which may not be paralleled, biochemically, at low doses. To detect a significant statistical difference in response of control (chemical absent) group versus test group (chemical added) at low doses, one would have to employ a kilomouse or megamouse procedure. However, the use of various large animal size groups may be counterproductive since the response from the control group, reflecting a background of exposures, may be equivalent to the test group response. That is, the background response from the control group may be equal to or greater than the response to the chemical of animals on test.

Using large doses to enhance the sensitivity of the test has been practiced widely. Unfortunately, it has been applied with little reflection and examination of overt toxicity brought about by the effect such large doses have on the metabolic processes and the defense mechanisms. Indeed, in many cases overt toxicity has been observed, resulting in a high incidence of mortalities but without any induction of neoplasia.

A comparison of the potencies of carcinogens is difficult. Many compounds would have to be tested under comparable conditions simultaneously in many test systems. From this general impression on toxic chemicals, which may be classified as carcinogens or alleged carcinogens, one arrives at the dictum that there is absolutely no safe level for exposure to a so-called carcinogen; low exposures involve a small, but not a zero order of risk. This hypothesis, in a way, is a reflection of our level of ignorance for biochemically following and pharmacologically predicting mechanisms taking place at low levels of insult. Mantel and Schneiderman (1975) and others have excluded trace substances; indeed many endogenous chemicals and biological intermediates may fit this category.

Concern about massive doses or routes of administration that may not be relevant is reflected in the following statement of the American Conference of Governmental Industrial Hygienists (1976):

> No substance is to be considered an occupational carcinogen of any practical significance which reacts by the respiratory route at or above 100 mg/m^3 for the mouse, 2000 mg/m^3 for the rat; by the dermal route, at or above 1500 mg/kg for the mouse, 300 mg/kg for the rat; by the gastrointestinal route at or above 500 mg/kg/day for a lifetime or equivalent to about 100 grams T.D. for the rate and 10 grams T.D. for the mouse.

Thus, under these limitations of dosage, dioxane and trichloroethylene would be excluded from consideration as carcinogens.

Safety margin susceptible members of the population. Previous reference has been made to selection of an inbred susceptible strain of rodent which will respond to the challenge of the chemical within a range of doses. This technique is used to simulate the probable role of susceptible individuals in the human population with variant thresholds of 10^6, 10^7, or 10^8 molecules as described by Rall (1975).

People may be more or less variable than inbred strains of rodents. The variability seems to occur in the enzymes that are involved in activating environmental carcinogens. The variability in the rodent could be of the order of 10% while in man it could be an order of magnitude of several thousand. The variability could explain why some cigarette smokers never develop bronchiogenic carcinoma.

Another aspect that should be considered when discussing susceptibility is that of multiple stress from carcinogens, i.e., PCB, chlorinated hydrocarbons, drugs, and tobacco, to name but a few. As laudable as these concepts may be, the heterogenity of the human population with its genetic patterns, disease profiles, and variant exposures during a lifetime, may not necessarily permit any general extrapolations. The risk could be overstated (Cuthbertson et al., 1976). Of course, this same perspective applies to the broad inherent problem of extrapolating toxicity data on metabolic patterns and biochemical behavior to man. Extrapolating no-adverse effect in animal to man falls within this category. Finally, extreme caution must be exercised in dealing with the matter of susceptibility extrapolation since the risk could be overstated or understated. We need more data on comparative pharmacology and comparative mechanisms.

Time-to-tumor formation. When some chemicals are administered continuously to animals, tumors may be induced within a short interval of time at a specified dose. There may be, in most of the cases of a potent carcinogen, a dose-dependent relationship. However, if the insult is applied infrequently, the time-to-tumor formation is advanced, sometimes approaching a two-year period (equivalent to 72 years in man) or even beyond the normal life expectancy. A low potency carcinogen, with a small number of animals, and at a low level of exposure, may not reveal tumor formation within the lifetime of the animal. By using a kilomouse experiment, one may perceive a significant tumor incidence; but perhaps not even then.

Despite the above, there are chemicals of low toxicity which, even when administered at massive doses, may still not have a sufficient induction period and thus exceed the lifetime for response. In comparing this to man, estimates have been made that the induction period would fall beyond a lifespan of 100 years, or, as once stated, beyond the age of Methuselah (Jones & Grendon, 1975). In any such events, certainly, the order of risk is almost negligible.

Threshold envisaged: mathematically defined safe doses. One of the unrelenting precepts among oncologists is that a biological threshold no longer holds for a chemical once it is defined by whatever evidence as a carcinogen. At least, it is contended that there is no scientific method available to establish such a threshold. This thesis is advanced drawing a parellelism from radiation carcinogenesis to chemical carcinogenesis. However, a chemical differs from radiation hits. It comes in contact with receptors in the intact animal where biochemical mechanisms with metabolic transformations are involved. Claims are made as to the irreversibility of this primary observed reaction and response, and the potential for synergizing this action at the cell level by other additives. Falk (1975) supported by others, has indicated that one single molecule may not cause a permanent change which, either alone or with other agents acting additively or cumulatively over a lifetime could produce a cancer.

Flamm (1975) indicates that on a certain biostatistical and theoretical basis less than one tenth of a puff from one cigarette in an entire lifetime could be responsible for the development of lung cancer. Thus, the application of the one-hit biomathematical hypothesis asserts that one individual in 100 million, where each individual was to inhale one tenth puff of a cigarette in his life-time, could acquire lung cancer as a consequence of such exposure. This illustrates the stringency of the one-hit theory; but, in the events of the real world one may never know the validity of these mathematical assumptions.

In line with Falk's reasoning, Roe (1972) noted that animals exposed to very low doses of a carcinogen did not respond as expected when the challenge was interrupted for a few months before a promoter was administered. The cells originally insulted had either disappeared or would no longer respond. It may be appropriate to speculate on the possible factors associated with tumor induction and the body's defense mechanisms then insulted by an agent which could be a carcinogen under certain biochemical/physiological conditions. Some of these factors are outlined in Table 7. Implicit in these concepts is the possibility that certain cell injury and the sequence of the neoplastic process is conditioned by the presence or absence of a homeostatic mechanism which will arrest or accelerate the proliferative process. A case in point here would be the experimentally proven effect of chloroform at high doses (Dept. of HEW, 1976) and the probable lack of an inductive process at micro levels in an environmental exposure. The no-threshold concept, of course, permits no reconciliation with such factors prevailing in the mammalian system.

Studies with bacterial and human cells indicate that there is a repair of genetic damage (DNA alteration and cell transformation). Thus, the reaction of a carcinogen or mutagen with DNA is not necessarily irreversible, as indicated by Morgan et al. (1973), Cleaver (1968), and Dinman (1972). Dinman shows that there is a finite level for an essential element. Below the threshold, there is indeed an adverse effect on the physiology or a disease state due to a deficiency. Tables 8 and 9 address the question whether there is a threshold for orally administered arsenic which has heretofore been implicated as a carcinogen or cocarcinogen in occupational exposures (Kraybill, 1976; Nielsen et al., 1975).

Several investigators (Friedman, 1972; Henschler, 1974; Kraybill, 1976) have attempted to calculate a threshold concentration for a carcinogen. Henschler

TABLE 7

FACTORS THAT MAY INFLUENCE TUMOR INDUCTION
AND PROBABLE EXISTENCE OF THRESHOLD

TUMOR INDUCTION

A. INSULT TO LIVER (OTHER ORGANS?)

IRREVERSIBLE DESTRUCTION OF HEPATOCYTES

NUTRIENT STATUS   PROBABLE

HOMEOSTATIC REQUIREMENT   THRESHOLD

GENETIC INFLUENCE ON ENZYME PROFILE

B. HORMONAL STATUS (INTERACTION)

PROMOTION AND ACCELERATION   –   NO THRESHOLD

HORMONE ACTING PHYSIOLOGICALLY   –   PROBABLE
  IN THE MILIEU   THRESHOLD

C. MOLECULAR INTERACTION

CONJUGATION TO MACROMOLECULES   NO THRESHOLD

DNA ALTERATION AND BINDING

D. VIRAL GENOME AND INTERACTION

ALTERATION OF DEFENSE MECHANISM   –   PROBABLY NO
                THRESHOLD

TABLE 8

PROBABLE THRESHOLD FOR ORALLY INGESTED ARSENIC (MAN)

A. ENVIRONMENTAL LEVELS

  1. AVERAGE ARSENIC IN DIET   400-500 µG/DAY

  2. AVERAGE LEVELS IN WATER   10 µG/DAY

  3. AVERAGE AIR LEVELS   2 µG/DAY

B. BIOLOGICAL LEVELS

  1. SERUM LEVELS (FASTING)   3.5 TO 7.2 µG/100 ML

  2. HAIR LEVELS   3.1 TO 3.2 µG/100 GMS

C. STANDARDS AND TOLERANCES

  1. BRITISH STATUTORY LIMIT   1 PPM

  2. U.S.A. LIMIT   2.6 PPM

  3. U.S.A. DRINKING WATER STANDARD   .01 MG/L

  4. OSHA & NIOSH OCCUPATIONAL STANDARD   .05 MG/M^3

KRAYBILL, H. F. (1975) PROC. 19TH MTG. OF THE INTERAGENCY
COLLABORATIVE GROUP ON ENVIRONMENTAL CARCINOGENESIS, 8-14-75.

TABLE 9

PHYSIOLOGICAL BASIS FOR PROBABLE THRESHOLDS FOR ARSENIC

A. ARSENIC AS A CARCINOGEN

1. IN TROUT - TESTING CARBARSONE IN DIET   480 MG/100 GMS

2. IN MAN - TAIWAN DRINKING WATER   1820 µG/LITER
DAILY INTAKE

B. PHYSIOLOGICAL REQUIREMENTS (RATS)

1. GROWTH PROMOTION

2. COMPETES WITH AND CONTROLS SELENIUM TOXICITY

3. CATALYST FOR PHOSPHORYLATION (METABOLISM)

4. INFLUENCES IODINE REQUIREMENT

5. ESSENTIAL IN HEMATOPOIETIC SYSTEM

C. ADVERSE EFFECTS - DEFICIENCY STATES (RATS)

1. ROUGH HAIR COAT

2. GROWTH RETARDATION

3. DECREASED HEMATOCRITS

4. ENLARGEMENT OF SPLEEN

5. INCREASE IN ERYTHROCYTE FRAGILITY

KRAYBILL, H. F. (1975) PROC. 19TH MEETING OF THE INTERAGENCY
COLLABORATIVE GROUP ON ENVIRONMENTAL CARCINOGENESIS, 8-14-75
NIELSEN ET AL, FASEB ABSTRACT, 1975

made such a calculation on the basis of a 70 kg man assuming 6×10^{13} cells in the body and using Avogadro's number of 6.02×10^{23} molecules per mole and 10^4 molecules per cell or 10^{-8} molar concentration per kg as the estimate of threshold, he calculated the threshold as 5 parts per billion for the molecular weight of a chemical carcinogen given at 500. These values are shown in Table 10.

Restating the issue, this means that the threshold for a carcinogen falls within the range of minimal concentrations of essential endogenous chemicals such as nutrients and hormones. The magnitude of the probable threshold and its applicability to compliance requirements in achieving a socioeconomic, low-level residue or exposure is thus indicated and obvious.

Eckhardt (1973) has maintained that sensitivity of analytical methods automatically establishes a tolerance for all substances, including a carcinogen. Thus, zero is not a precise value but an undefined tolerance. Rall (1975) indicates that even some potent carcinogens may be safe at exposure levels of 1 molecule, 10 molecules, 100 molecules, or more. If it were possible to design an experiment to show that very low concentrations would have a low probability of showing a deleterious effect, we might find a spectrum of signposts for different individuals in the population where the threshold could be 10^4, 10^6, 10^{10}

TABLE 10
ESTIMATION OF A THRESHOLD FOR A CARCINOGEN[a]

PART 1	
BODY WEIGHT OF REFERENCE MAN	70 KG
NUMBER OF CELLS IN BODY	6×10^{13} CELLS
AVOGADRO'S NUMBER	6.02×10^{23} MOLECULES/MOLE
THRESHOLD VALUE/CELL	10^4 MOLECULES
THRESHOLD VALUES MOLECULES/KG	8.6×10^{15}
MOLAR CONCENTRATION/KG	1×10^{-8}
PART 2	
ASSUMING MOLECULAR WEIGHT OF CHEMICAL	500
CALCULATED THRESHOLD	5 PPB

[a]DINMAN (1972); HENSCHLER (1974); FRIEDMAN (1972); KRAYBILL (1975).

and so on, up to 10^{20} molecules (see Figures 1, 2, 3). Thus each individual could have a different threshold. The question then arises: Whom are we going to protect in the population, realizing the susceptibility? Therefore, he concludes, one should consider the aspect of added risk since one may be considering a pool of carcinogens, each with its own threshold. Thus, basically, he feels the primary emphasis should not be placed on the debate of threshold or no thresholds per se.

$$10^0 10^1 10^2 10^3 \dots\dots\dots\dots\dots\dots\dots 10^{20} 10^{21} 10^{22} 10^{23}$$

NUMBER OF MOLECULES

FIGURE 1

THRESHOLDS FOR CHEMICALS THAT CAUSE CHRONIC
IRREVERSIBLE DAMAGE.

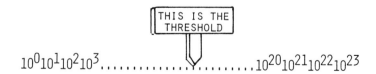

$$10^0 10^1 10^2 10^3 \dots\dots\dots\dots\dots\dots 10^{20} 10^{21} 10^{22} 10^{23}$$

NUMBER OF MOLECULES

FIGURE 2

THRESHOLDS FOR CHEMICALS THAT CAUSE CHRONIC
IRREVERSIBLE DAMAGE.

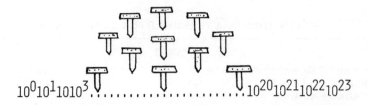

$10^0 10^1 10^1 10^3 \ldots\ldots\ldots\ldots\ldots\ldots\ldots 10^{20} 10^{21} 10^{22} 10^{23}$

NUMBER OF MOLECULES

FIGURE 3

THRESHOLDS FOR CHEMICALS THAT CAUSE CHRONIC
IRREVERSIBLE DAMAGE.

Source: Rall, (1975)e.

The World Health Organization (1974) Scientific Group, in the conclusions to their report, "Assessment of the Carcinogenicity and Mutagenicity of Chemicals," states that the possible existence of a threshold to the effects of both chemical carcinogens and mutagens should be envisaged.

Metabolic overloading. Experimentally, as previously discussed, it is common practice to challenge the animal with a dose schedule that far exceeds the exposure levels that would be received by the human population. Indeed, in many instances the dose to the animal, on a relative basis, far exceeds even the calculated exposure for man in the workplace. A previous example of this situation was cited in the case of the pesticide DDT/DDE that was tested in the mouse. The rationale for this was also previously mentioned.

In some instances, this procedure biases the tests in favor of highly toxic compounds. For example, chemicals with a low acute toxicity could be tested under the typical procedure of using a maximum tolerated dose at levels of 100 to 10,000 times the dose of a high toxicity chemical. A paper by Burchfield et al. (1975) described the results of using a MTD (maximum tolerated dose) and one half MTD, determined during a six-week subchronic test, to assess the carcinogenicity of some pesticides in a lifetime study. The levels were too high and resulted in excess mortalities and incomplete experiments. A total of 175 dose changes had to be made because of the metabolic overload to prevent further excessive losses of animals in the experiments. In Table 11 the comparisons on the starting and final levels of the test compound, percent of starting dose and the wide range in doses are presented from the report of Burchfield, Storrs, and Kraybill (1975). The high level noted was for the male Osborne-Mendel rat.

The organochlorine and organophosphorus nerve poisons were obviously more toxic than the herbicides, the latter designed to kill plants not animals. The metabolism of these compounds under test, or lack of it, could, therefore, be a misleading factor. Heptachlor, for example, is never found in human tissues as such, but as the epoxide; aldrin occurs as dieldrin. Thus, while the human

38

TABLE 11

COMPARISON OF STARTING AND FINAL LEVELS OF TEST CHEMICAL PESTICIDES

Group	Compound	Starting Dose (ppm)	Final Dose (ppm)	% of Starting Dose
	Aldrin	120	0	0
	Dieldrin	80	0	0
	Endrin	15	7.5	33
	Photodieldrin	10	10	100
A	Chlordecone	60	10*	17
	Heptachlor	160	20	13
	Chlordane	800	100	13
	Lindane	640	320	50
	Toxaphene	2,560	640	25
	Parathion	80	60	75
	Azinphos-methyl	250	125	50
	Phosphamidon	160	160	100
B	Dimethoate	500	250	50
	Dichlorvos	1,000	300	33
	Gardona (R)	16,000	8,000	50
	Malathion	16,000	8,000	50
	Captan	16,000	4,000	25
C	Daconil	20,000	10,000	50
	Picloram	20,000	10,000	50
	Amiben	20,000	20,000	100

A. chlorinated hydrocarbon insecticides;
B. organophosphate insecticides; and
C. phytocides.

Source: Burchfield, Storrs and Kraybill (1975). Lectures on Pesticides - Env. Quality and Safety Book, Suppl. Vol. III, Thieme Publ. Stuttgart, Germany.

population would not be exposed to significant amounts of the parent compound, in these experiments, the rodents were exposed to high levels of them. Obviously, in high dosing, the enzyme systems of rodents designed to epoxidize these compounds would be swamped.

It is interesting to compare the doses in animals which could be relevant exposures in man. Aldrin was tested at an average dose of 5 ppm compared to 1,100 ppm for toxaphene on computation of weighted doses over the experimental period. Thus, there was a 220-fold difference. The most toxic compounds are, therefore, most likely to escape detection as potential carcinogens due to overdosing, precluding induction of neoplasia. The most alarming feature in these dose selections is that the MTD is, in no way, related to potential environmental or industrial exposure in man. In one case, the dose indicated for a lifetime study in the rodent calculated to a total requirement exceeding in pounds the annual production by a manufacturer. The foregoing discussion emphasizes the fact that potential exposure should be given a high priority when selecting compounds and doses for testing. If such is not done, problems are created not only in the conduct of the experiment but in the final interpretation of data and scientific assessment.

In other areas of research, in either long-term nutritional or pharmacological studies, the aspect of metabolic overload has long been recognized. Even with biological intermediates such as the amino acids, vitamins, minerals, and metabolites from common biochemical pathways, adverse effects have been noted from overdosing and metabolic overload. A few examples of these are given in Table 12. The first is calcium tetany from overload of oxalic acid, which was noted in the feeding of 35% solids of irradiated spinach to rats in a toxicity study (Read, Kraybill, & Witt, 1958). The physiologically essential metal micro-nutrient, calcium, induced ultimobranchial tumors and nutritional hypercalcitoninism in bulls when fed in the ration at a rate of 3.5 to 5.7 times the National Research Council RDA (recommended daily allowance). Cows on the same ration with the same high calcium did not reveal these neoplasias since the lactation process excreted the excess (Krook, Lutwak, & McEntee, 1969). The tumor incidence of 30% in the bulls was higher than that of any organ in any domesticated animal. The maximum amount administered in these studies reported by Krook et al. was 87.92 g. Thus, the hypercalcitoninism with high levels of calcitonin in the blood leads to a hyperplastic or neoplastic thyroid gland. In rats, this leads to increased bone density and ultimately some decreased bone resorption (Foster et al. 1967).

In the consideration of lipids, especially under processing conditions, a certain peroxidation and epoxidation of unsaturation can occur. Vitamin E destruction was observed in long-term feeding experiments with irradiated beef that was treated at 6 megarads and fed to rats at the high level of 35% solids in the diet (Kraybill & Whitehair, 1967). Similarly, the formation of hydroxy-hydroperoxides led to some destruction of vitamin K and the occurrence of hemorrhagic diathesis accentuated by the fact that copraphagy (recycling of feces) did not take place (Kraybill & Whitehair, 1967).

Many studies have been done on overfeeding of sucrose in the diet of rats and man. A review of these studies by Kraybill (1975) shows that even this seemingly innocuous dietary chemical can induce hypertriglyceridemia, hypercholesterolemia, hypertension (due to accretion of extracellular fluid) and kidney lesions. For the amino acids, all of which play a role, physiologically, at the correct level in the milieu for homeostasis, overloading with these essential nutrients, especially as an imbalance, can lead to a series of aberrant biochemical effects and a toxicity. A complete review of the literature on these observations is presented by Harper, Benevenga, and Wohlhueter, (1970); a few of these observations are presented in Table 12.

For one to analyze, statistically, toxicity data obtained from experimental studies in animals where large doses of a chemical were given, and then predict what percent of humans may be adversely affected by a challenge at a lower dose is not valid, biochemically or pharmacologically. This assumes a priori that the ability to detoxify a chemical on a dose-dependency relationship is not altered. Piper et al. (1973) have demonstrated that the pharmacokinetic data have for different doses of 2,4,5,-T support the conclusion that at high doses the detoxication process, such as excretion, are altered. Other chamicals behave similarly, including thallium (Gehring & Hammond, 1967), ethyleneglycol (Gessner, Parke & Williams, 1961) and many organic acids (Wagner, 1971). Considering the metabolism of ethyleneglycol, it transforms to glycoaldehyde, glycolic acid and then to glyoxylic acid and, ultimately, to formic acid and carbon dioxide by the major pathway.

Weinhouse (1955) has shown that glyoxylic acid conversion to oxalate in

TABLE 12

ADVERSE EFFECTS OF CHEMICALS FROM METABOLIC OVERLOAD

CHEMICAL	ADVERSE EFFECT	REFERENCE
Oxalic Acid (in spinach)	Calcium Tetany (Rats)	Read, Kraybill and and Witt, 1958
Calcium (in bovine ration)	Ultimobranchial Tumors in Bulls	Krook et al, 1969
Hydroxyhydroperoxides (in irradiated beef)	Vitamin E and K Destruction Hemorrhagic Diathesis	Kraybill and Whitehair, 1967
Sucrose	Hypertriglyceridemia (Rats and Man) Hypercholesterolemia (Rats and Man) Hypertension (Rats) Kidney Lesions (Rats)	Kraybill, 1975 " " " " " "
Methionine	Lowered Fetal Weight – Growth Depression (Rats)	Harper et al, 1970
Tryptophane	Nephrotoxic Effects (Rats)	" " " "
Phenylalanine	Seritonin Depression (Rats)	" " " "
Tyrosine	Nephrotoxic Effects (Rats) Suppression, antibody response (Rats)	" " " " " " " "

rat liver homogenates is dependent on dose. At low dose the oxidation is entirely to carbon dioxide; however, at high doses, there is a partial oxidation to oxalate, as shown in Fig. 4. Such examples should caution the investigator on probable effects of overdosing and the errors in drawing conclusions on carcinogenicity assessment when dose-dependency and overload intervene. In such instances, a metabolite formed a high dose could be the proximate carcinogen which will not appear in the tissues at the lower dose.

Extrapolation of pathological alterations: animal to man. In a review report on environmental health criteria on DDT and its derivatives, the World Health Organization (1977) sets forth some interesting intercomparisons on liver changes in the rodents from administration of organochlorine compounds and the lack of such predictability to man. Kuwabana and Takayama (1974) elicited the marked differences between 2,7-FAA and DDT and BHC. In the first case, the final lesion was hepatocellular carcinoma while in the latter two cases the lesion was an adenoma. Alpha-feto protein was formed in the first instance while this was not true for DDT or BHC. Hanada, Yutani, and Miyaji (1973) also failed to find alpha-feto protein in mice treated with chlorinated hydrocarbon insecticide.

Both chlorinated hydrocarbon insecticides and phenobarbital do not produce in animals, other than rodents, the early visible changes in the endoplasmic reticulum which are indeed characteristic of rodents, and progress from this stage to tumors. Thus, it was recognized that such a progression of events to tumor formation could probably be predicted from early changes characterized by hyperthrophy, margination, and lipospheres.

As will be indicated later, there does not appear, thus far, to be any good evidence that the chlorinated hydrocarbon insecticides and phenobarbital have

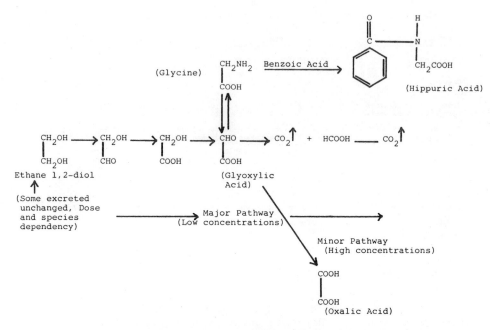

PROBABLE FATE OF ETHYLENE GLYCOL IN THE BODY
(Influence of Dose on Metabolites Formed and Excreted)

FIGURE 4

Source: Gessner et al (1961) Biochem. J. 79: 482-489.

any tumorigenic action in man for heavily exposed populations. As indicated above, one of the early changes from the smallest effective dose is that involving the endoplasmic reticulum. The initial change is reversible and it is peculiar to rodents. In essence then, evidence is lacking that those rodent changes—from an increase in endoplasmic reticulum to final development of nodular liver with some displacement of cells to the lung—really have any significance to man or other animals where the endoplasmic reticulum does not respond similarly.

Predictive value for short-term bioassays (mutagenicity). Many reports have been issued on the applicability of the so-called rapid bioassays or mutagenicity screens to predictions on associated carcinogenic activity using various test systems.

No attempt will be made to comment in detail on the validity of these procedures. DeSerres (1975) has indicated that the battery of tests used in a prescreen may not be completely comprehensive and that some chemicals will yield false negative and false positive results. Nevertheless, the short-term tests

42

can be useful to establish priorities for testing in higher organisms. More extensive data should be forthcoming in enhancement of carcinogenicity-mutagenicity correlations and the ultimate predictive value to human hazard situations.

In commenting on the lack of correlation between mutagenicity and carcinogenicity of certain chemicals, Rubin (1976) has stated the following: "To use this kind of test (mutagenicity) as a test for carcinogenicity is a bit like looking under the lampost for a coin lost a block away, because of the availability of the light." Mutagenicity correlates well with carcinogenicity for many groups of compounds but not in the case of the organohalogen compounds ($CHCl_3$, CCl_4, dieldrin, etc.), which may be carcinogenic to mice but not mutagenic under current methods for testing. Future tests may be developed for evolving the metabolic conversion of these compounds into ultimate electrophiles.

Statistical considerations in prediction of risk. Statistical considerations and the use of mathematical models play a great role, especially where biological data on dose-response is lacking. Certainly, quantitative extrapolations from test systems to man should be based not simply upon single dose tests but, instead, upon dose-response curves. Certain assumptions are extant in plotting the dose-response curve beyond certain points, concluding that the relationship is linear and that the line could extrapolate to the spontaneous rate at zero dose. However, curvilinear relationships may prevail and the response curve could be asymptotic to zero risk axis, and thus approach a zone of insignificance or even a true threshold. Thus, if there is a threshold or deviation from linearity then the procedure will overstate the risk. What is needed is more data in the low dose-response area to revise more accurately the true effect and mechanism. Such information would, of course, be more helpful to the statistician in computation of risk factors.

Many of the assessments for potential carcinogenic hazard to man, which are dependent on experimental data, usually involve evaluation of risk at low-level insults in the environment. These estimates have been made for a spectrum of chemicals. Usually, a finite level derived or a standard which is promulgated is extremely conservative, in many instances approaching zero. With a decreased level of risk, experimentally, in order for the assay to measure a carcinogenic response a vast increase in the number of animals is required.

The procedure requires tremendous resources. However, this additional resource may only provide a minor incremental increase in the degree of confidence in any decision that must be made on the results of the chronic toxicity tests. The complexities of such planning have been previously described in relation to kilomouse or megamouse experiments and the difficulties associated with these approaches.

The acceptance of risk and the decision-making process on risk factors ultimately are societal ones beyond the realms of the scientific community. These are judgmental areas wherein maximum levels of risk are changed from 1 cancer in 100 million to 1 cancer in 1 million. The decisions are difficult in terms of socioeconomics and technical feasibility. However, it should be remembered that the mathematical approaches with certain models involving different slopes on a dose-response curve are at best crude and full of assumptions. Thus, the biological scientist has his assumptions and theoretical forecasts on the metabolic fate and response of a chemical insult at low concentrations. His presentation should be heeded equally well in the decision-making process on establishment of probable carcinogenic hazard to man.

Until we begin to collect data quantitatively and qualitatively that is compatible with extrapolation from experimental animal situations to human situations or exposures, we will probably never be able to reconcile the disproportionality of the so-called acceptable risk (i.e., 1 in 100 million, 1 in 1 million, etc.) in the case of cancer. The statistical approaches fill in this void created by our level of ignorance on the mechanism of carcinogenesis and the probabilities prevailing on the different levels of exposure, species variation, and other factors. The question thus arises: Are the mathematical model projections within a species of sufficient validity to provide judgements as to human significance, especially where human exposure situations are vastly different from the experimental animal exposures scheduled in the test for carcinogenicity?

Epidemiological verification of experimental studies. Verification of experimental observations by cancer incidence in man is irrevocable evidence. While almost all chemicals found to induce cancer in man, with the exception of arsenic or arsenic compounds, have been shown to be carcinogenic in animals, the reverse situation frequently cannot be proven out. Variations in species, strain, sex, and in pharmacological response, as well as susceptibility to toxic agent, are some of the factors that preclude achievement of a correlation in response from animal to man.

The fact that man is exposed to multiple insults and, thus, additive effects, should introduce some caution in attempting to intrepret even a single agent negative response as to the implication for human risk. On the other hand, as Roe (1968) has emphasized, there is a need to distinguish between primary effects of a chemical as to whether it is a carcinogen or is merely acting synergistically as a cocarcinogen. This situation could be applicable to DDT and other chemicals. It is most important to delineate those differences experimentally.

Extrapolation of findings in an experimental system to man always raises questions and is a complex issue. Causality may not be established but when cancer induction in animals is observed, unfortunately, the publicity such information receives automatically impugns this chemical despite any inadequacies in the study; to the general public, the implications may be set that such is the case in man. Once a positive result is released from even questionable animal tests, and despite the subsequent appearance of negative findings in several well-designed studies, the isolated positive test result assumes greater significance in its applicability to human risk than perhaps is warranted. Thus, care must be taken in the development of accurate tests and some balance must be achieved in the testing program lest we misapply data and mislead public health officials in these matters. One case in point here, emphasized by several authors, is that of the debate on safety of DDT. The divergent views on this chemical are exemplified by the action taken on banning of DDT in the United States, while the World Health Organization supported the continued use of this pesticide for the benefit of the majority of the world population.

Not all cases are as convincing as that for vinyl chloride which was not only shown to produce the rare lesion of angiosarcoma of the liver in man, but was quite appropriately shown to produce cancer in several animal species on a dose-dependency basis and, at lower doses revealed cancers at organ sites other than the liver. DDT, on the other hand, is one of those controversial environmental chemicals which was established as a carcinogen only to the mouse. The human population has received an exposure to DDT/DDE since 1940 and thus far, even after a long induction period of 36 years, there is no evidence that this pesticide is a carcinogen to man. Although studies on man are limited, well-designed studies on those of high exposures over the years, such as pesticide formulators and applicators, should finally establish whether there are any excess cancers associated with DDT/DDE exposure. For the general population such a study would not be feasible, since DDT is ubiquitous and no cohort exists in the world which would be free of DDT exposure.

Deichmann (1975) has stated that "the effects in mice are, in general, not without reservation predictive of other rodents as well as man." He attempted to show that deaths from liver disease, including malignant neoplasms of the liver and biliary passages, were declining from 1940 to 1972. In the first column of Table 13 these trends are shown. In 1968 the ICDS (International Classification of Diseases) (Dept. of HEW, 1968) redesignated their coding of liver neoplasms and the ancillary cancers of contiguous organs. Table 13 (Columns 2,3,4 and 5) reflects rates calculated on this basis by the National Cancer Institute's Field Studies and Statistics Program for the years specified (Dept. of HEW, 1975). In this same comparison, from 1968 to 1972 there does not appear to be an increase in cancers from these organ sites which could be expected after 28-32 years' exposure.

While one cannot generalize on the aggregate cancer deaths for organ sites shown in Table 13, nevertheless, thus far in the time frame of some 30 years there does not appear to be the expected liver cancer excess unless the rates are "worked out," so to speak, in the large population of the USA and thus obscured.

For this reason, as stated earlier, a restricted study of a selected group on "high exposure" cohorts might be examined. Thus, future studies might be able to show any specific rates and trends for liver cancer associated with exposures to DDT/DDE. It is tempting, at this time, to assume a negative causal relation-

TABLE 13

LIVER DEATH RATE (1939-72) AND AGE ADJUSTED CANCER RATES
FOR NEOPLASMS OF LIVER, GALL BLADDER AND BILE DUCT
(Rate/100,000 in Total United States)

Year	Liver Deaths	Liver and Intrahepatic[1]	Liver Unspecified[2]	Gall Bladder Bile Duct[3]	All Sites Intra and Extrahepatic[2]
1939	9.6				
1940	7.4				
1949	6.7				
1950	6.5				
1960	5.4				
1968		1.06	1.4	2.2	5.3
1969		1.06	1.4	2.0	5.3
1970	4.7	1.08	1.3	1.9	5.2
1971	4.7	1.09	1.3	1.9	5.2
1972	4.7				

ICDA Codes: [1] = 155; [2] = 197.8; [3] = 156; [4] = 155, 156, 197.7 and 197.8.

Data from Deichmann (1975); Bureau of Census (1943); and National Cancer
  Institute (1975)

ship for DDT/DDE and, by analogy, other organochlorine pesticides with reference to man where liver is the target organ. Accordingly, thus far the risk for
these chemicals is stated in terms of experimental animal evidence and concerns
are based strictly on that base of reference.

III. SUMMARY

Neoplasia depends invariably on multiple factors acting concurrently or sequen-
tially, and the impact could vary at different stages of the disease process.
Kolbye (1976) in his report speaks of four dimensions, the first two dealing with
the insult and the response, and the third really referring to the multiple factors
mentioned above that influence the induction of cancer. The fourth dimension,
of course, is the time factor. At each stage in the development of neoplasia,
there is the complex interaction of genetic factors and the external environmental factors that have been described previously. The action of the recognized
carcinogenic insult, either initiator or promoter, is obviously conditioned by permissive factors at the cell level or in the milieu. Thus, these genetic and physiological factors, which influence homeostasis, play a role in transport and
initiation action of the carcinogen either at target organs or the micromolecellar
foci in a qualitative and quantitative manner. Other factors control the responsiveness of the target cells, the organ and tissue composed of these cells, or the
basic effects on DNA.

According to some, assessment of carcinogenesis becomes a statistical exercise in that one is measuring tumor incidence of the test group against an in-

cidence for a control group. These statistical relationships frequently obscure, especially where dose-response studies are carried out, the biological factors that impact so much on the end results. Thus, if responses are noted at high dose challenge, one should perceive the possibility that these may be absent at a low dose level. The adaptive response, for example, at a low dose as is true with trace elements, should not be misconstrued as an injury but more as a biological defense mechanism, or indeed, a conditioned response that is physiologically essential. Selenium is a good case in point here.

Smyth (1967) in his excellent treatise on "sufficient challenge" emphasizes some important pharmacological considerations in deliberations on dose-response and the concepts on risk. From several of his significant statements one can emphasize the following: "Any effect from our high doses which is statistically validated we accept. Any apparent benefit from our low doses which may be statistically validated we discount because it is not dose-related." He chides toxicologists for ignoring the manifestations of the sufficient challenge hypothesis (the concept that low-level insult may have apparent benefits) when they observe it in the laboratory, whereas nutritionists searching for dietary supplements are biased the other way, looking for benefits at low-level insult. The admonition in the field of carcinogenesis is self-evident. He goes on to state that nonspecific responses at low dosage are, in fact, readjustments or adaptations to sufficient challenge. The mammalian system is adequate to maintain homeostasis; but, when overwhelmed with stress, injury results. Moreover, not every adaptive response is a manifestation of injury. The question arises then whether a low-level insult, for instance, to chloroform, carbon tetrachloride, and others categorized as carcinogens, would not indeed fall within his concept of sufficient challenge.

As previously mentioned, an array of factors can modify upwards the incidence of cancer in test animals which is statistically greater than that for the control group. Again, these extraneous factors are too often overlooked. When they are recognized then the question arises: what weight should they be give in risk assessment? If they enhance susceptibility to cancer and are not carcinogenic *per se,* then certainly one must comprehend and interpret appropriately the role of such contributors in the neoplastic process.

There are a host of other variants that perhaps have not been fully evaluated in assessment of risk and in the extrapolation of data from experimental systems to their probable significance in man. For example, the unique toxicological properties of a chemical may condition the organ and cells to extensive injury as an antecedent to the ultimate formation of malignant cells. As stated earlier, we must ask: Will a decrease in dose negate the possibility of such biochemical, pharmacological, and pathological alterations? There are substances that are retained in the body, others that are rapidly metabolized or deactivated, some that are activated by enzymes in the liver, some that undergo placental transfer, some that are excreted in breast milk (i.e., PCB, DDT, etc.), while others appear to respond to certain defense mechanisms or interect with certain inhibitors. When experimental observations focus on carcinogenic activity of various agents, can we really equate all such events of equal significance as to any human significance unless we have fully explored the condition and the modifiers involved in the mechanisms wherein the stated chemical or agent was shown to be carcinogenic in a test system? Potency indices are rarely applied since some consider all carcinogens in the same risk class, yet, subconsciously, most would agree that the potent hepatocarcinogen, aflatoxin, could not be equated with a pesticide such as DDT insofar as potential risk to human health is concerned.

The dose-response relationships, especially in experimental situations where metabolic overload is achieved, certainly do not have a counterpart in human events, and thus the relevance to predicting human health hazard may be in doubt. In many situations where the exposure situations applicable to man are not reflected in the experimental dose-response patterns, mathematical extrapolation models are resorted to in order to provide a basis for judgment on risk factors. Lacking biological information in the area of the shallow or flat slope dose-response curve, the mathematical model is the alternative. Many assumptions underlie the use of such models; therefore, can such extrapolative mathematical projections, for example in the rodent, be assigned that much validity in application to probable hazard in man where indeed the exposures are different, the metabolism may be different, and the repair phenomena may present a different biochemical pharmacological reaction in the insult at the cell level?

Before extrapolation of experimental data to particular human usage can be made, it is generally recognized that additional studies must be made. A few cases worth mentioning which reinforce the preceding arguments are as follows:

1. Bioassays where test animals are subjected to grossly unphysiological and nonrelevant conditions in addition to challenge from the test chemical; under such conditions tumor induction may be enhanced.
2. Bioassays conducted by an unusual route of administration, such as bladder implantation, resulting in an effect which may not be due to the test compound.

The plea is made that one must resort to the best scientific judgment in the appraisal of risk in the areas of uncertainties and that bioassays which are conducted under designs that are not compatible with sound biochemical and pharmacological reasoning should be rejected. Our understanding of the mechanisms of carcinogenesis is limited, but, first and foremost, chemicals introduced into a mammalian system may be expected to produce a certain biological effect, one of which, under a unique set of conditions, could be carcinogenesis. However, the response achieved is mediated and limited by certain biochemical, metabolic, and pharmacokinetic relationships. Such boundaries must not be exceeded in biological testing and assessment of carcinogenesis, lest irreconcilable implications are left with the scientific community and the public which result, in the long run, in a waste of national resources in the interest of public health.

REFERENCES

Adamson, R. H., Correa, P., Sieber, S. M., McIntire, R. K., & Dalgard, D. W. Carcinogenicity of aflatoxin B_1 in rhesus monkeys: Two additional cases of primary liver cancer. *J. Natl. Cancer Inst.*, 1976, *57:* 67-78.

Allison, A. C. & Law, L. W. Effects of antilymphocyte serum on virus oncogenesis. Proc. Soc. Exptl. Biol. 1968, *127,* 207.

American Conference of Governmental and Industrial Hygienists. *Threshold limit values for chemical substances and physical agents in the Workroom Environment with Intended Changes for 1976.* Cincinnati, Ohio, 1976, Pp. 394-402.

Berg, J. W. (1975). Diet (Environmental Factor). In E.J. Fraumeni (Ed.), *Persons at High risk of cancer and Approach to Cancer etiology and control.* New York: Academic Press, 1975.

Burchfield, H. P., Storrs, E. E. Kraybill, H. F. The maximum tolerated dose in pesticide carcinogenicity studies. In F. Coulston and F. Korte (eds.), *Environmental Quality and Safety,* Vol. III. Stuttgart, Germany: Thieme Publ., 1975.

Cleaver, J. E. Defective repair replication of DNA in Xeroderma Pigmentosum. Nature, 1968, *218,* 652.

Cuthbertson, W. F. J., Laursen, A. C. & Pratt. D. A. H. Effect of groundnut meal containing aflatoxin on cynomolgus. *Brit. J. Nutr.,* 1967, *21,* 893-908.

Deichmann, W. B. The market basket: Food for thought. Cummings Memorial Lecture. *Am. Ind. Hyg. Assoc. Journ.,* June, 1975, 411-429.

DeSerres, F. J. The prediction of chronic toxicity from short-term studies. *Proc. of European Soc. of Toxicology,* 1975, *17,* 113-116. (Reprinted from Exerpta Medicus Int. Congress Series, No. 376, Amsterdam, The Netherlands)

DHEW, Public HEalth Service, National Center for Vital Statistics. *International Classification of Diseases (ICDA).* Government Printing Office, 8th Revision, Washington, D. C. 1968.

DHEW Public Health Service, National Cancer Institute. *Calculations on liver cancer rates in the USA by age adjustment.* (Rept. furnished by Field Studies and Statistics Program to author on October 2, 1975), 1975.

DHEW, National Cancer Institute, Division of Cancer Cause and Prevention. *Report on carcinogenesis bioassay of chloroform, carcinogenesis program.* 1976.

Dinman, D. B. "Nonconcept" of "no threshold." Chemicals in the environment. *Science* 1972, *1975,* 495.

Eckhardt, R. E. The Delaney Amendment. *Prevent. Med.,* 1973, *2,* 156-158.

Falk, H. L. Considerations of risks versus benefits. *Env. Health Perspectives.* 1975, *11,* 1-5.

Flamm, W. G. The need for quantifying risk from exposure to chemical carcinogens. *Proceedings of the Nineteenth Meeting of the Interagency Collaborative Group on Environmental Carcinogenesis.* National Cancer Institute, 1975.

Foster, G. V., Doyle, F. H., Bordier, P., Matrajt H. & Tun-Chot, S. Roentgenolgic and histologic changes in bone produced by thyrocalcitonin. *Am. J. Med.,* 1967, *43,* 691-695.

Friedman, L. Problems of evaluating the health significance of the chemicals present in food. *Proceedings of Fifth Int. Congress Pharmacol.,* San Francisco, Calif., 1972.

Gehring, P. J. & Hammond, P. B. The interrelationship between thallium and potassium in animals. *J. Pharmacol. Exp. Ther.* 1967, *155,* 187-201.

Gessner, P. K., Parke, D. V. & Williams, R. T. Studies on detoxification. *Biochem. J.,* 1961, *79,* 482-489.

Grant, G., Roe, F. C. J. & Pike, M. C. Effect of neonatal thymectomy on the induction of papillomata and carcinomata by 3,4-benzopyrene in mice. *Nature,* 1966, *210,* 603.

Hanada, M., Yutani, C., & Miyaji, T. Induction of hepatoma in mice by benzene hexachloride. *Gann*, 1973, *64*, 511-513.

Harper, A. E., Benevenga, N. J., & Wohlhueter, R. M. Effects of ingestion of disproportionate amounts of amino acids. *Physiol. Rev.*, 1970, *50*, 428-539.

Henschler, D. New approaches to a definition of threshold values for irreversible toxic effects. *Arch. Toxicol*, 1974, *32*, 63-67.

Hueper, W. C. & Ruchhoft, C. C. Carcinogenic studies on adsorbates of industrially polluted raw and finished water supplies. *Arch. Industr. Hyg. Occup. Med*, 1954, *9*, 488-495.

Innes, J. R. M., Ulland, B. M., Valerio, M. G., Petrucelli, I., Fishbein, L., Hart, E. R., Pallotta, A. J., Bates, R. R., Falk, H. L., Gart. J. J., Klein, M., Mitchell, I. & Peters, J. Bioassay of pesticides and industrial chemicals for tumorigenicity in mice. A preliminary note. *J. Natl. Cancer Inst.*, 1969, *42*, 1101.

Ito, N., Nagasaki, H., & Arai, M. Interactions of liver tumorigenesis in mice treated with technical polychlorinated biphenyls and benzene hexachloride (BHC). In F. Coulston, F. Korte & M. Goto (Eds.), *New methods in environmental chemistry and toxicology*, Academic Scientific Book, 1973.

Jones, H. B. & Grendon, A. Environmental factors in the origin of cancer and estimation of possible hazard to man. *Fd. Cosmet. Toxicol.* 1975, *13*, 251-268. Pergamon Press, Oxford England.

Kensler, C. J. Sugiura, K., Young, N. F., Halter, C. R. & Rhoads, C. P. Partial protection of rats by riboflavin with casein against liver cancer sauced by dimethylaminoazobenzene. *Science*, 1941, *93*, 308-310.

Kimbrough, R.D., & Linder, R. E. The induction of adenofibrosis and hepatomas of the liver in mice of the BALB/C_1 strain of polychlorinated biphenyls (Arochlor 1254). *J. Natl. Cancer Inst.*, 1974, *53*, 547-552.

Kline, B. E., Rusch, H. P., Baumann, C. A., & Lavik, P. S. The effect of pyridoxine on tumor growth. *Cancer Res.* 1943, *3*, 825-829.

Kolbye, A. C. Cancer in humans: Exposures and responses in a real world. *Oncology*, 1970, *33*, 90-100.

Kraybill, H. F. Carcinogenesis associated with food. *Clin. Pharmacol. and Therapeutics*, 1963, *4*, pp. 73-87.

Kraybill, H. F. Food contaminants and gastrointestinal or liver neoplasia. Survey of experimental observations. *Env. Res.*, 1969, *2*, (No. 4) 231-246.

Kraybill, H. F. Illustrations of probable thresholds. *Proceedings of the Nineteenth Meeting of the Interagency Collaborative Group on Environmental Carcinogenesis, National Cancer Institute*, 1975.

Kraybill, H. F. The questions of benefits and risks of sugar. *Academy forum on sweeteners; issues and uncertainties*. Washington, D. C.: Natl. Academy of Sciences, 1975, 59-76.

Kraybill, H. F. Carcinogencity of arsenic: experimental studies. In B. W. Carnow, (Ed.), *Proceedings of Symposium on Health Effects of Occupational Lead and Arsenic Exposure*. DHEW/USPHS/CDC/NIOSH. Chicago Ill. Washington, D.C.: U. S. Gov. Printing Office, 1976.

Kraybill, H. F. & Shimkin, M. B. Carcinogenesis related to foods contaminated by processing and fungal metabolites. In (eds.) *Advances in Cancer Research, 8*, New York: Academic Press, 1964.

Kraybill, H. F. & Whitehair, L. A. Toxicological safety of irradiated foods. *Ann. Rev. of Pharmacology*, 1967, *7*, 357-380.

Krook, L., Lutwak, L., & McEntee, K. Dietary calcium, ultimobranchial tumors and osteoporosis in the bull. *Am. J. Clin. Nutr.*, 1969, *22*, (No. 2), 115-118.

Kuwabana, N. & Takayama, S. (1974). Comparison of histogenesis of liver of mice administered respectively, BHC, DDT and 2,7-FAA. *Proc. Jap. Cancer Assoc.*, 1974, *33*, 50.

Maltoni, C. & Lefemine, G. Carcinogenicity bioassays on vinyl chloride. I. Research plans and early results. *Env. Res.*, 1974, *7*, 387-405.

Mantel, N., & Schneiderman, M. A. Estimating "safe" levels; a hazardous undertaking. *Cancer Research*, 1975, *35*, 1379-1386.

McLean, A. E. M. Diet and the chemical environment as modifiers of carcinogenesis. In Doll & Vodopiya, (Eds.), *Host environmental interactions in the etiology of cancer in man. IARC Sci. Publ.*, 1973, No. 7, 223-230.

Michigan State Dept. of Health Survey. *Mother's milk in quarantined areas of PBB contamination,* October, 1976.

Morgan, K., Hastings, P. J. & von Borstel, R. C. A potential hazard: Explosive production of mutations by induction of mutators. *Environ. Health Perspectives*, 1973, *6*, 207.

Nielsen, F. H., Givand, S. & Myron, D. Evidence of a possible requirement for arsenic by the rat. *Fed. Proceed.*, 1975, *34*, Abstract 3987, 923.

Penn, I. Malignant tumors in organ transplant recipients. In *Recent results in cancer research* Berlin: *35*, 1-51, Springer Verlag, 1970. Pp. 1-51.

Piper, W. N., Rose, J. Q., Leng, M. L., & Gehring, P. J. The fate of 2,4,5-trichlorophenoxyacetic acid (2,4,5-T) following oral administration to rats and dogs. *J. Tox. Appl. Pharmacol,,* 1973, *26*, (No. 3), 339-351.

Rall, D. Extrapolating environmental toxicology: The costs and benefits of being right and wrong. *Proceedings of the nineteenth meeting of the interagency collaborative group on environmental carcinogenesis.* National Cancer Institute, 1975.

Read, M. S., Kraybill, H. F., & Witt, N. I. Short-term feeding studies with gamma irradiated food products. I. Frozen stored foods. *J. Nutrition*, 1958, *65*, 39-52 (specific reference, p. 47).

Roe, F. S. C. Carcinogenesis and sanity. *Food Cosmet. Toxicol.*, 1968, *6*, 485.

Roe, F. S. C. On the persistence of tumor initiation and the acceleration of tumor progression in mouse skin tumorigenesis. *Int. J. Cancer*, 1972, *9*, 264.

Roe, F. J. C., & Tucker, M. J. Recent developments in the design of carcinogenicity tests on laboratory animals. *Proc. of Europ. Soc. for the Study of Drug Toxicity*, 1974, *15*, 171-197.

Rubin, H. Carcinogenicity tests. *Science*, 1976, *19*, 241.

Salmon, W. D., & Copeland, D. H. Liver carcinoma and related lesions in chronic coline deficiency. *Ann. N. Y. Acad. Sci.*, 1954, *57*, 664-677.

Salmon, W. D., Newberne, P. M. & Prickett, C. O. Hematomas in rats fed diets containing commercial peanut meal. *Fed. Proc.*, 1963, *22*, 262, Abstr. 609.

Smyth, H. F. Sufficient challenge. *Fd. Cosmet. Toxicol.*, 1967, *15*, 51-58.

Tannenbaum, A. Nutrition and cancer. In F. Homberger (Ed.), *The diets physiopathology of cancer.* New York: Hoeber, 1959, 517-562.

Tannenbaum, A., & Silverstone, H. The genesis and growth of tumors. IV. Effects of varying the proportion of protein (casein in the diet). *Cancer Res.*, 1949, *9*, 162-173.

Tomatis, L., Turusov. V., Day, N., & Charles, R. T. The effect of longterm exposure to DDT on CF$_1$ mice. *Int. J. Cancer*, 1962, *10*, 489.

Tulpule, P. G., Madhavan, T. V., & Gopalan, C. Effect of feeding aflatoxin to young monkeys. *Lancet*, 1964, *1*, 926-963.

U. S. Environmental Protection Agency. *Progress report of pesticide program, Colorado State University survey.* August, 1976.

Wagner, J. G. (1971). *Biopharmaceutics and Relevant Pharmacokinetics.* Hamilton, Illinois. Drug Intelligence Publications, 1971.

Weinhouse, S. (1955). In W. D. McElroy & H. B. Glass, (Eds.), *Amino Acid Metabolism.* Baltimore, Md., The Johns Hopkins Press, 1955.

White, J., White, F. R., & Mider, G. B. Effects of diets deficient in certain amino acids on the induction of leukemia in DBA mice. *J. Natl. Cancer Inst.,* 1947, *7,* 199-202.

World Health Organization. Report of scientific group on assessment of the carcinogenicity and mutagenicity of chemicals. *Tech. Rept. Series, 546,* Geneva, WHO, Switzerland, 1974. Pp. 11-12.

World Health Organization. *Draft report of the environmental health criteria program. Environmental health criteria for DDT and its derivatives,* 1977.

Discussion

DR. UPHOLT: In all of these discussions, it seems inevitable that some question comes up about threshold levels: whether or not there is such a thing as a threshold. I submit that a discussion of threshold may be very useful, but only if we define exactly what we are talking about. I have heard all of these discussions, but I don't remember anybody ever stating exactly what he means by a threshold. I don't like to put Herman on the spot, but I wonder if he or anybody else in the group would like to give such a definition.

DR. COULSTON: I think this is a very legitimate point that you are making, but I'm so simplistic. A threshold to me means the point at which nothing is really happening or just about to happen. I'd rather call it a no-effect level if I mean nothing happens, and a threshold level where just borderline effects occur. Herman, let's hear your view.

DR. KRAYBILL: What I'm thinking about is what Fred said. Below a certain point there may be no effect physiologically, pharmacologically, or pathologically, and that's why I used the cases of things that react homeostatically, and as to support homeostasis, like a vitamin or a hormone. It may be that we can go beyond such things as selenium, arsenic, and other things at low levels. They're acting, as Morris Diamond said, in a beneficial sort of way. But then you go on the other side of the mountain and you're getting into an adverse effect. I don't think this shocks me because in the noncarcinogenic field we see many cases, many examples. The other thing we didn't mention here is that I look upon all these things as chemicals, and once we give it the tag of a carcinogen, it takes on a whole new aura. But we've got to think first of these as chemicals that go through certain metabolic pathways and certain biochemical mechanisms. That, to me, is important. I haven't defined it, but I think I'm defining what I think is the effect below a certain level, if you don't have a physiological effect.

DR. UPHOLT: A definition such as either of you have given does not specify how long after exposure you're looking at it, it does not specify what you mean by the size population; you're talking about "no effect" in any organism in the population, and if so, a population of what size? It does not talk about how you detect an effect.

If you're talking about detection by visual means, if you're talking about it by biochemical means, by electron microscopic method, or whether you're talking about a desirable effect or undesirable effect, these things all have to be considered and defined before I think we can really talk intelligently about whether there is or is not an effect at any particular level.

DR. COULSTON: This is, of course, the crux. We could almost do away with the papers at this point, and just go into a discussion for two days on this question alone. But I would hope and I would ask you again to bring this up in the discussion period which will occur very shortly after this paper.

It's a very crucial point and it needs to be resolved. I am thinking of no effect, in the lifespan of a mouse, that could be discerned by an technique that we use in our laboratories, including electron microscopy. We can find such levels with dieldrin, DDT, and methoxychlor. We have done this with mirex, and with many other chemicals, even with phenobarbital. There is a point where nothing can be observed. It may be below a useful level, if you add a safety factor, for the intended use of the chemical in society. But at least let's find the point and see if that point has any relationship to other species of animals, and then determine what the projection is to man.

We have to get into this discussion. There are all kinds of chemicals. If I'm talking about a nitrogen mustard, a very strong alkylating agent, it is a different story. But if I'm talking about so-called carcinogens like cyclamate, saccharin, DDT, and phenobarbital, these are not strong carcinogens like nitrogen mustard any way you look at it. These changes caused by the mentioned chemicals in a cell occurred because some eager scientist in the laboratory added chemicals day in and day out in enormous amounts until the physiologic state of the animal broke down and he got a pathologic condition.

This is just nonsense! It's like hitting a man on the head once or hitting him on the head daily for his lifespan. Obviously, if you hit him on the head every day something is going to happen, and I don't know if this is toxicity or not. This is what we have to discuss later. Thank you, very much.

Now we're ready for the hext speaker. It gives me pleasure to introduce Dr. Conney who will present his paper entitled "The Effects of Environmental Factors and Nutrition on Human Drug Metabolism."

3. Effects of Environmental Factors and Nutrition on Human Drug Metabolism

A. P. Alvares
Uniformed Services
Bethesda, Maryland

A. H. Conney
Hoffmann-La Roche
Nutley, New Jersey

E. J. Pantuck
College of Physicians and Surgeons
Columbia University

A. Kappas
The Rockefeller University
New York

Large differences occur in the intensity and duration of action of drugs in different individuals. One individual may have a toxic side effect, whereas another individual may not have any response to the drug. This variability in drug response is caused at least in part by differences in the rates of metabolism of drugs in different individuals. Because of similarities in the enzyme systems that metabolize drugs and chemical carcinogens, it is not surprising that there are also large differences in the metabolism of carcinogens in different people, and it is possible that individuality in the metabolism of a carcinogen may, in part, explain differences in the response of different members of a population to the carcinogen. A 35-fold difference in the plasma concentrations of the antidepressant drug desmethylimipramine was found in several individuals given the same dose (Hammer et al., 1967), and ten-, six- and sevenfold interindividual differences in plasma half-lives of bishydroxycoumarin (Vesell & Page, 1968a; Weiner et al., 1950), phenylbutazone (Burns et al., 1953; Vesell & Page, 1968b), and antipyrine (Kolmodin et al., 1969; Vesell & Page, 1969), respectively, also have been observed. In addition, marked interindividual differences have been observed in the metabolism of the carcinogen 2-acetylaminofluorene in man (Weisburger et al., 1964). The marked individuality in rates of metabolism of foreign chemicals is caused by genetic and environmental factors. Studies by Vesell et al., (1968b, 1969) have shown that interindividual variations in the metabolism of antipyrine and phenylbutazone were greater in fraternal than in identical twins, and similar results have been observed in twins administered nortriptyline (Alexanderson et al., 1969).

Although there have been only a few studies on the influence of diet and other environmental factors on the metabolism of foreign chemicals in man, the effects of environmental factors on drug metablism have been studied extensively in experimental animals. More than 25 years ago, Gerald Mueller and James Miller (1950) at the University of Wisconsin found that riboflavin adenine dinucleotide was required for the reductive cleavage of a carcinogenic aminoazo dye to noncarcinogenic metabolites by enzymes in rat liver. This observation provided an explanation for the protective effect of dietary riboflavin on aminoazo dye hepatocarcinogenesis observed earlier by Kensler et al. (1941), and for the observation that the overall rate of destruction of Aminoazo dyes by rat liver slices was dependent on the concentration of riboflavin in the liver (Kensler, 1949). Additional studies in the laboratory of James Miller demonstrated enhanced hepatic metabolism of an aminoazo dye when rodents were switched from a synthetic diet to a chow diet (Brown et al., 1954). These investigators found that hepatic aminoazo dye metabolism was markedly stimulated by certain peroxides and sterols present in the diet (Brown et al., 1954). The above pioneering studies on the influence of dietary factors on the metabolism of aminoazo dyes were the first to show that changes in diet can alter the metabolism and action of foreign chemicals, and this research has been extended by many investigators.

Substances present in man's diet that may influence the metabolism of foreign chemicals include macronutrients (carbohydrate, protein, fat), trace substances important to human health (vitamins, trace metals, etc.) and numerous nonnutrient, lipid-soluble foreign chemicals. Although the latter very diverse group of substances has not been well characterized, the presence of these chemicals in foods is receiving increasingly more attention (Committee on Food Protection, 1973; Crosby 1969) and, indeed, nonnutrient substances in foods are probably the greatest source of human exposure to foreign chemicals. Substances in man's environment which have been shown in animals to stimulate the metabolism of foreign chemicals include halogenated hydrocarbon insecticides, polychlorinated biphenyls, urea herbicides, volatile oils, polycyclic hydrocarbons, dyes used as coloring agents, nicotine, food preservatives, safrole, xanthines, and organic peroxides. Substances in man's environment which have been shown in animals to inhibit the metabolism of foreign chemicals include organophosphate insecticides, carbon tetrachloride, ozone, carbon monoxide, and certain heavy metals such as lead and cadmium. Studies on the effects of environmental substances on drug metabolism in man showed that occupational exposure to DDT (Poland et al., 1970), Lindane (Kolmodin et al., 1969), or polychlorinated biphenyls (Alvares et al., 1977) results in a marked enhancement in the metabolism of antipyrine and/or phenylbutazone and that acute exposure of children to the environmental pollutant lead results in a significant inhibition of antipyrine metabolism (Alvares et al., 1975).

EFFECTS OF CIGARETTE SMOKING
ON DRUG METABOLISM

Polycyclic aromatic hydrocarbon carcinogens such as benzo(a)pyrene, dibenz-(a,h)anthracene, and benz(a)anthracene, are widespread in man's environment as products of incomplete combustion (Committee on Biologic Effects of Atmospheric Pollutants, 1972). Particularly high concentrations of polycyclic hydrocarbons occur in tobacco smoke, coal tar skin ointments, mineral oils, certain smoked foods, and in polluted city air. Twenty years ago, it was found that many environmental polycyclic hydrocarbons have a potent stimulatory effect on the metabolism of certain drugs and carcinogens in rats (Conney et al., 1956, 1957, 1959). Subsequent studies in our laboratory revealed that cigarette smokers have markedly increased activity of enzymes in human placenta which hydroxylate benzo(a)pyrene (Welch et al., 1968, 1969) and zoxazolamine (Kapitulnik et al., 1976), N-demethylate 3-methyl-4-monomethylaminoazobenzene (Welch et al. 1969), and O-dealkylate 7-ethoxycoumarin (Jacobson et al., 1974; see Table 1). The induction of these enzymatic activities is probably the result of the systemic absorption of polycyclic hydrocarbons present in cigarette smoke and the transport of these substances to the placenta. A stimulatory effect of cigarette smoking on placental benzo(a)pyrene hydroxylase activity

TABLE 1
EFFECT OF CIGARETTE SMOKING ON THE METABOLISM OF
CARCINOGENS AND DRUGS BY HUMAN PLACENTA[a]

	Enzyme activity in placenta	
Reaction measured	Nonsmokers	Cigarette smokers
	nmol product/g placenta/hr.	
1. Benzo(a)pyrene hydroxylation	0.7 ± 0.1[b]	28 ± 8
2. 3-Methyl-4 monomethylaminoazobenzene N-demethylation	< 4[c]	26 ± 5
3. Zoxazolamine hydroxylation	0.4 ± 0.1[d]	5.8 ± 1.5
4. 7-Ethoxycoumarin 0-dealkylation	29 ± 3[e]	46 ± 5

[a]All cigarette smokers smoked 7-30 cigarettes daily during pregnancy. Data from studies by Welch et al. (1968, 1969), Jacobson et al. (1974), and Kapitulnik et al. (1976).

[b]nmol 3-hydroxybenzo(a)pyrene formed/g placenta/hr.

[c]nmol 3-methyl-4-aminoazobenzene formed/g placenta/hr.

[d]nmol tritiated water formed/g placenta/hr.

[e]nmol 7-hydroxycoumarin formed/g placenta/hr.

also has been observed by others (Juchau, 1971; Nebert et al., 1969; Pelkonen et al., 1972). Placental tissue from different smokers who smoked the same number of cigarettes exhibited marked individuality in the metabolism of benzo(a)pyrene in vitro. Among the subjects who smoked 15-20 cigarettes daily, placental benzo(a)pyrene hydroxylase activity varied more than 70-fold (see Table 2). Since the metabolism of benzo(a)pyrene is required for its carcinogenic activity, it would be of interest to determine whether or not the marked differences in rates of metabolism of benzo(a)pyrene in different people might be of predictive value in the identification of individuals who are particularly susceptible to benzo(a)pyrene or to other chemical carcinogens present in the environment.

Recent studies in our laboratory have shown that cigarette smoking increases the metabolism of orally administered phenacetin (Pantuck et al., 1974b), a widely used analgesic. Nine smokers and nine nonsmokers were administered 900 mg of phenacetin orally; blood was drawn at various time intervals, and the plasma concentration of phenacetin and of N-acetyl-p-amino-phenol (APAP), its major metabolite, were determined. The plasma levels of phenacetin were considerably lower in cigarette smokers than in nonsmokers (Table 3), and the ratios of the concentrations of N-acetyl-p-aminophenol to those of unchanged parent drug were markedly increased in the cigarette smokers (Table 4). Interestingly, the plasma half-life of phenacetin was not influenced by cigarette smoking. Investigations in rats revealed the presence of an enzyme

TABLE 2
VARIABILITY IN THE INDUCTION OF
BENZO(A)PYRENE HYDROXYLASE
ACTIVITY IN HUMAN PLACENTA[a]

Subject	Hydroxybenzo(a)pyrene formed ng product/g placenta/hr.
A	0.9
B	1.0
C	2.0
D	2.5
E	4.7
F	6.9
G	16.4
H	61.7
I	63.8

[a]All subjects in this study smoked 15-20 cigarettes daily during pregnancy. Little or no hydroxylase activity was found in placentas from nonsmokers. Variability in enzymatic activities was not related to medication taken during or prior to delivery. Data from studies by Welch et al. (1968, 1969)

TABLE 3

PLASMA LEVELS OF PHENACETIN IN CIGARETTE SMOKERS AND
NONSMOKERS AT VARIOUS INTERVALS AFTER THE ORAL
ADMINISTRATION OF 900 MG PHENACETIN[a]

Subjects	Phenacetin in plasma ($\mu g/ml$) at intervals after administration (hr)			
	1	2	3.5	5
Nonsmokers	0.81 ± 0.20	2.24 ± 0.73	0.39 ± 0.13	0.12 ± 0.04
Smokers	0.33 ± 0.23	0.48 ± 0.28*	0.09 ± 0.04[b]	0.02 ± 0.01[b]

[a]Each value represents the mean ± S. E. for 9 subjects. Data from Pantuck et al (1974b).

[b]Values significantly different from that obtained with nonsmokers ($p < 0.05$).

TABLE 4

RATIOS OF MEAN CONCENTRATIONS OF TOTAL
N-ACETYL-p-AMINOPHENOL (APAP) TO MEAN
CONCENTRATIONS OF PHENACETIN IN PLASMAS
OF CIGARETTE SMOKERS AND NONSMOKERS[a]

Subjects	Total APAP/phenacetin in plasma at hr after administration			
	1	2	3.5	5
Nonsmokers	7.7	6.0	35.3	85.4
Smokers	17.2	23.7	127.1	374.5

[a]Subjects were administered 900 mg of phenacetin orally and plasma concentrations of phenacetin and total (conjugated & unconjugated) APAP were determined at various time intervals. The ratio of the mean concentration of total APAP to the mean concentration of phenacetin was calculated. Each value represents the mean from 9 subjects. Data taken from Pantuck et al. (1974b).

system in the wall of the small intestine which is capable of metabolizing phenacetin to N-acetyl-p-aminophenol (Pantuck et al., 1974a, 1974b; Welch et al., 1972), and it was shown that the activity of this enzyme system is increased in rats exposed to cigarette smoke (Pantuck et al., 1974a; Welch et al., 1972) and in rats pretreated with either benzo(a)pyrene (Table 5)—a constituent of cigarette smoke—or with the polycyclic hydrocarbon carcinogen 3-methylcholanthrene (Pantuck et al., 1974a; Welch et al., 1972). Our results demonstrate that cigarette smoking markedly decreases the bioavailability of phenacetin and suggest that cigarette smoking enhances the metabolism of phenacetin during its first pass through the liver and/or in the gastrointestinal tract. Ciga-

TABLE 5
EFFECT OF PRETREATMENT OF RATS WITH
BENZO(A)PYRENE ON THE METABOLISM OF
PHENACETIN BY INTESTINE IN VITRO[a]

Treatment	N-acetyl-p-aminophenol formed ($\mu g/10cm$ intestine/90 min)
Control	3.6 ± 1.0
Benzo(a)pyrene	31.6 ± 4.4[b]

[a]Male Long-Evans rats weighing 250 ± 10 g were given benzo (a)pyrene (40 mg/kg p.o.). The rats were killed 24 hours later and their intestines excised and assayed for phenacetin 0-dealkylating activity. Each value represents the mean ± S.E. for 4 rats. Data taken from Pantuck et al. (1974a).

[b]Value significantly different from control value ($p < 0.001$).

rette smoking decreases the action and/or stimulates the metabolism of several other drugs and carcinogens in man, and these effects are summarized in Table 6.

EFFECT OF CHARCOAL-BROILED BEEF ON DRUG METABOLISM

Charcoal-broiled beef, a food which contains high concentrations of polycyclic hydrocarbons (Lijinsky & Shubik, 1964), is eaten by large numbers of people. To determine whether this food affects drug metabolism, we studied the intestinal metabolism of phenacetin in rats fed charcoal-broiled beef. The in vitro metabolism of phenacetin by intestine was stimulated severalfold when rats were fed a diet containing charcoal-broiled beef (Pantuck et al., 1975; see Table 7). To determine if these findings extended to man, phenacetin was administered to nine normal volunteers after they had been fed (1) a control hospital diet for 7 days, (2) the control hospital diet for 3 additional days and a charcoal-broiled beef diet for 4 days, and (3) the control hospital diet for another 7 days. The control hospital diet contained hamburger at lunch and steak at dinner, and these meats were cooked over burning charcoal with aluminum foil placed between the meat and the burning charcoal. The charcoal-broiled beef diet was identical to the control hospital diet, except that the meat was cooked directly over the burning charcoal. The details of this study are given elsewhere (Conney et al., 1976; Pantuck et al., 1976a). After each of the three dietary regimens, the subjects were administered 900 mg phenacetin orally. Plasma samples were obtained after various time intervals and were analyzed for phenacetin and N-acetyl-p-aminophenol content. Feeding the charcoal-broiled beef diet for 4 days markedly lowered the plasma concentrations of phenacetin (Table 8). Feeding the charcoal-broiled beef did not have a significant effect on plasma N-acetyl-p-

TABLE 6

EFFECTS OF CIGARETTE SMOKING ON THE METABOLISM AND/OR ACTION OF DRUGS

Parameter measured	Compound	Reference
Lowered blood levels	Phenacetin	Pantuck et al. (1974b)
	Theophylline	Jenne et al. (1975)
	Imipramine	Perel et al. (1975)
	Antipyrine	Vestal et al. (1975); Hart et al. (1976)
Decreased urinary excretion	Nicotine	Beckett & Triggs (1967)
Decreased effectiveness	Pentazocine	Keeri-Szanto & Pomeroy (1971)
	Propoxyphene	Boston Collaborative Drug Surveillance Program (1973a)
Decreased drowsiness	Chlorpromazine	Swett (1974)
	Diazepam	Boston Collaborative Drug Surveillance Program (1973b)
	Chlordiazepoxide	Boston Collaborative Drug Surveillance Program (1973b)
Enhanced metabolism by placenta	Benzo(a)pyrene	Welch et al. (1968, 1969)
	3-Methyl-4-mono-methylaminoazobenzene	Welch et al. (1969)
	Zoxazolamine	Kapitulnik et al. (1976)
	7-Ethoxycoumarin	Jacobson et al. (1974)
Enhanced metabolism by pulmonary alveolar macrophages	Benzo(a)pyrene	Cantrell et al (1973)

TABLE 7
EFFECT OF DIET CONTAINING CHARCOAL-BROILED GROUND BEEF ON THE METABOLISM OF PHENACETIN BY INTESTINE IN VITRO IN THE RAT[a]

Diet	N-Acetyl-p-aminophenol formed (μg/5 cm intestine/90 min)
Control	1.35 ± 0.17
Ground beef cooked on aluminium foil	1.95 ± 0.38[b]
Charcoal-broiled ground beef	15.88 ± 4.11[c]

[a]Adult male Long-Evans rats were fed for 7 days a nutritionally complete semi-synthetic diet or a 3:1 ratio of beef in semisynthetic diet. The small intestines were excised and their drug metabolizing activity measured. Each value represents the mean $\pm$ S.E. for three rats. Data taken from Pantuck et al. (1975).

[b]Value not significantly different from control value ($p > 0.05$).

[c]Value not significantly different from control value ($p < 0.05$), and from ground beef cooked on foil value ($p < 0.05$).

aminophenol levels. The ratio of the mean N-acetyl-p-aminophenyl concentration to the mean phenacetin concentration was markedly higher after the subjects ate charcoal-broiled beef, and the ratio decreased when the subjects returned to the control hospital diet (Table 9). These results suggest that feeding charcoal-broiled beef stimulates the metabolism of phenacetin in the gastro-intestinal tract and/or during its first pass through the liver, causing a marked decrease in the bioavailability of phenacetin.

TABLE 8
EFFECT OF FEEDING CHARCOAL-BROILED BEEF ON THE PLASMA CONCENTRATION OF PHENACETIN IN HUMANS[a]

Intervals after phenacetin administration (hr)	Plasma concentration of phenacetin (ng/ml)		
	Control hospital diet (1st time)	Charcoal-broiled beef diet	Control hospital diet (2nd time)
1	1328 ± 481	319 ± 90	1827 ± 661
2	925 ± 166	163 ± 32	623 ± 128
3	313 ± 60	74 ± 17	271 ± 76
4	149 ± 27	34 ± 9	99 ± 24
5	66 ± 14	15 ± 4	40 ± 11
7	17 ± 4	7 ± 2	14 ± 4

[a]Plasma concentrations of phenacetin were measured following the administration of 900 mg of phenacetin after each dietary regimen. Each value represents the mean $\pm$ S.E. for 9 subjects. The plasma levels of phenacetin after the charcoal-broiled beef diet were significantly lower than the plasma levels after either of the control hospital diets. Data taken from Conney et al. (1976).

TABLE 9
EFFECT OF FEEDING CHARCOAL-BROILED BEEF ON THE RATIO
OF THE CONCENTRATION OF APAP IN PLASMA TO THE
CONCENTRATION OF PHENACETIN IN PLASMA[a]

Intervals after phenacetin administration (hr)	Ratio of total APAP : Phenacetin		
	Control hospital diet (1st time)	Charcoal-broiled beef diet	Control hospital diet (2nd time)
1	4.7	25.1	4.3
2	11.1	69.4	16.7
3	31.7	138.2	37.4
4	56.2	236.5	83.2
5	106.5	412.7	170.3
7	219.4	505.7	276.4

[a]Subjects were administered a 900 mg dose of phenacetin orally after each dietary regimen. Each value represents the mean concentration of total APAP to the mean concentration of phenacetin for the 9 subjects. Data taken from Conney et al. (1976).

Marked differences were observed among the subjects in their responsiveness to the diet containing charcoal-broiled beef. Switching the subjects from the control hospital diet to the charcoal-broiled beef diet resulted in a significant decrease in the area under the plasma concentration of phenacetin-time curve for 7 of the 9 subjects (Fig. I). Two of the subjects, MJ and GO, did not show a lower area under the plasma concentration of phenacetin-time curve when placed on the charcoal-broiled beef diet. These subjects had very low plasma concentrations of phenacetin while they were eating the control hospital diet. The reasons for the nonresponsiveness of these 2 subjects to the stimulatory effects of eating a charcoal-broiled beef diet are unknown but may be due to genetic and/or environmental factors.

ALTERATION IN DRUG METABOLISM BY CHANGES IN THE PROTEIN AND CARBOHYDRATE CONTENT OF THE DIET

Man's diet is a complex point of daily interaction with the environment. Considerable variability among individuals occurs in this environmental exposure both because of the variety of foods chosen for their diet by healthy individuals and because of dietary restrictions imposed by certain disease states. We have recently reported on the effects of changes in the protein and carbohydrate content of the diet of six healthy male subjects (Alvares et al, 1976; Kappas et al, 1976). Smokers and heavy drinkers of alcohol were excluded from the study, and no medication, except for occasional aspirin, was permitted for at least three weeks prior to and during the study. In addition, no smoked foods, brussels sprouts, cabbage, or other known inducers or inhibitors of drug metabolism were

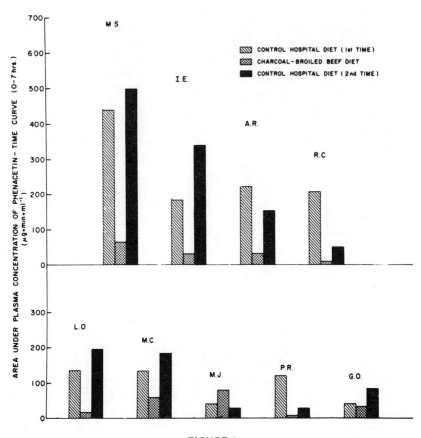

FIGURE 1

Area under the plasma concentration of phenacetin-time curve (0→ 7 hr) in nine subjects administered a 900-mg dose of phenacetin after eating a control hospital diet, a charcoal-broiled beef diet, and the control hospital diet for a second time. Data taken from Cooney et al. (1976).

eaten by the subjects during the course of the study. During the first two weeks of the study, subjects were on their usual home diet (Home Diet 1). During the next two weeks, the same subjects were maintained on a low carbohydrate-high protein diet, the composition of which was 44% protein, 35% carbohydrate, and 21% fat. During the third two-week period, the same subjects were maintained on a high carbohydrate-low protein diet. The composition of this diet was 10% protein, 70% carbohydrate and 20% fat. The caloric intake during each of the above two test diets was 2,400 to 2,500 calories per day per subject. Thus, the fat and total caloric intake remained unchanged during the two test diet periods. For comparative purposes, the macronutrient composition of the average American diet is 15% protein, 50% carbohydrate, and 35% fat (Goodhart et al.,

64

1968). In the final two weeks of the study, the subjects returned to their customary home diet (Home Diet 2). Each subject was administered an oral dose of antipyrine (18 mg/kg) on Day 10, and theophylline (5 mg/kg) on Day 14 of each of the four study periods. The plasma concentrations of antipyrine and theophylline were determined at various time intervals following the administration of the drugs.

The effects of changes in the protein and carbohydrate content of the diet on the plasma half-lives, volume of distribution, and metabolic clearance rates of antipyrine and theophylline are shown in Tables 10 and 11. The six subjects, when fed a low carbohydrate-high protein diet, showed a 35-40% decrease in plasma half-lives of antipyrine and theophylline as compared to the half-lives obtained when the subjects were fed their usual home diets. A change from a low carbohydrate-high protein diet to a high carbohydrate-low protein diet resulted in a 50-60% increase in the half-lives of the two drugs. The drug half-lives at the end of the high carbohydrate-low protein diet period were not significantly different from the half-lives obtained at the end of the two home diet test periods.

A review of the subjects' home diets revealed that their normal home diets were relatively high in carbohydrate compared to protein. There was no significant change in the volume of distribution for antipyrine or theophylline when

TABLE 10
EFFECTS OF VARIOUS DIETS ON MEAN PLASMA HALF-LIFE,
VOLUME OF DISTRIBUTION AND METABOLIC CLEARANCE
RATE OF ANTIPYRINE IN HUMANS[a]

Measurement	Home diet I	Low CHO-high PRO diet	High CHO-low PRO diet	Home diet II
Plasma half-life, in hr	16.22 ± 1.59	9.55[b] ± 0.40	15.62 ± 1.74	14.20 ± 0.60
Volume of distribution, in liters	52.00 ± 6.0	47.8 ± 3.4	49.9 ± 4.9	48.8 ± 3.4
Metabolic clearance rate, in ml/min	37.0 ± 1.4	58.0[b] ± 3.6	38.7 ± 4.3	39.9 ± 2.6

[a]Each value represents the mean ± S. E. for 6 subjects. Each subject was maintained on his usual home diet (Home Diet I) for 2 wks, followed by 2 wks on the low carbohydrate (CHO)-high protein (PRO), followed by 2 wks on the high CHO-low PRO diet, followed by 2 wks on the usual home diet (Home Diet II). Data taken from Alvares et al. (1976) and Kappas et al. (1976).

[b]The value for the low CHO-high PRO diet is significantly different from home diet I and from the high CHO-low PRO diet ($p < 0.01$). The values for Home Diets I and II and the high CHO-low PRO diet are not significantly different from each other. The values for volume of distribution are not significantly different from each other.

TABLE 11
EFFECTS OF VARIOUS DIETS ON MEAN PLASMA HALF-LIFE, VOLUME OF DISTRIBUTION AND METABOLIC CLEARANCE RATE OF THEOPHYLLINE IN HUMANS[a]

Measurement	Home diet I	Low CHO-high PRO diet	High CHO-low PRO diet	Home diet II
Plasma half-life, in hr	8.12 ± 0.99	5.23[b] ± 0.39	7.62 ± 0.66	7.53 ± 0.66
Volume of distribution, in liters	33.0 ± 1.2	33.8 ± 2.3	33.4 ± 1.9	33.8 ± 1.9
Metabolic clearance rate, in ml/min	49.2 ± 4.2	75.7[b] ± 4.5	52.3 ± 4.4	52.1 ± 2.4

[a]The protocol for the study is described in the legend for Table 10. Data taken from Alvares et al. (1976) and Kappas et al. (1976).

[b]The value for the low CHO-high PRO diet is significantly different from Home Diet I and from the high CHO-low PRO det ($p < 0.01$). The values for Home Diets I and II and the high CHO-low PRO diet and not significantly different from each other. The values for volume of distribution are not significantly different from each other.

the subjects were maintained on either of their home diets or on the two test diets. As anticipated from the changes in plasma half-lives of the two test drugs, there was a significant increase in the mean metabolic clearance rates for the two drugs when the subjects' diets were changed from their usual home diets to the low carbohydrate-high protein diets, and there was a significant decrease in the mean metabolic clearance rates when the subjects' diets were changed from the low carbohydrate-high protein diet to a high carbohydrate-low protein diet. The changes in clearance rates without changes in volumes of distribution indicate that the test diets change the rate of metabolism of the two drugs. Studies in rats have shown that increases in the dietary protein content result in increased rates of metabolism of drug substrates by liver microsomes (Campbell & Hayes, 1974; Kato et al., 1968). Similarly, feeding a high carbohydrate diet to mice decreases liver monooxygenase activities and prolongs barbiturate-induced sleeping time (Strother et al., 1971). Our present studies demonstrate that changes in the carbohydrate and protein content of the diet can markedly influence the oxidative biotransformation of drugs in man.

EFFECT OF BRUSSELS SPROUTS AND CABBAGE ON DRUG METABOLISM

Studies by L. Wattenberg and his associates (1971) showed that feeding rats a diet containing brussels sprouts, cabbage, cauliflower, or certain other vegetables markedly stimulates benzo(a)pyrene hydroxylase activity in the intestine. It was subsequently demonstrated that certain indoles present in brussels sprouts and cabbage are strong inducers of benzo(a)pyrene hydroxylase activity in the rat (Loub et al., 1975). In collaborative studies with L. Wattenberg, we found that brussels sprouts and cabbage stimulate the intestinal metabolism of several drugs in rats (Pantuck et al., 1976b). The stimulatory effects of these vegetables on the intestinal metabolism of phenacetin, 7-ethoxycoumarin, hexobarbital, and benzo(a)pyrene are summarized in Table 12. The most marked stimulatory effects of these vegetables occurred for the metabolism of 7-ethoxycoumarin and benzo(a)pyrene. Smaller increases were observed for the metabolism of phenacetin and hexobarbital. Feeding cabbage was about half as effective as feeding brussels sprouts. Studies are in progress to determine whether or not these vegetables can stimulate drug metabolism in man.

SUMMARY

Microsomal monooxygenases metabolize a variety of drugs, carcinogens, and other foreign compounds, as well as endogenous substrates such as steroid hormones. In experimental animals, the activities of these monooxygenases are markedly influenced by environmental chemicals and nutritional factors. The results described here demonstrate that many of these factors can influence the rates of biotransformation of drugs in man. We have shown that cigarette smoking enhances the in vitro metabolism of the carcinogen benzo(a)pyrene, as well as certain drugs in human placenta, and that cigarette smoking increases the in vivo metabolism of phenacetin. We have shown that charcoal-broiled meat, which contains polycyclic hydrocarbons, markedly lowers the plasma levels of orally administered phenacetin, and our results demonstrate marked influences of dietary carbohydrate and protein content on the oxidative biotransformation rates of antipyrine and theophylline. In addition, we have presented the results of studies which show that brussels sprouts and cabbage enhance the intestinal metabolism of benzo(a)pyrene and several drug substrates in the rat.

A major point of direct contact between man and his environment is the diet he ingests. It is likely that dietary factors contribute to variability in the metabolism and action of drugs in different individuals and in the same individual given a drug on different occasions. Individuals who manipulate their diets to lose weight or to manage certain disease states, and those who observe special dietary restrictions (such as vegetarians), may have a different response to drugs and environmental carcinogens from that of the general population.

Since microsomal monooxygenases that metabolize drugs also are involved in the metabolism of endogenous steroid hormones and other normal body substrates (Conney, 1967; Conney & Kuntzman, 1971), it would be of importance to determine if the metabolism of normal body constituents in man is altered by changes in the composition of the diet. Many chemical carcinogens in man's environment require metabolism by monooxygenases to a reactive inter-

TABLE 12
EFFECT OF DIET CONTAINING CABBAGE OR BRUSSELS SPROUTS ON THE METABOLISM OF PHENACETIN, 7-ETHOXYCOUMARIN, HEXOBARBITAL AND BENZO(A)PYRENE[a]

Diet	N-Acetyl-p-aminophenol formed (nmol/5cm intestine/90 min)	7-Hydroxycoumarin formed (pmol/mg intestine/min)	3-Hydroxy-hexobarbital formed (nmol/5cm intestine/90 min)	3-Hydroxybenzo-(a)pyrene formed (pmol/mg intestine/min)
Control	214 ± 2	0.66 ± 0.10	161 ± 19	0.19 ± 0.06
Cabbage	408 ± 25[b]	6.35 ± 0.71[c]	254 ± 14[b]	2.23 ± 0.44[c]
Brussels sprouts	615 ± 93[d]	13.23 ± 1.54[c]	351 ± 21[d]	5.40 ± 0.99[c]

[a]Rates were fed a nutritionally complete semisynthetic diet or 25% dry vegetable powder in semisynthetic diet for seven days. The small intestines were excised and their drug-metabolizing activity measured. Intestinal strips were used for the determination of phenacetin and hexobarbital metabolism, and homogenates were used for studies on the metabolism of 7-ethoxycoumarin and benzo(a)pyrene. A higher substrate concentration (1 mM) was used to determine phenacetin metabolism in this study than in the studies reported in Tables 5 and 7. Each value represents the mean ± S.E. for four rats. Data taken from Pantuck et al. (1976b).

[b]$p < 0.001$; [c]$p < 0.005$; [d]$p < 0.01$; vaules significantly different from control values.

mediate that exerts a carcinogenic effect, and these monooxygenase systems also participate in the detoxification of carcinogens. Epidemiological studies suggest that nutritional factors can influence the incidence of certain human cancers (Wynder et al., 1978). It would be important to know whether changes in the composition of the diet can influence the formation of human cancers by altering the activity of enzymes that metabolize environmental chemicals to detoxified products and/or to ultimate carcinogens, cocarcinogens, and promoters. Additional research is needed to evaluate the biochemical and physiological significance of dietary changes for the metabolism of foreign chemicals and normal body constituents.

ACKNOWLEDGMENTS

The authors wish to thank Dr. Karl Anderson for assistance in the clinical studies. The authors also wish to thank Miss Elizabeth Dunn and Mrs. Nanci Brice for secretarial assistance. These studies were supported in part by USPHS grant ES 01055 and NIGMS grant GM 09069.

REFERENCES

Alexanderson, B., Evans, D. A. P., & Sjöqvist, F. Steady-state plasma levels of nortripyline in twins: influence of genetic factors and drug therapy. *Brit. Med. J.,* 1969, *4,* 764-768.

Alvares, A. P., Kapelner, S., Sassa, S., & Kappas, A. Drug metabolism in normal children, lead-poisoned children and normal adults. *Clin. Pharmacol. Ther.,* 1975, *17,* 179-183.

Alvares, A. P., Anderson, K. E., Conney, A. H., & Kappas, A. Interactions between nutritional factors and drug biotransformations in man. *Proc. Nat. Acad. Sci. U.S.A.,* 1976, *73,* 2501-2504.

Alvares, A. P., Fischbein, A., Anderson, K. E., & Kappas, A. Alterations in drug metabolism in workers exposed to polychlorinated biphenyls. *Clin. Pharmacol. Ther.,* 1977, *22,* 140-146.

Beckett, A. H., & Triggs, E. J. Enzyme induction in man caused by smoking. *Nature,* 1967, *216,* 587.

Boston Collaborative Drug Surveillance Program. Decreased clinical efficacy of propoxyphene in cigarette smokers. *Clin. Pharmacol. Ther.,* 1973(a), *14,* 259-263.

Boston Collaborative Drug Surveillance Program. CNS Depression Due to Benzodiazepines: Relation to Smoking and Age. *New Engl. J. Med.,* 1973(b), *288,* 277-280.

Brown, R. R., Miller, J. A., & Miller, E. C. The metabolism of methylated aminoazo dyes. IV. Dietary factors enhancing demethylation in vitro. *J. Biol. Chem.,* 1954, *209,* 211-222.

Burns, J. J., Rose, R. K., Chenkin, T., Goldman, A., Schulert, A., & Brodie, B. B. The physiological disposition of phenylbutazone (Butazolidin) in man and a method for its estimation in biological materials. *J. Pharmacol. Exp. Therap.,* 1953, *109,* 346-357.

Campbell, T. C., & J. R. Hayes. Role of nutrition in the drug-metabolizing enzyme system. *Pharmacol. Rev.*, 1974, *26*, 171-197.

Cantrell, E. T., Warr, G. A., Busbee, D. L., & Martin, R. R. Induction of aryl hydrocarbon hydroxylase in human pulmonary alveolar macrophages by cigarette smoke. *J. Clin. Invest.*, 1973, *52*, 1881-1884.

Committee on Biologic Effects of Atmospheric Pollutants. Particulate Polycyclic Organic Matter, National Academy of Sciences, Washington, D. C., 1972.

Committee on Food Protection, Food and Nutrition Board, National Research Council. *Toxicants Occurring Naturally in Foods*, Washington, D.C.: Natl. Acad. Sci., 1973.

Conney, A. H., Miller, E. C., & Miller, J. A. The metabolism of methylated aminoazo dyes. V. Evidence for induction of enzyme synthesis in the rat by 3-methylcholanthrene. *Cancer Res.*, 1956, *16*, 450-459.

Conney, A. H., Miller, E. C., & Miller, J. A. Substrate-induced synthesis and other properties of benzpyrene hydroxylase in rat liver. *J. Biol. Chem.*, 1957, *228*, 753-766.

Conney, A. H., Gillette, J. R., Inscoe, J. K., Trams, E. R., & Posner, H. S. Induced synthesis of liver microsomal enzymes which metabolize foreign compounds. *Science*, 1959, *130*, 1478-1479.

Conney, A. H. Pharmacological implications of microsomal enzyme induction. *Pharmacol. Rev.*, 1967, *19*, 317-366.

Conney, A. H., & Kuntzman, R. Metabolism of normal body constituents by drug-metabolizing enzymes in liver microsomes. In B. B. Brodie & J. Gillette (eds.), *Concepts in Biochemical Pharmacology*. Springer-Verlag, 1971, pp. 401-421.

Conney, A. H., Pantuck, E. J., Hsiao, K.-C., Garland, W. A., Anderson, K. A., Alvares, A. P., & Kappas, A. Enhanced phenacetin metabolism in humans fed charcoal-broiled beef. *Clin. Pharmacol. Ther.*, 1976, *20*, 633-642.

Crosby, D. G. Natural toxic background in the food of man and his animals. *J. Agric. Food Chem.*, 1969, *17*, 532-538.

Goodhart, R. S. Criteria of an adequate diet. In M. C. Wohl & R. S. Goodhart (Eds.), *Modern nutrition in health and disease*. Philadelphia, Pa.: Lea & Febiger, 1968, pp. 587-599.

Hammer, W., Ideström, C. M., & Sjöqvist, F. Chemical control of antidepressant drug therapy. In *Proceedings of the First International Symposium on Antidepressant Drugs, Milan, 1966*. Amsterdam: Excerpta Medica, 1967, pp. 301-310.

Hart, P., Farrell, G. C., Cooksley, W. G. E., & Powell, L. W. Enhanced drug metabolism in cigarette smokers. *Brit. Med. J.*, 1976, *2*, 147-149.

Jacobson, M., Levin, W., Poppers, P. J., Wood, A. W., & Conney, A. H. Comparison of the O-dealkylation of 7-ethoxycoumarin and the hydroxylation of benzo(a)pyrene in human placenta. *Clin. Pharmacol. Ther.*, 1974, *16*, 701-710.

Jenne, J., Nagasawa, H., McHugh, R., MacDonald, F., & Wyse, E. Decreased theophylline half-life in cigarette smokers. *Life Sci.*, 1975, *17*, 195-198.

Juchau, M. R. Human placental hydroxylation of 3,4-benzpyrene during early gestation and at term. *Toxicol. Appl. Pharmacol.*, 1971, *18*, 665-676.

Kapitulnik, J., Levin, W., Poppers, P. J., Tomaszewski, J. E., Jerina, D. M., & Conney, A. H. Comparison of the hydroxylation of zoxazolamine and benzo(a)pyrene in human placenta: Effect of cigarette smoking. *Clin. Pharmacol. Ther.*, 1976, *20*, 557-564.

Kappas, A., Anderson, K. E., Conney, A. H., & Alvares, A. P. Influence of dietary protein and carbohydrate on antipyrine and theophylline metabolism in man. *Clin. Pharmacol. Ther.*, 1976, *20*, 643-653.

Kato, R., Oshim, T., & Tomizawa, S. Toxicity and metabolism of drugs in relation to dietary protein. *Jap. J. Pharmacol.*, 1968, *18*, 356-366.

Keeri-Szanto, M., & Pomeroy, J. R. Atmospheric pollution and pentazocine metabolism. *Lancet*, 1971, *1*, 947-949.

Kensler, C. J., Sugiura, K., Young, N. F., Halter, C. R., & Rhoads, C. P. Partial protection of rats by riboflavin with casein against liver cancer caused by dimethylaminoazobenzene. *Science*, 1974, *93*, 308-310.

Kensler, C. J. The influence of diet on the riboflavin content and the ability of rat liver slices to destory the carcinogen N,N-dimethyl-p-aminoazobenzene. *J. Biol. Chem.*, 1949, *179*, 1079-1084.

Kolmodin, B., Azarnoff, D. L., & Sjöqvist, F. Effects of environmental factors on drug metabolism: Decreased plasma half-life of antipyrine in workers exposed to chlorinated hydrocarbon insecticides. *Clin. Pharmacol. Ther.*, 1969, *10*, 638-642.

Lijinsky, W., & Shubik, P. Benzo(a)pyrene and other polynuclear hydrocarbons in charcoalbroiled meat. *Science*, 1964, *145*, 53-55.

Loub, W. D., Wattenberg, L. W., & Davis, D. W. Aryl hydrocarbon hydroxylase induction in rat tissues by naturally occurring indoles of cruciferous plants. *J. Nat. Cancer Inst.*, 1975, *54*, 985-988.

Mueller, G. C., & Miller, J. A. The reductive cleavage of 4-dimethylaminoazobenzene by rat liver: Reactivation of carbon dioxide-treated homogenates by riboflavinadenine dinucleotide. *J. Biol. Chem.*, 1950, *185*, 145-154.

Nebert, D. W., Winker, J., & Gelboin, H. V. Aryl hydrocarbon hydroxylase activity in human placenta from cigarette smoking and nonsmoking women. *Cancer Res.*, 1969, *29*, 1763-1769.

Pantuck, E. J., Hsiao, K. -C., Kaplan, S. A., Kuntzman, R., & Conney, A. H. Effects of enzyme induction on intestinal phenacetin metabolism in the rat. *J. Pharmacol. Exp. Ther.*, 1974(a), *191*, 45-52.

Pantuck, E. J., Hsiao, K. -C., Maggio, A., Nakamura, K., Kuntzman, R., & Conney, A. H. Effect of cigarette smoking on phenacetin metabolism. *Clin. Pharmacol. Ther.*, 1974(b), *15*, 9-17.

Pantuck, E. J., Hsiao, K. -C., Kuntzman, R., & Conney, A. H. Intestinal metabolism of phenacetin in the rat: Effect of charcoal-broiled beef and rat chow. *Science*, 1975, *187*, 744-746.

Pantuck, E. J., Hsiao, K. -C., Conney, A. H., Garland, W., Kappas, A., Anderson, K., & Alvares, A. P. Effect of charcoal-broiled beef on phenacetin metabolism in man. *Science*, 1976(a), *194*, 1055-1057.

Pantuck, E. J., Hsiao, K. -C., Loub, W. D., Wattenberg, L. W., Kuntzman, R. & Conney, A. H. Stimulatory effects of vegetables on intestinal drug metabolism in the rat. *J. Pharmacol. Exp. Ther.*, 1976(b), *198*, 278-283.

Pelkonen, O., Jouppila, P., & Karki, N. T. Effect of maternal cigarette smoking on 3,4-benzpyrene and N-methylaniline metabolism in human fetal liver and placenta. *Toxicol. Appl. Pharmacol.*, 1972, *23*, 399-407.

Perel, J. M., Shostak, M., Garne, E., Kantor, S. J., & Glassman, A. H. In L. Gottschalk & S. Marlies (Eds.), *Pharmacokinetics, Psychoactive Drug Blood Levels and Clinical Outcome*. New York: Spectrum-John Wiley, 1975, pp. 229-241.

Poland, A., Smith, D., Kuntzman, R., Jacobson, M., & Conney, A. H. Effect of intensive occupational exposure to DDT on phenylbutazone and cortisol metabolism in human subjects. *Clin. Pharmacol. Ther.*, 1970, *11*, 724-732.

Strother, A., Throckmorton, J. K., & Herzer, C. The influence of high sugar consumption by mice on the duration of action of barbiturates and in vitro metabolism of barbiturates, aniline and p-nitroanisole. *J. Pharmacol. Exp. Ther.*, 1971, *179*, 490-498.

Swett, C., Jr. Drowsiness due to chlorpromazine in relation to cigarette smoking. *Arch. Gen. Psychiat.*, 1974, *31*, 211-213.

Vesell, E. S., & Page, J. G. Genetic control of dicoumarol levels in man. *J. Clin. Invest.*, 1968(a), *47*, 2657-2663.

Vesell, E. S., & Page, J. G. Genetic control of drug levels in man: phenylbutazone. *Science*, 1968(b), *159*, 1479-1480.

Vesell, E. S., & Page, J. G. Genetic control of the phenobarbital-induced shortening of plasma antipyrine half-lives in man. *J. Clin. Invest.*, 1969, *48*, 2202-2209.

Vestal, R. E., Norris, A. H., Tobin, J. D., Cohen, B. H., Shock, N. W., & Andres, A. Antipyrine metabolism in man: Influence of age, alcohol, caffeine and smoking. *Clin. Pharmacol. Ther.*, 1975, *18*, 425-432.

Wattenberg, L. W. Studies of polycyclic hydrocarbon hydroxylases of the intestine possibly related to cancer. Effect of diet on benzpyrene hydroxylase activity. *Cancer*, 1971, *20*, 99-102.

Weiner, M., Shapiro, S., Axelrod, J., Cooper, J. R., & Brodie, B. B. The physiological disposition of dicoumarol in man. *J. Pharmacol. Exp. Therap.*, 1950, *99*, 409-420.

Weisburger, J. H., Grantham, P. H., Vanhorn, E., Steigbigel, N. H., Rall, D. P., & Weisburger, E. K. Activation and detoxification of N-2-fluorenylacetamide in man. *Cancer Res.*, 1964, *24*, 475-479.

Welch, R. M., Harrison, Y. E., Conney, A. H., Poppers, P. J., & Finster, M. Cigarette smoking: Stimulatory effect on metabolism of 3,4-benzpyrene by enzymes in human placenta. *Science*, 1968, *160*, 541-542.

Welch, R. M., Harrison, Y. E., Gommi, B. W., Poppers, P. J., Finster, M., & Conney, A. H. Stimulatory effect of cigarette smoking on the hydroxylation of 3,4-benzpyrene and the N-demethylation of 3-methyl-4-monomethylaminoazobenzene by enzymes in human placenta. *Clin. Pharmacol. Ther.*, 1969, *10*, 100-109.

Welch, R. M., Cavallito, J., & Loh, A. Effect of exposure to cigarette smoke on the metabolism of benzo(a)pyrene and acetophenetidin by lung and intestine of rats. *Toxicol. Appl. Pharmacol.*, 1972, *23*, 749-758.

Wynder, E., et al. Present symposium.

Discussion

DR. TRUHAUT: My remarks are about carcinogens. I was interested about what was said by Dr. Conney about interference of nutritional factors, and this requires my making a remark about the differences between animal species and man, and to recall papers published. I think in 1968 or 1969 one appeared in *Nature* in which it was shown that if you give rats a human diet of average composition you get indirect harmful effects, and if you give chicken and green beans to dogs you also obtain harmful effects.

We have to think this over, because in experimental design one must not forget that sometimes nutrition which is good to man is bad for laboratory animals. It is all that I wanted to say.

DR. COULSTON: Dr. Wynder, please. Would you just identify yourself and then talk please.

DR. WYNDER: Dr. Wynder, from the National Health Foundation. I would just like to make two general points to consider at the beginning. Number one: We are somewhat of a mutual admiration society, we're all in the same area, and I'm sure we're going to get a lot of intellectual discussions out of this meeting. But I would like to think that we are going to see beyond this meeting and determine whether we as a group can indeed have a societal effect.

For some time now we have felt that some 60-90% of all cancers relate to environmental factors. Do we, in fact, do something about it, and do we in environmental carcinogenesis indeed deal with the major issues?

I recently attended a meeting on cobalt, and I think there were some 250 researchers who were all engaged and interested in studying the mechanism. I asked whether anyone there was involved in alcoholism, which I think is one of the better known human promoting agents, and in fact nobody was. I then wrote to my friends at the NCI and I said, "Can I hear from your computer whether any contract or grant for fiscal year '76-'77 is funded to take on this major human lead which we have known for 30 years?" The answer came back that not a single grant or contract was currently being carried out studying this major human lead.

It seems to me that we ought to ask ourselves whether we, in fact, are covering the major epidemiological clues that have been available to us for some time. And so I would like to end up with two specific recommendations that we should perhaps consider over the next three years.

Dr. Shubik and we have discussed for some time that what we think this country needs are centers for environmental carcinogenesis. I'm a great believer in the idea that we would advance the cause of environmental cancer work better if we could bring together in one institution the epidemiologists, the chemists, and the biologists so they can work together and think together, so that we do not have to come together in a meeting like this and review what we think ought to be done. And, of course, Dr. Shubik and I know, we have a question of significant priority evaluation with the National Cancer Institute.

The last point I want to make is that now that we have a new leadership at the National Cancer Institute, perhaps this group ought to decide that we should establish a committee to meet with the new director who, I believe, is friendly to cancer prevention and discuss with him the state of the art, or the lack of support for work in environmental carcinogenesis.

As it now stands, there's tremendous emphasis in the international cancer board on so-called basic research. There's great support for clinical activity, and, I must say, being a clinician myself, clinicians could eat up the entire national cancer budget for doing things for which Blue Cross and other health insurance industries already pay a great deal of money. So I think we ought to consider to what extent we can influence the government—the national campaign—to put proper support into these environmental cancer programs, and, we, as scientists in this area, ought to consider whether we ourselves take up the major priorities first.

DR. GREENWALD: (Albany.) I was glad to hear that, because I was thinking along the same lines. I think one of the issues which was initially pointed out was how can epidemiology and toxicology be brought together or with other laboratory sciences, and when I think about what we epidemiologists can really be working on, what we see as priorities, we choose them first because they're numerically important as causes of death from cancer, and we figure from that what is the most likely productive direction to go.

Secondly, we tend to pick things where there's enough information, so that there's a high likelihood of success. The more cynical way of putting that is that there's a tendency to jump on the bandwagon. A third thing we do is tend to take advantage of the uniqueness of our own situations. What I'd really like to ask of the toxicologists is how they determine their priorities, because I think if there's some effort toward a resolution of this we may actually be able to collaborate more. It seems from what I've heard thus far, priority tends to fall in the area of chemicals of industrial importance, or consumer products or drugs which may have a potential for harm in the future—those that are related to the big illnesses, and probably our life-style may be more important than some of the chemicals. So I'd really be curious about how the toxicologists really choose what to work on.

DR. COULSTON: This will be an important point for discussion I'm sure before we're done with this meeting. Thank you very much, Dr. Greenwald. I would like to address myself back to Dr. Wynder's point. You suggested the creation of a committee. Did you mean from this meeting? May I then appoint you chairman of such a committee, and select your own members and we would put in into our minutes and make recommendations. If you would care to do so Dr. Wynder, I think we all would agree.

DR. WYNDER: Well, from discussing this with various members, including Jim Miller, I think we all feel the same need, and since I have learned with age, I recognize that you must not only be scientifically correct, but you must be politically on target, and the old phrase of Bismarck applies to science just as well. I think the timing is right, with the new leadership in the NCI, and because there is a limit to the amount of monies we can spend in cancer and other research. When our leadership considers the economics of health care, I think prevention will have an unusual appeal.

I would be glad to accept your offer, and there may be those of you who would like to join me on this particular committee. It would be good, I believe, if it had on it experts from various groups, let's say chemical carcinogenesis or basic carcinogenesis—Jim Miller, others from toxicology—and if all of you would come forward to join is in this effort, we would be delighted to meet with you.

DR. COULSTON: I would suggest that this statement be incorporated into the proceedings of this meeting. This statement can then be sent to the proper people, government or wherever, politicians, senators, and congressmen; we could see that it gets wide publicity. I think it's a great idea and to come so early in our meeting makes me feel very good. Thank you. Dr. Shubik?

DR. SHUBIK: I would think it's very important that we make sure this very much needed effort that Ernie suggests is not directed just at the National Cancer Institute. It should not be directed at the National Cancer Program but also to toxicology in general in the entire country, the Environmental Protection Agency, and the various other agencies concerned.

The National Cancer Institute at the moment—speaking as a member of their board—is of the opinion that they are under violent attack already from the environmental carcinogen people, and they seem to feel that they've already been told to spend most of their money in that area, which, of course, they're not by any manner of means doing. But, there has been a series of suggestions from congressional committees that there should be a large-scale change, and I think it's very important that this be an overall approach to the health problem.

Can I bring up one other side issue? I'm sorry to sidetrack things entirely, but Herman Kraybill's paper was really wonderful today. I'd like to congratulate him. I'd also like to make one small observation, and that is there was once upon a time in the *British Journal of Pathology and Bacteriology,* an article the title of which was "The Use of the Egg as a Unit of Measurement in Pathology." This was in the good old days when pathologists used to talk about things being the size of seagull eggs and blackbird eggs, and so on. Well, there's a new unit that seems to have crept into toxicology, and that is the use of the pop bottle as a unit of measurement. And I'm merely observing in your paper, Herman, when you talk about 5% saccharin cyclamate being equivalent to 520 bottles of pop per day, or 800. Since the ratio of the use of saccharin cyclamate is 1:10, there may be a slight error there somewhere down the line, and I think that the amount of cyclamate that is actually tested would be more in the region of maybe 50 bottles of pop. Somehow, rather, I don't think that's terribly unreasonable when you remember that the ADI of cyclamate was 5 grams a day, which a lot of us thought was too much anyhow.

DR. COULSTON: Thank you. Dr. Truhaut, please.

DR. TRUHAUT: I speak enthusiastically about the proposal of Dr. Wynder, and I listen too, with enthusiasm, to the proposal of Professor Shubik to extend the recommendation from environmental carcinogenesis to general toxicological evaluation.

May I as a man from France suggest that we expand your proposal from one restricted to the United States to a worldwide proposal, because I admire the thoughts of my American colleagues, and very often I am enthusiastic about their actual efforts and their reasons? But scientists from the other countries of the world should join them to provide an international forum for extending the research in such a way as to obtain results to decrease our area of ignorance, and at the same time to make people all over the world—and especially the politicians and some scientists—be more reasonable. Thank you, Mr. Chairman.

DR. COULSTON: You see, the International Academy that sponsors this meeting has a mechanism to go worldwide from Russia to China to Japan to South Africa, because literally we have members in all of these countries.

It would be a proper statement to come out of this meeting, which Dr. Goto as a secretary of the Academy would distribute worldwide immediately, reaching the top people in every country that are interested in science. But you made the original proposal; are you interested in advancing the international proposal or just for the States?

DR GOTO: Well, there are two points. I obviously agree with Dr. Shubik that the problem is bigger than cancer, and indeed many of the factors that we discuss are not only toxic in terms of carcinogenesis, but they affect other diseases as well.

DR WYNDER: Now, obviously I appreciate the international interest in this problem, since it *is* an international problem, and those of us who are epidemiologists have, of course, gotten our major leads from the epidemiology of diseases throughout the world, which is one's best proof that diseases are environmentally related. My concern now is not that we make a statement which appears on page 15 in the *New York Times,* but indeed, that we have a specific impact.

All of us know that a big problem in preventive medicine historically is the apathy of man himself, and all of us for instance, who have been in clinical cancer research, know that we get calls from all over the world from people when they have cancer to ask our advice to see whether we can get them into the cancer hospital. And these are the same people who have ignored us all these years in our long-term fight in cancer prevention.

So I want to make sure that the proposals that we have coming from this committee are realistic, and politically doable. I think we have, unfortunately, to take one step at a time. We've got to recognize that the problems that we have indeed in the world out there—for instance, if you look at the *New York Times.* The *New York Times* will take a story on asbestos and vinyl chloride, and it will be a page-one representation. And yet when you come to say "Listen, last year, we had again 100,000 deaths from lung cancer, and we certainly know that most of them are related to smoking," you get the reply, "What else is new?"

The reason I emphasize this is because it is not just a scientific problem, it is a problem that we have with man himself, it is a problem that we have with ourselves. Therefore, I am pleased to undertake the assignment, but I would hope that those of you who will join us in this effort will recognize the difficult time that we have had historically in preventive medicine because of, for example, vested commercial interests. I remind you that John Snow, in 1849 in his famous essay in the *Medical Gazette* in London said, "My proposal should be accepted because it does not involve commercial intercourse." Well, you and I know he was wrong, because it involved a private water company.

So, yes, but I like us to be political realists in terms of what can be done.

DR COULSTON: Thank you very much. There were two hands; Dr. Farah first, please.

DR. FARAH: I just want to reiterate what you have said. I had an experience recently with a congressman who blamed the medical profession for not doing anything about the general health of the public; I pointed out to him the cigarette business and it was quite clear he was on the defensive there.

However, I think, as you have said, it's a social problem we are dealing with and not a problem we can solve here in this group. We have to attack some very powerful political and economic factors, namely, the government spent $3 million dollars advertising that you should not smoke but it spends $80 million supporting the tobacco-growing industry. Too, I think the other factor to be kept in mind is that some of the most powerful chairmen of the various congressional committees are southerners coming from the tobacco states; therefore, I think it's a formidable task that Dr. Wynder has accepted, and I wish him very well.

DR. KRAYBILL: Perhaps you know as well as the rest that we've been trying to interdigitate the people in the carcinogenesis program of experimental cancer and also the statisticians and epidemiologists, particularly in our division of epidemiologists and statisticians and people in the bioassay program. We're making some strides in that direction. We had a meeting one day and I thought this was interesting. We looked to them to give us a statistical answer to the problem, and lo and behold, the meeting broke up soon thereafter. What they gave us was a biochemical answer to the problem. So what I'm saying is that sometimes we can't see the trees for the forest.

DR. PLUMLEE: (EPA.) This isn't really a criticism of the agenda, it's really more of a question, and I don't know whom to direct the question to. It's my impression that there is a wide variation in the human population in immunologic competence, and that extrapolating from animal data to man would have to take these immunologic factors into account. Yet I don't see them addressed on the agenda, and I don't know quite how they fit, or what we know about them, or perhaps our knowledge is so primitive that immunology doesn't therefore deserve a place on the agenda of the people concerned with this interspecies extrapolation, but I wondered if anyone here had reflections on that.

DR. COULSTON: Yes, I would like to speak first, because in my Institute we spend a great deal of effort on immunological aspects, and at the recent Society of Toxicology meeting in Toronto we presented our first paper showing clearly the effects of chemicals like PCB on immunological competence of mice and rats and monkeys, so what I'm saying in essence, is that we as a group feel very certain what you've said is correct.

I would recognize the need for discussion in this area and I promise we will get it in. Too bad it doesn't appear on the program because it's too new. Very few laboratories do the kind of work I just described as being done in Albany by Dr. Loose and his group. If you read some of the reports coming out of this group, I don't know how to interpret them yet, but it's startling. There is an effect on immunological competency of these rats and mice.

DR. KRAYBILL: About this immunology question, there is in the May issue of *Scientific American* a review article by an employee of Sloan-Kettering on cancer immunology, and I recently heard Allan Goldstein speak on immunology as related to the hypothalamus gland. He made a comment that immunosuppressive factors have been identified as involved in the effects of cigarette smoking and certain other carcinogens.

DR. COULSTON: Especially when inhaled. Charlie, you look like you're going to have apoplexy if you don't speak.

DR. KENSLER: I thought it's exciting for Ernie, who's already set up this program in Valhalla, to get it endorsed at the Inn of the Mountain Gods.

Second, I certainly enjoyed Dr. Kraybill's talk. When he got to dealing with Marvin Schneiderman on "How much will you give me from this one, if I give you this one?" I'd like to mention that there are anticarcinogens. There are interrelationships which protect us. Weak carcinogens prevent the actions, or at least diminish the actions of strong carcinogens. I can remember the famous experiment of Howard Richardson who put some aromatic hydrocarbon carcinogen on the cervix of a rat and protected the rat against azodye carcinogenesis. He thought this was due to an effect on the adrenal gland, but which Jim Miller and his colleagues said was mediated through hepatic metabolism.

And with respect to Dr. Farah and vested interests, I would like to mention that in 1972, the government of this country of ours was collecting over $5 billion dollars from cigarette smokers, and the cigarette industry isn't where the politicians get that kind of money.

Just a point I wanted to make on this question of immunology, and the concept of immunological surveillance. We talked about it, but it doesn't seem to be holding up at all as far as biomedical carcinogenesis goes, and one of the main items of evidence against this are the recent studies on the nude mouse.

People are not able to keep them alive for a very long time. It does not have an increased incidence of cancer at all. And it doesn't respond to the more sensitive cancer carcinogens. Of course, as you all know, the nude mouse has no T cells at all; therefore, this seems to cause a lot of doubt on the concept of immunological surveillance as a defense mechanism against early cancer induced by chemicals.

I know there's evidence in the case of biocarcinogenesis, but as far as chemical carcinogenesis is concerned (which is what we're discussing), the recent evidence is that this is not a very important factor.

DR. COULSTON: It's a very important view you give, and I'm sure we'll discuss that further before the day is out. We've been sitting here, and Dr. Mrak has indicated he'd like to say some final words.

DR. MRAK: I sound like Mohammad Ali. I would just like to say: "Dr. Wynder, if you go into this, I think you'd better define very well what you had in mind. Because if you talk in generalities, I don't know where you'll get."

DR. COULSTON: It just shows that when you get a group of amiable people around a table, who know their business, we can have the finest discussions possible, and we will have more I'm sure before the week is out. But Dr. Cranmer, you should say something.

DR. CRANMER: I think I should say, "Let's go to lunch."

* * *

DR. COULSTON: I'd like then to start this afternoon with the first paper listed as "Chemical Reactions of Halogenated Hydrocarbons in the Mammalian Body." Unfortunately, as most of you know, Prof. Korte has the flu and could not come, but he sent his good assistant, Dr. Klein.

DR. KLEIN: Thank you very much, Dr. Coulston.

4. Chemical Reactions of Halogenated Hydrocarbons in the Mammalian Body

Friedhelm Korte and Werner Klein
Institut für Ökologische Chemie der
Gesellschaft für Strahlen- und Umweltforschung mbH München
and
Institut für Chemie der Technischen Universität München

The assessment of the fate of potential harmful chemicals in organisms reached some focus of interest in toxicology and ecotoxicology during the last decade. This is mainly a consequence of the evidence that metabolization and metabolites of chemical agents are involved in the mechanism of toxic action. Regarding drug efficacy, this has been known for a long period of time. On the other hand, we have to realize today that the elucidation of a complete chemical metabolic pattern might not be sufficient as a basis for toxicological evaluation. This is due to the fact that unstable, active, and chemically hardly detectable metabolic intermediates may be formed and that the mode of metabolite formation ought to be known also. Furthermore, the speed of metabolic conversion or persistence may not be indicative as regards unwanted effects.

Both hexachlorobenzene and saccharin are not easily metabolized in the mammalian body, but for different reasons: HCB is rather resistant to metabolic attack, whereas saccharin, together with chlorofluoromethanes, is eliminated from the body so quickly that it hardly undergoes metabolism. In general, the detailed investigation of metabolic pathways includes the following two aspects, apart from specific questions: (1) elucidation of the mode of action; and (2) establishment of a sufficient number of models for the development of structure-activity correlations and to predict for unknown substances. When concerned with chemical carcinogenicity, both aspects are of special significance. It is generally accepted today that chemicals can react with the DNA system, and that these reactions may lead to cytotoxic effects if the repair mechanisms are quantitatively insufficient.

79

Generally, from the biochemical point of view of transport and chemical balances, the major processes in the body may be classified as: (a) energy-producing reactions, which form the whole complex of intermediary metabolism; (b) reactions for the biosynthesis of internal regulators (hormones); and (c) reactions for the detoxication of internal xenobiotic toxic substances. Within our topic, we may disregard (a) and (b), and I would like to summarize quickly the biochemical processes involved in foreign compound metabolism. They are generally divided into two types, namely, (1) the metabolic changes of the structure of the chemical under investigation (primary processes), and (2) bonding reactions with abundant molecules, especially as conjugations (secondary processes). Primary processes in the metabolism of xenobiotics often result in the introduction of polar functional groups into nonpolar parent compounds. The main reactions are direct oxidation, hydration, and reduction.

The oxidation processes are among the best-known enzymatic processes today and are claimed to play a role in chemical carcinogenesis. Direct oxidation is achieved by unspecific or mixed function oxidases which are found in the microsomal fraction of mammalian livers; in the intact liver, they are located in the endoplasmic reticulum. These oxidases are involved in the biosynthesis of steroids and amino acids as well as in the conversion of heme to biliverdin and in the ω-oxidation of fatty acids. Some of these enzymes are capable of attacking xenobiotics. It has not been finally established whether this is really due to their low specificity or to their ability of quick adaptation to foreign substrates.

For the direct oxidation of organic molecules, molecular oxygen must be activated. This can be effected by binding the oxygen molecule to free ligand positions of metal complexes, and most of the mixed function oxidases contain iron (II) or copper (I) complexes are reactive sites. In some bacterial oxidases, flavoproteins are utilized instead of metal complexes.

The best known and most frequently encountered mixed-function oxidases contain iron bound in cytochrome P_{450} as oxygen-activating component. Cytochrome P_{450} is a hemoproteide which forms a carbon-monoxide compound with a maximum of light absorption at 450 nm. This is what the name P_{450} comes from.

Cytochrome P_{450} has been found in mammals, insects, yeasts, and bacteria. In almost all cases an interaction in hydroxylation was attributed to its presence; thus it may be regarded as the most important prosthetic group in mixed function oxidases, whereas the role of cytochrome P_{448} is not yet completely established. According to the proposed mechanism, the cytochrome component of the enzyme complexes with molecular oxygen to form an "activated oxygen" intermediate. One atom of the activated oxygen molecule is then transferred to the substrate, and the other is reduced to water.

Hydroxylation of substituted aromatic compounds follows clearly the rules of electrophilic aromatic substitution; intramolecular rearrangement of chlorine, bromine, tritium, or deuterium, which is familiar to the organic chemists as NIH-shift (because it was first discovered in the National Institute of

Health), leads to the suggestion that arene oxide is an intermediate of the reaction. The suggestion that the active oxygen is added to the π-system is supported by the formation of epoxides from isolated double bonds. Based upon this evidence, an oxenoid structure has been postulated for the active oxygen.

After the oxygen transfer, the oxidases enzyme must be reactivated by some reducing agent. All mixed function oxidases with cytochrome P_{450} seem to require NADPH or NADH for this purpose. Some oxidases which contain other prosthetic groups are reduced by ascorbic acid or tetrahydropteridins, as for example dopamine-β-monooxygenase or phenylalanine-4-monooxygenase. The reducing agents are not always (very) specific, or may even be interchanged in related systems.

By attachment of carbon monoxide to the free ligand position of the iron-porphyrin complex, enzymes with cytochrome P_{450} are inhibited. They can be reactivated in vitro by irradiation with light of 450 nm, which dissociates the CO complex. This specific reaction may be utilized to verify the presence of cytochrome P_{450}.

The question arises whether the mixed function oxidases responsible for the direct oxidation of xenobiotics are entirely unspecific. Induction experiments showed that there is at least a certain group specificity. Induction experiments with drugs or other foreign substances result in an increase of mixed function oxidase activity. Barbiturates mainly increase the oxidation of aliphatic substrates, whereas pretreatment with polycyclic hydrocarbons strongly increases the hydroxylation of aromatic compounds.

Epoxidation of double bonds does not result in a marked detoxication of xenobiotics. The epoxides are only little more polar than the corresponding unsaturated compounds, and there is consequently no substantial increase of excretion. In the class of cyclodiene insecticides, the epoxides are sometimes even more active than the original dienes. We will come back to this question later.

Enzymatic hydration has been found to be the mechanism of epoxide elimination. In 1964, we isolated trans-6,7-dihydroxy-dihydro-aldrin from the urine of rabbits which had been treated with dieldrin. Brooks isolated a solubilized cyclodiene epoxide hydrase from livers of pigs, rabbits and rats, and from some insects, which hydrates dieldrin and heptachlor epoxide in vitro. The hydration of heptachlor epoxide in vivo had not been found so far. The hydration of endrin, the endo-endo stereoisomer of dieldrin, has also been reported recently.

Several groups studied the enzymatic oxidation of benzene and naphthalene. They found benzene oxide and naphthalene-1,2-epoxide to be the primary intermediates, which are converted into the corresponding trans-dihydro-diols by an epoxide hydrase in rabbit liver microsomes. Chemical rearomatisation to form phenols, accompanied by NIH-shift, competes with the enzymatic hydration for the arene oxides: competitive blocking of naphthalene-1,2-oxide hydrase by styrene oxide results in increased formation of 1-naphthol.

Reductive conversion is another pathway of metabolism. The best known examples of enzymic reduction of xenobiotics are those effected by the so-called "nitroreductase" enzymes which appear to be present in most living organisms and are responsible for the reduction of aromatic nitro-groups, and by the azo-reductases responsible for the reduction and cleavage of azo-compounds. Mammalian liver and kidney contain both microsomal and soluble enzymes that can reduce nitro-groups under anaerobic conditions in the presence of NADPH or NADH.

The replacement of chlorine by hydrogen in the conversion of DDT into DDD has been described for a number of biological systems. This reductive dechlorination was shown to be effected by dilute solutions of reduced iron-prophyrin complexes. The anesthetics halothane and methoxyflurane are dechlorinated in the presence of liver microsomes, NADPH, and oxygen, to the derivatives containing hydrogen in place of chlorine. The enzyme activity is stimulated by the classic inducing agent, phenobarbital, and also by subanaesthetic doses of methoxyflurane vapor to the animals.

After the introduction of functional groups into the molecule of a xenobiotic, its excretion can be greatly increased by conjugation to more hydrophilic compounds. Most of our knowledge on conjugation reactions has been derived from drug metabolism studies in mammals. From these investigations, certain generalizations have been established, which appear to be of evolutionary origin and can doubtless be extended to xenobotics. Conjugation with sugars, for example, takes the form of glycosides in plants, bacteria, mollusca, and insects, but in most vertebrates the mechanism is modified to give glucuronides instead, glucuronic acid being activated by uridine diphosphate. The conjugation—using coenzyme A—of foreign acids with endogenous amino acids to form peptides, also differs between species. Conjugation with glycine to form hippuric acids occurs in all terrestrial animals. In addition, man and primates employ glutamine, the amino acid employed being related to the mode of nitrogen metabolism of the species. The conjugation of glutathione to xenobiotics often involves its direct interaction with the unchanged molecule, and might therefore be regarded as a primary process, whereas the glutathione conjugation of aromatics requires their preceding oxidation to arene-oxide intermediates by mixed function oxidases, and must be regarded as a secondary process. Different S-transferases effect the transfer of glutathione to various xenobiotics, with two groups of reactions involved: first, the addition of GSH to double bonds and epoxides by glutathione-S-alkene- and S-epoxide transferases, and second, the substitution by GSH catalyzed by S-alkyl-, S-aralkyl-, and S-aryl-transferases, *replacing*, for example, the halogens of methyl iodide, benzyl chloride, or chloronitrobenzene, respectively. Glutathione conjugation is, for example, involved in the metabolism of the hexachlorocyclohexane isomers, which results, among others, in γ-penta chlorocyclohexene and in 2-, 4-dichlorophenylglutathione for lindane. Whereas the lindane metabolism consumes glutathione, the dehydrohalogenation of DDT to DDE requires it as a catalyst, GSH-levels remaining unchanged during the reaction.

Similar to the glutathione conjugation, the "covalent binding" to DNA, which is discussed today with regard to carcinogenicity, must be classified as a primary process if the unchanged xenobiotic is bound, and as a secondary reaction if a primary metabolite is bound. The latter case would represent a good example for the importance of the study of *primary metabolism* for carcinogenicity research. A special representative of secondary reactions is the methylation of natural cell constituents by xenobiotics. In this case the methyl group may be regarded as the "primary metabolite" reacting with the cell macromolecules.

Which correlations exist between the above discussed reactions and the potential for undesired effects, especially carcinogenicity?

Today, it is assumed that the epoxides which are formed from chlorinated solvents, aliphatic olefines, and aromatics are active to be covalently bound to endogenous biomolecules, especially DNA. This binding is being recognized as a cause for the cytotoxicity of some of these chemicals. The fact that not all epoxides are active in this sense is explained by differences in membrane permeability, organotropism, and elimination.

Another term for cytotoxic chemical is "alkylating agents," a term as unprecise as "active epoxides" regarding their action: any chemical with an alkyl moiety in its structure can be used chemically, in principle, as an alkylating agent. In the discussion of carcinogenicity, however, only those should be included which have activated alkyl groups and are subject to transport mechanisms which allow their reaction with DNA.

Regarding the metabolism of chlorinated solvents and its significance in their carcinogenic potential, I would like to refer the work of Prof. Henschler's group at Würzburg University.

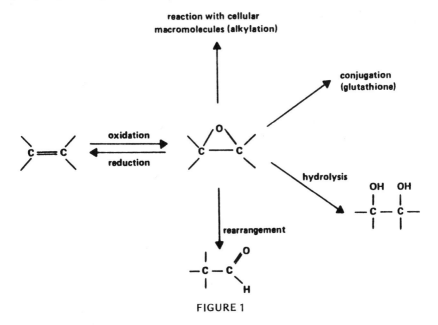

FIGURE 1

Chlorinated ethylenes are metabolically converted predominantly to the respective alcohols and acids via the respective epoxides (oxiranes) as shown schematically in this slide. With increasing number of chlorines, the rate of monooxygenase conversion to oxiranes is decreased. Acute as well as chronic toxicity of this type of compounds has been correlated with alkylating activity, whereas the other reactions like reduction, hydrolysis, and conjugation, and chemical rearrangements, are regarded as detoxications. According to this synopsis, trichloroethylene is metabolized to its oxide which is further converted to chloral. This is further converted partly to trichloroethanol, partly to trichloroacetic acid. The unstable oxirane intermediate could be spectroscopically substantiated for this compound.

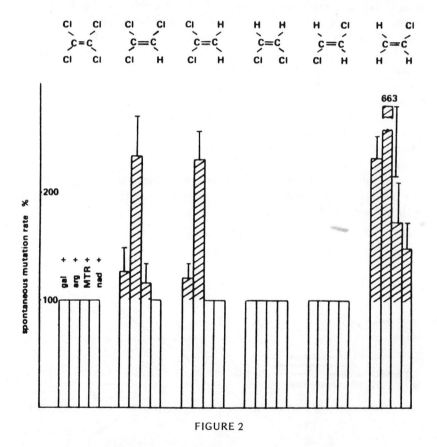

FIGURE 2

Three chlorinated ethylenes are claimed to be mutagenic: vinyl chloride, vinylidene chloride, and trichloroethylene. The explanation in this case—three of the six shown chloroethylenes are mutagenic and the others not—is the difference in the stability of the metabolically derived oxiranes.

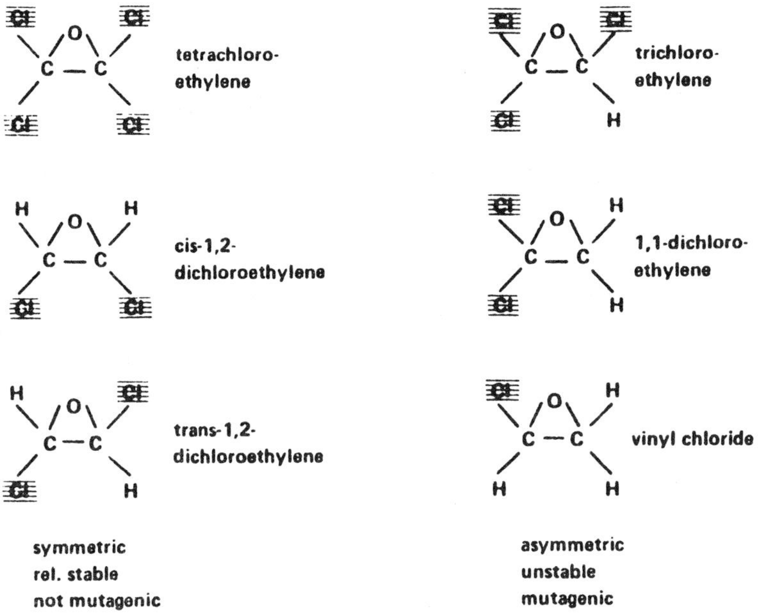

tetrachloro-ethylene	trichloro-ethylene
cis-1,2-dichloroethylene	1,1-dichloro-ethylene
trans-1,2-dichloroethylene	vinyl chloride
symmetric rel. stable not mutagenic	asymmetric unstable mutagenic

FIGURE 3

As seen from this slide the mutagenic chlorinated ethylenes form asymmetric oxiranes which are unstable. The nonmutagenic compounds give symmetric relatively stable oxiranes. If the reaction of the oxiranes with constituents of the animal cell is the basis for genotoxic effects, this correlation between symmetry/asymmetry and stability/instability could be a criterion to predict biologic activity.

For both groups, epoxides and alkylating agents, scientific assessment is difficult to achieve, since the final experimental proof for their covalent binding to DNA has been given in a few cases only. In most publications, it is concluded from nonseparability, nonextractability, or differences in the chromatographic behavior, as compared to the blanks, that covalent binding exists. This conclusion, however, is not allowed for macromolecular systems. A reliable approach for the final experimental proof of covalent binding to macromolecules is the partial chemical degradation and identification of the degradation products. This procedure, however, is difficult to perform with the low amounts of "covalently bound" chemicals which can be isolated. Examples published with good evidence for DNA binding are the 7-N- and 6-O-alkylation of DNA-guanine by dimethyl-methane-sulfonate, the alkylation by di-alkyl-nitrosamines, and the reaction with propylene oxide. In these investigations with alkylating agents, isolates from in vivo or in vitro experiments have been separated by paper chromatography, the spots corresponding to the expected alkylguanines were

85

subject to direct-inlet mass-spectrometry, and the calculated parent peaks could be detected.

I would like to emphasize that metabolic characteristics *are* an important basis for toxicological assessment, but that even labile structural intermediates, if they are formed, do not allow for conclusions unless the mode of action is known. For demonstration, I would like to discuss metabolism and carcinogenicity of organic chemicals with two examples of experiments we have done in the International Center of Environmental Safety in a joint program with our colleagues of Albany Medical College. I would like to emphasize that this does not implicate these model chemicals as being carcinogens in man.

Cyclic organochlorine compounds are the best known environmental chemicals today regarding metabolism and fate. The metabolism of DDT, and, to a comparable extent, of aldrin and dieldrin, has been most thoroughly investigated in a number of different species. Furthermore, we have a good knowledge in this respect on the other cyclodienes, the PCB's, hexachlorobenzene, and chlorinated solvents.

HEXACHLOROBENZENE (HCB)

Dehydrochlorination, as first demonstrated with DDT, seems to be a well-established metabolic reaction. Elimination of chlorine from aromatic molecules has been reported for several substances. In our experiments with hexachlorobenzene orally administered to Rhesus monkeys, we found pentachlorobenzene as a major fecal metabolite and pentachlorophenol as the major urinary metabolite, besides pentachlorobenzene and tetrachlorobenzenes.

Regarding the balance of metabolism, we may ignore metabolites in tissues since mainly HCB is present. Consequently, both pentachlorobenzene and pentachlorophenol are major metabolites. The significant formation of pentachlorobenzene suggests a reductive dechlorination process without arene oxide

Quantitative Estimation of Total Excreted Radioactivity Following 550 Days Dosing of 110 μg/day Hexachlorobenzene to 10 Male Rhesus Monkeys (in % of total applied radioactivity)

	Urine	Feces
Hexachlorobenzene	< 1.5	51.8
Pentachlorobenzene	1.5-2	0.5
Pentachlorophenol	3-4.5	traces
Tetrachlorobenzenes	traces	n.d.
total	6.0	52.4

FIGURE 4

intermediate. It cannot be concluded from the data available whether the penta-chlorophenol is formed via pentachlorobenzene as an intermediate, or whether the first step is an oxidative attack. The primary intermediate and, therefore, the mechanism of metabolism remain to be assessed.

There is one further phenomenon which still needs an explanation, namely, the increase in the excretion of metabolites during the HCB feeding experiment from about 0.5% in the urine in early stages up to more than 5% in the urine after 550 days (% based on daily applied radioactivity). MFO-enzyme induction seems to be no explanation for this effect: liver-P_{450} of a sacrificed animal and, furthermore, SGOT (serum glutamate oxalacetate transaminase), SGPT (serum glutamate pyruvate transaminase), and SLDH (serum lactate dehydrogenase) were within normal values. It could be mentioned that metabolism in rats seems to be different from that in monkeys. Another group investigating rat metabo-lism found additionally chlorine substitution by SR. In sum, HCB, however, is metabolized only to a small extent, as are the chlorofluoromethanes, but for different reasons, as discussed above.

ALDRIN/DIELDRIN

Finally, I would like to discuss the insecticide, aldrin, the carcinogenic potential of which has been discussed during recent years. Aldrin is easily converted to its exo-epoxide, dieldrin, which is used as insecticide itself. Dieldrin is a stable epoxide and should not be genotoxic according to the chloroethylenes scheme discussed. This conversion is possible under biotic and abiotic conditions. Metabolism studies with both chemicals have been carried out in a large number of animal, insect, plant, and microbial species.

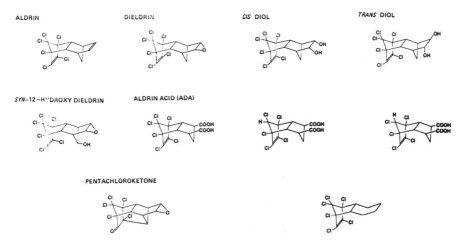

FIGURE 5

We can assume that all significant metabolites constituting more than 0.5% in the balance are known, with the exception of unstable intermediates and non-solvent-extractable portions.

In the context of aldrin metabolism, I would like to mention for comparison metabolic conversion of another experimental cyclodiene insecticide with extremely low toxicity, namely β-dihydroheptachlor. This compound is very easily metabolized to its mono- and dihydroxy derivatives without intermediate epoxide formation, which generally increases persistence for this type of chemicals. Consequently, only very low amounts in the form of derivatives remain in organs and tissues following administration of β-dihydro-heptachlor. This slide shows the kinetics of residue distribution in rats.

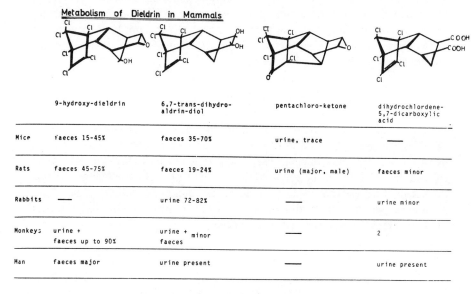

Metabolism of Dieldrin in Mammals

	9-hydroxy-dieldrin	6,7-trans-dihydro-aldrin-diol	pentachloro-ketone	dihydrochlordene-5,7-dicarboxylic acid
Mice	faeces 15-45%	faeces 35-70%	urine, trace	——
Rats	faeces 45-75%	faeces 19-24%	urine (major, male)	faeces minor
Rabbits	——	urine 72-82%	——	urine minor
Monkeys	urine + faeces up to 90%	urine + minor faeces	——	2
Man	faeces major	urine present	——	urine present

FIGURE 6

With the aim of correlating hepatoma formation with metabolic conversion, we carried out an investigation of the comparative metabolism of dieldrin in different animal species. This investigation had to be done experimentally, since published data for different species were derived from different experimental conditions. According to our knowledge, this is the only example where a reliable comparison of metabolism in different species is available: qualitatively, metabolism in mice and rats is identical, but in mice, the 6-, 7-trasdiol is the major product, whereas in rats the 9-hydroxydieldrin prevails. Rabbits are similar to mice, and Rhesus monkeys are similar to rats. This would indicate that the diol formation is involved in the development of hepatoma in mice. The fact that rabbits do not develop hepatomas can be explained by the low rate of diol formation, which in turn results in low liver concentrations.

At the fourth international symposium on "Chemical and Toxicological Aspects of Environmental Quality," a report was given on a comparative study of hepatoma formation in CF-1 mice, CFE-rats, and Rhesus monekys Hepatomas were found only in CF-1 mice, as has been expected. However, with respect to the correlation between so-called DNA-binding and carcinogenic activity, the results indicate a negative correlation: three times as much dieldrin was bound to DNA in rats as in mice (mice 0.58, rats 1.52 molecule equivalent dieldrin per 10^9 nucleotide units). It should be emphasized that DNA binding in this experiment was determined by methanol extraction, but nonextractability is not a proof of chemical binding.

I would like to conclude this presentation with these facts, which are self-explanatory but which require the investigation of reactions of so-called carcinogens at the subcellular level with reliable methods, if we are to get a real understanding of the relevant processes.

Discussion

DR. COULSTON: As I listened to this, there were several points made, that if true, could keep us here all week discussing them. If I understand what you're saying, Dr. Klein, you say there's very little evidence for covalent binding, except in one case that you were able to find.

DR. KLEIN: In alkylating agents.

DR. COULSTON: But this concept that covalent binding is necessary for carcinogenesis, you are questioning very much.

DR. KLEIN: We would just say, at least for the more complicated chemicals and for the chlorinated chemicals, that there is no proof that covalent binding exists.

DR. MILLER: I think what Dr. Klein says about the chlorinated hydrocarbons is certainly correct. However, I think it's incorrect to give the impression that covalent binding has not been demonstrated for a wide variety of chemical carcinogens. It certainly has been and wherever any chemical carcinogen has been investigated adequately—and I emphasize the word adequately—covalent binding has been demonstrated, and for the polycyclic hydrocarbons, the aromatic amines, and a variety of alkylating agents as he's mentioned. There actually have been demonstrations of the chemical nature of the covalent binding, and I would like to emphasize also, or at least point out, that in addition to DNA binding you also find binding to RNA's and to proteins, not just DNA. And this has relevance to mechanisms of action. The important thing is that the active intermediates are electrophiles; they attack nucleophiles and macromolecules of all types. So now you've thrown a certain amount of doubt on retention of labeled molecules after exhaustive extraction by methanol, and I think there should be proper caution there. But, I think once again, wherever binding has been observed under that kind of condition and it has been investigated chemically, it's always turned out to be covalent.

DR. KLEIN: It's hard to comment on this. We made a real literature study and we found a number of applications, you are right, but when comparing them to all the plain covalent bindings, the number that has really been demonstrated is low. I might have overemphasized a bit, but the number really demonstrated is low. On the other hand, when talking about something else, the so-called nonextractable residues and from experimental investigations of the last two years on unextractable residues, we can conclude that there are many cases where it's not covalent binding, because we are just talking about nonextractable residues, for instance, of chlorinated anilines. We get them dissolved in a certain experimental procedure and we can isolate again the nonchanged anilines. We cannot generalize the identification of covalent binding.

DR. MILLER: I might point out that in many cases the physical extractions have been incomplete, there's no question of this. I might also point out that our feeling, and we stated this many times in print, is that while we feel covalent binding in general is necessary; it is not sufficient for carcinogenic action. I'd like to bring up the problem that hasn't been addressed at this meeting yet and that is stages in carcinogenesis. Binding appears to be primarily involved in initiation. And if proper promotion has not occurred, you're not going to see tumors.

90

DR. COULSTON: A very interesting point. Dr. Magee, I don't want to get into a big discussion now, or we won't have anything to do tonight, but I will recognize two or three more people on a very urgent issue here.

DR. MAGEE: I just wanted to ask Dr. Klein to what extent these various chlorinated derivatives that he's mentioned have been tested for mutagenicity with suitable activating systems. Presumably, that would imply an interaction with DNA of some kind, if we're going to get mutagenicity. Are these compounds mutagenic in general?

DR. KLEIN: No, not at all.

DR. MAGEE: Have they been studied in the Ames system or with adequate activation? And they're not mutagenic?

DR. KLEIN: Yes and they are not mutagenic.

DR. CRANMER: I'm commenting on whether a number of chlorinated hydrocarbon pesticides have been tested adequately with the Ames system and some other types of predictive mutagenic tests: hopefully these will act as screens for carcinogens. We all know that they're very effective for aromatic amines; however, the last time I looked at the problem, and I could be in error, but for DDT, aldrin dieldrin and heptachlore, chlordane, methyoxychlor, and a couple of others, the Ames system or equivalent was negative.

There may have more than one reason. One would be perhaps not actually producing mutagenic modes, another could be the very small solubility of these compounds in aqueous media as compared to the amounts necessary to drug the bug, that's the other side of it, or the greater affinity of the material for the cell membrane as opposed to penetrating across and getting into, say, DNA.

But quite aside from that, what is your opinion about the importance one can attach to the statement that in any of the studies on the chlorinated hydrocarbon pesticides conducted in laboratory animals (particularly in mice, but in mice and rats), one could argue that it was a perhaps a genetic as opposed to an epigenetic mechanism for induction of those lesions?

Since most of the animals do have fair spontaneous background rates—and that spontaneous background rate may be genetic, or it may be indeed a response to other carcinogens in the feed—can we separate the issue as to whether these compounds are acting as promoters? Until someone does, does it really make any difference from the standpoint of public health, categorizing them as percentages? To my knowledge that evidence isn't available.

DR. COULSTON: Thank you, Dr. Cranmer. Would you care to answer that, Dr. Magee?

DR. MAGEE: I think that is getting right to the point. Perhaps this particular group of carcinogens is acting rather more like phenobarbital, and they are really promoters and not initiators in the sense of cobalt reacting with DNA.

DR. COULSTON: They're not covalently bound—that's the problem. That's why with dieldrin Korte and Klein can find what they do and, make the statements they make. Dr. Thorpe, please, get to a microphone, introduce yourself to all of us, and say some words of wisdom.

DR. THORPE: I wish to address first of all Dr. Magee's question regarding dieldrin: We have done the Ames test ourselves. I know Ames himself has tried it, and I think one can endorse it, but he's tried very hard with a whole lot of hydrocarbons and has had a singular lack of success in showing mutagenic or mutotoxic effects. From other studies on DDT, I think the only animal test that I recall where there was a suggestion that chlorinated hydrocarbons did have a mutagenic effect was with, I think, a dominant lethal study in rats, and I think the effect was somewhat debatable. We have attempted to find out whether these compounds cause chromosomal damage, all with negative results.

So, I think in some way one can say, we have no evidence to support the proposition that dieldrin behaves as a mutagen. I was a little puzzled, if I can ask a question about something that Dr. Klein said about the covalent interactions. I think he may have been quoting some of the work from our laboratory, and my recall of that was that we got virtually negligible binding of any kind to DNA. This was in work done with two strains of mice and CAB rats, and again it didn't correlate at all with the responses that one saw in the liver in long-term studies.

Additionally, I think one can say that there is some work that's not yet published, and Professor Shubik might yet address this question of dieldrin in hamsters, long-term studies with again, I think, negative results. I don't know. Were any metabolic or interaction studies done in those studies?

DR. SHUBIK: I think not.

DR. THORPE: Work has been presented in a paper where, in fact, an attempt was made to study the effect on nonhuman primates with various chemical carcinogens, and one phenomenon observed was an elevation of α-feto protein. We have no evidence that there is an elevation of α-feto protein in any animal studies or exposed humans with dieldrin, which is another aspect of carcinogenicity. It does address the question of the genotoxic effects of these compounds.

DR. COULSTON: Thank you very much. We will talk more about the use of nonhuman primates in this kind of research, I'm sure, at another time. Dr. Kolbye, please.

DR. KOLBYE: I just wanted to make a comment related to the one that Dr. Cranmer made and not necessarily in opposition to what he said. I would say that, speaking in terms of the immediate future, it may be very difficult to isolate the promotion aspect, and it may not make much of an immediate pragmatic impact on the way regulatory agencies function, but I would simply like to urge that we continue and expand in that area for one very salient reason (and I think I may be wrong, that the dose-response relationships of a promoter might be considerably different from many of the electrophilic agents *per se*. One could question whether or not some of the extrapolation models that may have some relevance to electrophilic compounds have this same degree of relevance to promoting agents, which to my way of thinking, perhaps follow more classical toxicological relationships. Thank you.

DR. COULSTON: This whole question of using the word promoter in terms of these kinds of chemicals leaves a great question. I think the whole episode of DDT or dieldrin actually causing the tumor which can become a cancer in a small number of mice has nothing to do with promotion. It's a fact that changes in the hepatic cells are caused by a continual administration of the chemical. I can't see this as a covalent promoter or anything else, except just like the rat bladders in the Canadian saccharin animals.

DR. SHUBIK: The tumors were cancer of the bladder, and anybody who went and saw them agreed; there was absolutely no question among the group that saw them. How they occurred is another story, but they were cancer.

DR. COULSTON: Now Dr. Miller did ask for the floor again, and I would be very happy to give it to him.

DR. MILLER: I'd like to keep this brief. Comments were made about the Ames test, and I think it's important to point out that in the Ames test it's generally done with enzymatic activation of the microsomes, and those microsomes do not remain enzymatically active indefinitely. I'll try to tell tomorrow my story; this was quite interesting. We sent safrole and its carcinogenic metabolic, 1'-methoxysafrole and the synethic electrophile, 1'-acetoxysafrole, several years ago to be studied in the Ames test. We couldn't detect any one of those as mutagenic with the TA198 and 100. Then we got TA 98 and TA100. Even with TA100-plus microsomes, Ames could not detect the mutagenic activity of safrole or 1 hydroxy-safrole, and he just barely detected the mutagenic activity of the synthetic electrophile, 1'-acetoxysafrole.

Well, now we have studied the metabolism of the 1-hydroxysafrole, the carcinogenic metabolite, in vitro with liver microsomes, and we find that its epoxide and sulfate ester, for which we have enzymatic evidence, are formed at very slow rates. And the microsomes don't last much more than about a half hour after the agar overlay is made. Our feeling is that Ames can't just pick up the mutagenicity under these conditions, because the mutagen isn't made at a fast enough rate to permit detecting the mutagenicity. Only when we give him the synethic electrophile, the 1'-acetoxysafrole could he even find weak mutagenicity. So with your chlorinated hydrocarbons the mutagen may be made, but in far too small an amount to be picked up with the assay as it stands.

DR. BUECHEL: I'm going to comment on a different aspect. In the introduction, Dr. Klein made a statement which I want to support strongly. He said that metabolic studies of biologically active compounds and the establishment of their physiologic properties are an aid in structure-activity understanding. These results are indeed useful strategic tools for the design of new pesticides.

And this is used in practice, as a matter of fact, and I can speak here for my own bioresearch. On the other hand, metabolic data and related things are part of registration data, and these are open to the public, and I think that a comment in Dr. Klein's lecture strictly underlined that these data might be perfected. They are for continuing the discussion. The registration data need some protection, because they definitely include some confidential work.

5. Mammalian Metabolism of DDT and Related Chlorinated Hydrocarbons

Ralph Gingell
Eppley Institute for Research in Cancer
University of Nebraska Medical Center
Omaha, Nebraska

Much work has been done examining the major residues in biopsy and autopsy tissues of humans exposed either occupationally or environmentally to DDT, but little has been concluded concerning the toxic effects or the carcinogenicity of long periods of human exposure (IARC Monograph, 1974). We must consider data from several animal species exposed to high doses of DDT and see how these can help us evaluate the potential hazards of human exposure.

Since much has been published on various aspects of DDT metabolism in animals, I shall review mostly my own work, and try to show how this relates to the literature. I began a few years ago in this area by trying to determine if there were a metabolic basis that could explain the observed species differences in the acute and chronic effects of DDT in the mouse and the hamster. DDT was quite toxic to mice, inducing nervous tremors and then death, with an oral LD_{50} of about 300 mg/kg. Hamsters, however, were not killed by oral doses of DDT up to 2000 mg/kg, although they did exhibit nervous tremors. DDT and not a metabolite was the toxic agent, but we were unable to determine a metabolic difference, for example, in the rates of absorption, metabolism or excretion, which might account for this acute toxic effect (Gingell & Wallcave, 1974).

Table 1 illustrates the brain residue levels of DDT at 12 hours after an oral dose of 500 mg/kg, when they were double for the mouse than for the hamster, and also when we fed lethal doses to the mouse and the hamster. We had to feed up to 5000 mg/kg and only then succeeded in killing half of the hamsters. At death the brain residue levels were approximately equal in both species, so we assumed that there must be a species difference in the blood brain barrier to

DDT, and not a metabolic difference, which could explain the difference in acute toxicity.

TABLE 1
WHOLE BRAIN CONCENTRATIONS OF DDT AFTER
ACUTE ADMINISTRATION OF DDT[a]

Time after DDT administration	Sex	Brain DDT (ppm)	
		Hamster	Mouse
12 hr	M	24 ± 2	39 ± 10
	F	25 ± 4	46 ± 15
At death	M	53	49 ± 5
	F	56, 78	58 ± 14

[a]Brain DDT concentrations were determined 12 hrs after oral administration of 500 mg/kg of DDT to mice and hamsters, and after administration of lethal doses (mice 500 mg/kg, hamsters up to 5x1000 mg/kg). Except where indicated the results are the mean ± S.D. of 3 animals (Gingell & Wallcave, 1974).

Undaunted by this lack of success, we performed further experiments in an attempt to explain the species difference in the chronic effects of DDT in the mouse and the hamster in terms of metabolism. Briefly, at that time technical DDT had been shown by Tomatis's group in Lyon to induce hepatomas in CF-1 mice at doses of up to 250 ppm in the diet (Tomatis et al., 1972). Syrian golden hamsters, however, were not susceptible to these or to other tumors when maintained on diets containing 1000 ppm of DDT in the diet (Agthe et al., 1970). Technical DDT contains several impurities, which at this time we ignored, and performed a metabolic study of the pure p,p'-DDT isomer, the major insecticidal component.

We fed hamsters and mice for six weeks at 250 ppm of DDT in the diet, which is the maximal dose tolerated by the mice, and measured the residues of DDT and of the two major metabolites, DDD and DDE, in the liver (Table 2). Total residue levels were about 8 times higher in the mouse liver than in the hamster liver, and we found similar differences when we examined the fat, except that the residue levels were much higher in the fat of both these species. This species difference was partly due to the fact that the mice ate three times more DDT-containing food per kg body weight than did the hamsters, and also to the fact that after six weeks on the diet the metabolism of DDT was induced in the hamsters so that they excreted three times as much C-14 after a dose of C-14 DDT than did the mice (Gingell & Wallcave, 1974).

The surprising difference, however, was in the amount of DDE: levels of DDE were about 100 times higher in the mouse than in the hamster maintained on similar DDT-containing diets for a similar time. We decided to investigate

TABLE 2
LIVER RESIDUE LEVELS AFTER MAINTENANCE ON
DIETARY DDT, DDD, OR DDE[a]

Species	Residue in food	Sex	Liver Residue (ppm)		
			DDT	DDD	DDE
Hamster	DDT	M	2 ± 1	6 ± 2	0.2 ± 0.1
		F	4 ± 1	5 ± 2	0.1 ± 0
	DDT	M	21 ± 3	22 ± 3	12 ± 2
		F	34 ± 11	23 ± 1	13 ± 3
Mouse	DDD	M	0	3 ± 1	0
		F	0	1 ± 0	0
	DDE	M	0	0	62 ± 5
		F	0	0	54 ± 6

[a]Syrian golden hamsters and CF-1 mice were maintained for 6 weeks on diets containing 250 ppm DDT, DDD, or DDE. Results are the mean ± S.D. for three animals (Gingell & Wallcave, 1974).

the urinary metabolites of C-14 DDT in the hamster and the mouse in order to determine if this were due to a species difference in DDT metabolism.

The metabolism of DDT has been recently reviewed (Fishbein, 1974). DDT is metabolized in the rat to the primary metabolites DDD and DDE, which are not interconvertible. DDD can be further metabolized via a series of intermediates to the acid DDA, but DDE is not metabolized to any significant extent (Fig. 1). DDA can be excreted readily in the urine either unchanged or as various conjugates. Thus the conversion of DDT to DDD is rate limiting for further metabolism and excretion of DDT. When we gave DDE, no free or conjugated DDA was detected in the urine (Gingell & Wallcave, 1974). Essentially the same conclusions can be drawn from the liver residue levels after feeding these different compounds to the mouse (Table 2). When DDT was fed for 6 weeks in the diet, DDT as well as DDD and DDE were present in the liver. After feeding DDD, only low levels of DDD were detected, indicating that DDD is readily metabolized and excreted. When we fed 200 ppm of DDE for 6 weeks, quite high levels of DDE were detected, which is consistent with the fact that DDE is not metabolized and excreted.

Further metabolism of DDE was unknown until recently when Sundstrom (1977) reported various ring-hydroxylated metabolites of DDE in rat feces. The dichloro-ethylene part of the DDE remains intact in all the metabolites, but the ring hydroxylated metabolites indicate that possibly an NIH shift mechanism is operating, presumably through arene oxide intermediates (Fig. 2). Some of these intermediates would be chloro-epoxides, the possible significance of which will be mentioned later. These DDE metabolites only accounted for about 5% of the dose given to rats.

TABLE 3
INDUCTION OF DRUG METABOLISM BY DDT
AND METABOLITES IN MICE[a]

Treatment	Sex	Liver/body wt	Aminopyrine demethylase	Benzo(a)pyrene hydroxylase	Cytochrome P450	Hexobarbital sleep time
				% Control value		
Phenobarbital	M	135[b]	390[b]	520[b]	310[b]	35[b]
	F	165[b]	265[b]	170[b]	240[b]	30[b]
DDT	M	135[b]	290[b]	660[b]	190[b]	35[b]
	F	145[b]	210[b]	170[b]	150[b]	50[b]
DDD	M	105	95	150	120	105
	F	110	90	80	90	125
DDE	M	120	220[b]	340[b]	160[b]	50[b]
	F	155[b]	230[b]	160[b]	150[b]	70[b]

[a]CF-1 Mice were maintained for 6 weeks on diets containing 200 ppm DDT, DDD, or DDE. Phenobarbital (1 mg/ml in the drinking water) was administered for 5 days. Enzyme activities were determined per mg microsomal protein. Hexobarbital sleeping time was determined after the i.p. administration of 150 mg/kg Na hexobarbital. Results are the mean for four animals.
[b]Indicates significantly different from controls.

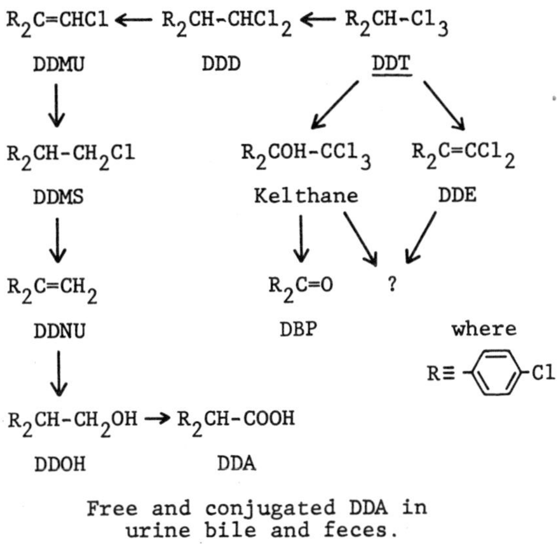

$$R_2C=CHCl \longleftarrow R_2CH-CHCl_2 \longleftarrow R_2CH-Cl_3$$

DDMU DDD DDT

$$R_2CH-CH_2Cl \qquad R_2COH-CCl_3 \qquad R_2C=CCl_2$$

DDMS Kelthane DDE

$$R_2C=CH_2 \qquad R_2C=O \qquad ?$$

DDNU DBP

where

$$R \equiv \text{—}\bigcirc\text{—}Cl$$

$$R_2CH-CH_2OH \rightarrow R_2CH-COOH$$

DDOH DDA

Free and conjugated DDA in
urine bile and feces.

FIGURE 1.

Metabolic pathways of DDT. After Datta and Nelson (1970), Peterson and Robinson (1964), Brown et al. (1969), and others.

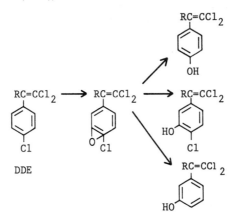

FIGURE 2

Metabolism of DDE in rats by epoxidation. After Sundstrom (1977).

We studied the metabolism of C-14 DDT in the mouse and the hamster. The urinary metabolites were divided into two fractions: that which was extracted by hexane and that subsequently extracted with ether. The ether extract of both species contained DDA, mostly conjugated with glucuronic acid. Small amounts of glycine, alanine, and serine congugates were also detected (Gingell, 1976; Wallcave, 1974) but, since the conjugates were present in both the urine of mouse and hamster, none of them is likely to be responsible for the tumorigenesis observed in mice by DDT. The hexane extract contained less than 1% of the dose; in the hamster urine this fraction consisted of small amounts of unchanged DDT and DDD, whereas in the mouse both DDT and DDD were found, together with relatively large amounts of DDE.

DDT is not tumorigenic in the mouse after a single dose, only when mice are maintained for long periods on dietary DDT. In order to determine if this species difference in metabolism were maintained after chronic administration of DDT, we determined the urinary metabolites when mice and hamsters were maintained on 250 ppm DDT in the diet (Fig. 3). The total of metabolites was somewhat proportional to the food intake, but in the hamster metabolites consisted mostly of free and conjugated DDA, whereas in the mouse urine initially there was DDA with a small amount of DDE. After four months on the diet, the proportion of DDE was quite markedly increased until it was almost as great as the polar DDA metabolites.

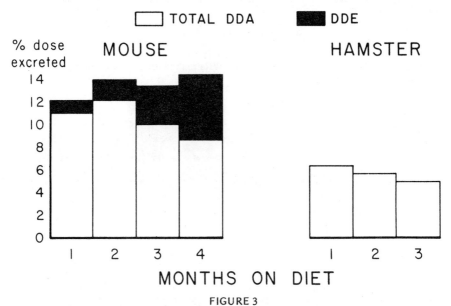

FIGURE 3

DDT metabolites in mouse and hamster urine. Animals were maintained ad libitum on food containing 250 ppm DDT. Urine was collected weekly for 24 hours. Total excretion is the integrated results from four animals (Wallcave et al., 1974).

At this time Thorpe and Walker (1973) in England confirmed, using pure DDT in CF-1 mice, that the hepatomas observed were not due to impurities in the technical DDT. Also Tomatis et al. (1974) observed liver tumors, which were more pronounced in the females, in the CF-1 mouse with 250 ppm dietary DDE. DDD in the diet caused no increase in the liver tumors in either sex. DDD did induce a small but significant increase of lung tumors in both sexes of CF-1 mice. It does seem possible that metabolic formation of DDE from DDT may be responsible for the induction of liver tumors by DDT in the CF-1 mouse. The rate of this formation, as I have shown from our studies, was much less in the hamster than the mouse, as measured by tissue residue levels and also by the urinary metabolites. This rate of formation may not be sufficient for tumor induction in the hamster. This, at least, was our tentative conclusion from these metabolic data.

The obvious experiment to perform, in order to test our ongoing hypothesis that DDT is tumorigenic in the mouse liver, but not in the hamster, due to metabolic conversion to DDE, is to bioassay DDE in the hamster. This is presently being done by Dr. Rossi of the Eppley Institute at dietary levels of DDE up to 1000 ppm. So far there is no evidence for tumorigenicity in the hamster.

We have performed some experiments in an attempt to exclude the complications of metabolism, and of impurities in the technical product, by testing for malignant transformation of mouse embryo cells in culture using pure DDT and metabolites (Langenbach & Gingell, 1975). We tested DDT, DDD, DDE, and DDA at various equimolar concentrations (Fig. 4). DDA was inactive in this system. DDT and DDE showed some slight activity at the higher dose levels, but the most active compound was DDD. These results may correlate with the ability of DDD to induce lung tumors in mice, but do not appear to be related to the ability of these compounds to induce liver tumors in the CF-1 mouse. However, the morphological transformation observed with these compounds was of the type 1 and type 2 as classified by Heidelberger, and not of the malignant type 3 as observed with the DMBA positive controls. When these morphologically transformed cells derived from DDT and metabolites were grown in culture and injected subcutaneously into irradiated syngenic mice, none gave rise to tumors, indicating that this is just a morphological transformation which is of doubtful significance to carcinogenesis.

Another activity of DDT and many of the related chlorinated hydrocarbon insecticides, which may be related to hepatoma induction in mice, is the ability of these compounds to induce hepatic drug metabolizing enzyme levels in the mouse and many other species. This can be conveniently measured as hexobarbital sleeping time. CF-1 mice were maintained on 200 ppm dietary DDT, DDD, or DDE for 6 weeks. Sleeping time was markedly decreased by DDT and DDE, but not by DDD (Table 3). Using in vitro assays of hepatic enzyme activity, the same results were obtained: DDT and DDE were about as effective inducers as phenobarbital, the positive control, whether measured as liver to body weight ratios, aminopyrine demethylase activity, benzo(a)pyrene hydroxylase activity, or cytochrome P450 content of the microsomal fraction, whereas DDD had no significant effect on any of these parameters.

Thorpe and Walker (1973) had suggested that these chlorinated hydrocarbon pesticides and phenobarbital, which induce hepatic microsomal enzymes in mice and other species, also induce, but only in the mouse, a liver cell hyperplasia. They had suggested that this induced mitosis makes the mouse liver DNA much more susceptible toward whatever endogenous factors, either biological or chemical, which are responsible for the fairly high level of so-called spontaneous

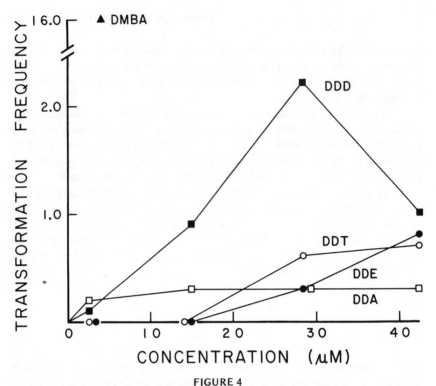

FIGURE 4

Oncogenic activity of DDT and metabolites to mouse embryo cells in culture. Test compounds were dissolved in DMSO and added to the cell cultures for 5 days. Morphological transformation was scored after 6 weeks in culture. Transformation frequency is the number of transformed colonies as a percentage of total colonies formed (Langenbach & Gingell, 1975).

tumors in mouse. However in these short-term studies we never observed any hepatic hyperplasia with these compounds (J. Cabral, personal communication).

Figure 1 summarizes the pathways of DDT metabolism. Most have been demonstrated only in the rat and some are hypothetical. DDT is metabolized through DDD and a series of intermediates, which are abbreviated according to a not very logical system. DD*MU*, for example, means *monochlorinated unsaturated*. This pathway to DDNU takes place in the liver, as shown by liver perfusion, and the conversion of DDNU through the alcohol to DDA apparently takes place in the rat kidney (Datta & Nelson, 1970). Apparently, DDA is absorbed from the kidney into the circulation, because DDA is secreted in the bile as the glucuronide conjugate, which can undergo extensive enterohepatic circulation (Gingell, 1975). The conversion of DDT to DDD can also take place in the microflora of the intestine, and this may be a nonenzymatic mechanism. As the previous speaker mentioned, reduced flavins can perform this conversion. Also DDT has been reportedly metabolized in some in vitro systems by hydroxylation to Kelthane, which also has some insecticidal activity; Kelthane can be further metabolized to the benzophenone and also to DDE. With a knowledge of

102

these possible pathways of metabolism of DDT, we have tried to postulate mechanisms for formation of reactive metabolites that might account for the tumorigenesis observed in the mouse (B. Gold, personal communication).

DDT is itself an analog of carbon tetrachloride, which does induce liver tumors in mice, and possibly a mechanism via a free radical similar to carbon tetrachloride is possible, but I think unlikely. Kelthane, if formed in vivo in mammals, may be further metabolized by acetylation (Fig. 5) forming a good leaving group—the acetate ion—which would leave an electrophile which could then react with cellular nucleophiles such as the bases of DNA, and thus possibly give rise to tumors. But we have been unable to demonstrate that Kelthane is formed from DDT in the mouse.

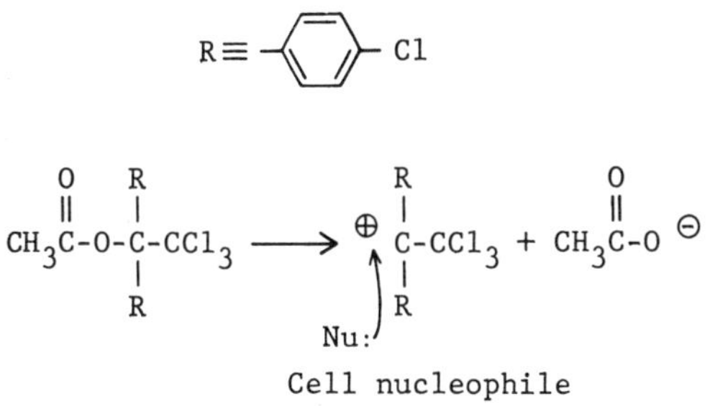

Cell nucleophile

FIGURE 5

Possible biological reactivity of Kelthane acetate.

It has been recently reported that p-chlorobiphenyl is mutagenic in the Ames mutagenicity assay (Wyndham, 1976). This author postulates that possibly a chloro-epoxide is an intermediate in the hydroxylation of p-chlorobiphenyl, which may be responsible for its mutagenicity. It may also be possible that the tumorigenicity of DDE in the mouse liver is due to metabolic formation of a chloro-epoxide, as mentioned earlier (Sundstrom, 1977), analogous to the mutagenic chlorobiphenyl arene oxide.

Recent reports implicating vinyl chloride and vinylidine chloride as carcinogens and mutagens (Elmore, 1976; Haley, 1975) have encouraged us to examine similar mechanisms for the DDT metabolites. Vinyl chloride is presumably mutagenic by epoxidation, although the chlore-epoxide has not been isolated. This could react with water, amines, sulfides, or other nucleophiles in the cell, such as the bases in the DNA to give bound products, or could rearrange to the chloroacetaldehyde which itself can react with nucleophiles in the cell, or be further oxidized to the urinary metabolite chloroacetic acid.

Fig. 6 shows a possible mechanism by which DDE and DDMU may be metabolized by epoxidation, strictly analogous to vinyl chloride, to forms which may react to cellular nucleophiles possibly resulting in neoplastic change. Rearrangement to the chloroacetaldehyde derivatives may occur, yielding acids which might be urinary metabolites. The chloro-epoxide primary metabolite, if

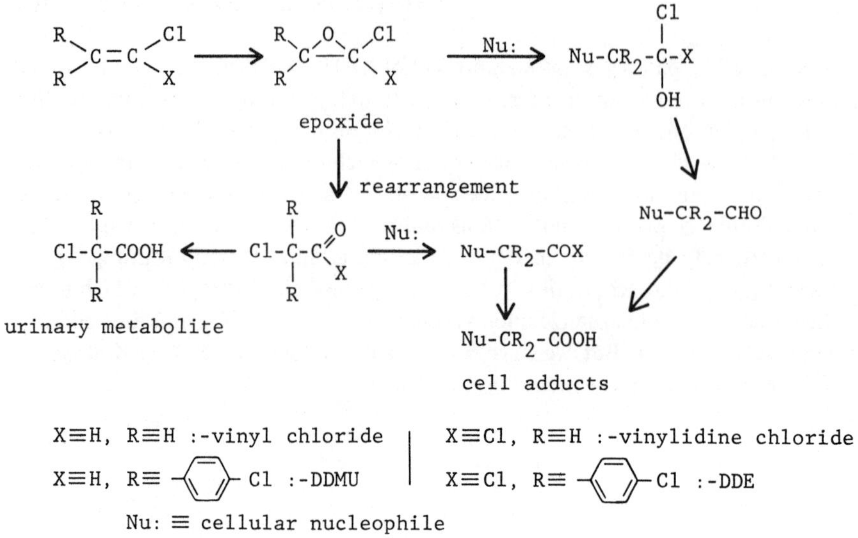

epoxide

rearrangement

$$R_2C=C(Cl)(X) \longrightarrow R_2C-C(Cl)(X) \text{ (epoxide)} \xrightarrow{Nu:} Nu-CR_2-C(Cl)(X)-OH$$

X≡H, R≡H :-vinyl chloride   X≡Cl, R≡H :-vinylidine chloride

X≡H, R≡ —⟨benzene⟩—Cl :-DDMU   X≡Cl, R≡ —⟨benzene⟩—Cl :-DDE

Nu: ≡ cellular nucleophile

FIGURE 6

Possible metabolism and reactivity of vinyl chloride and related chlorinated hydrocarbons.

formed, is probably not stable, but we may obtain some indirect evidence for its formation in vivo by examining urinary metabolites or by elucidating the structure of bound adducts. In order to determine the extent of binding of DDT to target organ macromolecules, we gave up to 75 microcuries of ^{14}C-DDT either singly or as 5 repeated oral doses to CF-1 mice and examined the binding to protein, DNA and RNA isolated from the liver (Table 4). Very little radioactivity was associated with the DNA or RNA, which implied that little if any covalent binding was occurring under these conditions, but possibly prolonged feeding would yield more definite results.

TABLE 4
BINDING OF ^{14}C-DDT TO MOUSE LIVER[a]

	Specific activity (dpm/mg)	
Liver fraction	Single dose	Repeated dose
Whole tissue	825	4450
Protein	30	1470
DNA	6	16
RNA	3	33

[a] ^{14}C-DDT (15 µCi/animal, 10 mg/kg in olive oil) was administered by gavage to male CF-1 mice, either singly, or once daily for 5 days. Six hrs after the last dose, the livers were removed and fractionated by the Kirby-Phenol method, and the extent of ^{14}C-binding determined.

Morgan and Roan (1974) have extensively studied the pharmacokinetics of DDT storage and excretion of human volunteers administered small acute or chronic doses of DDT and its various metabolites. Their conclusions are similar to those obtained from experimental animals. DDT was converted to DDD and to a very small extent to DDE. The DDD was slowly further metabolized and excreted in the urine as DDA and as some unreported conjugates, whereas the DDE tissue residues were very slowly decreased. No DDA was detected in the urine after DDE administration. These authors estimated that an average American with about 17 kg of fat has a body burden of 25 mg of DDT and 75 mg of DDE as a result of dietary exposure to environmental DDT residues. Assuming no further exposure, tissue DDT would be depleted in 10-20 years, but even over the normal lifespan DDE would still be present in the adipose tissue. The large amounts of DDE residues are not due to metabolite formation in man but due to the fact that DDT is partly decomposed to DDE in the environment, and most of the ingested residue is DDE.

It is my view that there are at least two kinds of carcinogens: strong carcinogens like nitrosamines and aflatoxin that can react directly, or be metabolized to forms which can react, with cell nucleophiles at relatively small doses, and are carcinogenic in several organ sites in several species; and there are also chemicals which are only carcinogenic at high doses given for long periods. These may act indirectly with the genetic material, or may be active through a very minor metabolite and induce tumors only in one organ, or possibly in only one or two species. I think DDT is probably one of the latter compounds, and the results of classical carcinogenesis experiments in animals where no specially reactive metabolites appear to be formed are very difficult, if not impossible, to extrapolate for human safety evaluation. Possibly my views may be changed if we can synthesize some of the epoxide derivatives mentioned, or at least show indirectly that they might be formed in vivo. The results of our own and other metabolic studies indicate that possibly DDE and not DDT may be the source of a reactive metabolite.

ABBREVIATIONS

DDT	1,1,1-trichloro-2,2-bis (p-chlorophenyl)ethane
DDD	1,1-dichloro-2,2-bis(p-chlorophenyl) ethane
DDE	1,1-dichloro-2,2-bis (p-chlorophenyl)ethylene
DDA	1-bis(p-chlorophenyl)acetic acid
DDMS	1-chloro-2,2-bis (p-chlorophenyl)ethane
DDMU	1-chloro-2,2-bis(p-chlorophenyl)ethylene
DDNU	1,1-bis (p-chlorophenyl)ethylene
DDOH	1,1-bis(p-chlorophenyl)ethanol
DBP	1,1-bis(p-chlorophenyl)benzophenone

ACKNOWLEDGMENTS

The work reported here is currently supported by Public Health Service Contract NO1 CP33278 from the National Cancer Institute, NIH. The author is grateful to Dr. Barry Gold for useful advice and discussion and to G. Meehan for technical assistance.

REFERENCES

Agthe, C., Garcia, H., Shubik, P., Tomatis, L. & Wenyon, E. *Proc. Soc. Exp. Biol. Med.*, 1970, *134*, 113-116.

Brown, J.R., Hughes, H. & Viriyanondha, J. *Toxicol., Appl. Pharmac.* 1969, *15*, 30-37.

Datta, P.R. & Nelson, M.J. *Ind. Med. Surg.*, 1970, *39*, 195-198.

Elmore, J.D., Wong, J.L., Laumbach, A.D. & Streips, U.N. *Biochem. Biophys. Acta*, 1976, *442*, 405-419.

Fishbein, L. *J. Chromat.*, 1974, *98*, 177-251.

Gingell, R. *Drug Metabl. Disp.*, 1975, *3*, 42-46.

Gingell, R. & Wallcave, L. *Toxicol. Appl. Pharmacol.*, 1974, *28*, 385-394.

Haley, T.J. *Br. J. Med. Sci.*, 1975, *145*, 633.

IARC Monograph (International Agency for Research on Cancer). DDT and associated substances. In *The Evaluation of the Carcinogenic Risk of Chemicals to Man*, Vol. 5: *Some Organochlorine Pesticides.* 1974, pp. 83-124.

Langenbach, R., & Gingell, R. *J. Natl. Cancer Inst.*, 1975, *54*, 981-983.

Morgan, D.P., & Roan, C.C. In W.J. Hayes (Ed.), *Essays in Toxicology* (Vol. 5). N.Y.: Academic Press, 1974, pp. 39-97.

Peterson, J.E., & Robinson, W.H. *Toxicol. App. Pharmac.*, 1964, *6*, 321-327.

Sundstrom, G. *J. Ag. Fd. Chem.*, 1977, *25*, 18-21.

Thorpe, E., & Walker, A.T. *Fd. Cosmet. Toxicol.*, 1973, *11*, 433-442.

Tomatis, L., Turusov, V., Charles, R.T., & Boichi, M. *J. Natl. Cancer Inst.*, 1974, *52*, 883-891.

Tomatis, L., Turusov, V., Day, N., & Charles R.T. *Int. J. Cancer*, 1972, *10*, 489-506.

Wallcave, L., Bronczyk, S., & Gingell, R. *J. Ag. Fd. Chem.* 1974, *22*, 904-908.

Wyndham, C., Devenish, J. & Safe, S. *Res. Comm. Chem. Path. Pharmacol.* 1976, *15*, 563-570.

6. Toxicological and Pathological Data on Polycyclic Aromatic Hydrocarbons and Automobile Exhaust Condensate

Ulrich Mohr
Medizinische Hochschule, Hanover, Germany

There is a wealth of information concerning the effects of polycyclic aromatic hydrocarbons on various tissues and organs of laboratory animals. However, in man exposure is usually not to an individual chemical, but rather to combinations of such as they occur in soot, coal tar, pitch, and mineral oils, as well as in tobacco smoke and automobile exhaust condensate. Exposure of man to these environmental chemical contaminants with carcinogenic potential usually involves frequent or continuous contact with minute quantities of these compounds over a lengthy period of time. This obviously limits the extent to which it is feasible, or indeed expedient, to simulate human experience. Moreover, to what extent the extrapolation to man of data obtained from experimental models is valid, is a question still requiring final resolution. Nevertheless, such studies do provide the simplest and most direct method of establishing what substances pose a carcinogenic threat to man and, in addition, the nature and extent of this hazard. Polycyclic hydrocarbons have long been established as being carcinogenic in laboratory animals, and as I would like to describe today, three distinct experimental approaches exist for the elucidation of more detailed toxicologic and pathologic data on this group of chemicals, and, in particular, on benzo(a)pyrene.

The first slide, please.

INSTILLATION

Here you can see represented the three main methods used for the testing of polycyclic hydrocarbons in the respiratory tract of laboratory animals: these are instillation, implantation, and inhalation. Instillation has long been the most common of all three techniques, although with the publication of a paper by Stanton et al. in 1968 the implantation method received favorable attention. This involves the direct injection of the carcinogenic substance mixed with a carrier vehicle into the surgically exposed lung. Surprisingly, the method most comparable to the human situation (that is, inhalation), has been examined by only a limited number of investigators.

I would now like to present a few experimental studies that have employed such techniques, in order to examine in more detail the various advantages and disadvantages implicit in each procedure and most importantly to assess their individual effectiveness.

Because benzo(a)pyrene has been emphasized as an important factor in environmental carcinogenesis, numerous investigators have examined the nature of respiratory tract carcinogenesis in the Syrian golden hamster after its intratracheal instillation. By using a surface active agent or a carrier dust as vehicles, relatively high tumor yields have been achieved. However, there is some evidence indicating that one of the most commonly used vehicle solutions, Tween 60, possesses tumor-promoting properties. Moreover, it would also seem that the carrier dust, ferric oxide, is to some extent cocarcinogenic. A few investigators have succeeded in inducing respiratory tract tumors in hamsters by the use of benzo(a)pyrene alone. However, such reports are relatively scarce; this fact is probably related to the difficulties in suspending benzo(a)pyrene in an aqueous medium suitable for intratracheal instillation.

In order to compare the effects of such vehicles on benzo(a)pyrene carcinogenesis, and thereby also the effects of different doses on the larynx, trachea, and lung, we conducted a series of studies using benzo(a)pyrene in Tris buffer, physiological saline, and bovine serum albumin. In these studies, benzo-(a)pyrene suspended in Tris buffer was significantly more effective than that given in 0.9% saline, following a single administration. A dose-dependent effect could not be established at levels between 4 and 16 mg. The overall tumor incidence in the respiratory tract ranged between 3% and 15% in benzo(a)pyrene and physiological saline-exposed hamsters, and between 10 and 40% in the benzo(a)pyrene and Tris buffer-treated animals. When bovine serum albumin was used, respiratory tumor incidences ranged between 20% and 40%.

It was also not possible to establish a clear dose-response relationship when benzo(a)pyrene was given in a mixture of tris and saline. Here, the highest incidence of respiratory tumors was found after multiple applications of 0.25 mg, whereas with doses higher than this, survival time and frequency of tumors decreased. The tumors of the larynx and trachea were mainly papillary polyps, whereas pleomorphic sarcomas occurred in the lungs, in addition to bronchiogenic adenomas.

From these investigations it can be learned that the solvent or the medium of suspension can well influence the frequency of respiratory neoplasms in the Syrian golden hamster. It would also appear that high doses (that is, more than 0.5 mg) when given chronically are rather more toxic than carcinogenic.

I would now like to turn to another study we conducted using this procedure of intratracheal instillation. Automobile exhaust, which results from the incomplete combustion of organic fuels, is known to contain a wide spectrum of polycyclic aromatic hydrocarbons. Since experimental studies using skin-painting techniques have demonstrated automobile exhaust condensate to be carcinogenic in mice, we decided to conduct an experiment using intratracheal installation to examine the effects of exhaust condensate on the lungs of Syrian golden hamsters. For this purpose, two groups each consisting of 6 animals were intratracheally instilled at two weekly intervals with either 5 or 2.5 mg per animal of exhaust condensate dissolved in 0.2 ml of Tris-saline mixture and EDTA. Control animals received the solvent solution only.

The next slide, please. The exhaust condensate contained the known polycyclic hydrocarbons listed in the present table. Animals were fixed in situ by perfusion when moribund, and tissues were prepared for routine histological and electron microscopic examination.

The next slide please. As shown in this table, survival times ranged between 30 and 60 weeks; this meant that the minimum total doses of benzo(a)pyrene received by the animals of the two groups were 25.5 or 11.56 micrograms per animal. All hamsters developed multiple pulmonary adenomas.

This slide illustrates the histological view of an adenoma found after 30 instillations of 5 mg of automobile condensate. Black deposits of the condensate are distinctly visible.

This next picture shows a semithin section taken from a hamster which received 40 instillations of 2.5 mg of the condensate. This illustrates quite clearly the bronchiogenic origin of the adenoma.

The next slide, please. This semithin section was taken from an animal in the twenty-second treatment week, and shows epithelial hyperplasia of the bronchus. This EM survey picture demonstrates that the adenomas were composed of well-differentiated ciliated and nonciliated cells.

The next slide, please. This electron micrograph illustrates a macrophage with phagocytized exhaust condensate in the pulmonary tumor. These results quite clearly prove that automobile exhaust condensate does exert a carcinogenic effect upon Syrian golden hamster lungs. Both dosage groups exhibited a 100% rate of multiple pulmonary tumors. Considering the relatively low total dose of benzo(a)pyrene contained in the condensate, this pronounced neoplastic response cannot be explained by the effects of this well-known carcinogenic hydrocarbon.

IMPLANTATION

As I have already mentioned, Stanton et al. reported in 1968 an experiment using an implantation method. Since then surprisingly few additional attempts have been made to induce lung cancer by direct injection of carcinogens into the lungs.

This schematic drawing illustrates the technique used by Stanton and his colleagues. Beeswax was selected as a vehicle, since it is reputedly noncarcinogenic, is easily mixed with polycyclic hydrocarbons, and is also sufficiently soft when gently heated to permit the injection of accurate quantities through a hyperdermic needle directly into the surgically exposed lung. Rapid solidification of the wax at body temperature results in a well-circumscribed pellet that is easily identifiable, so that tissue response at the margin of the pellet can be localized readily. Characteristically, a fibrous capsule can be observed upon macroscopic examination.

This slide shows the perfused lung of a Syrian golden hamster taken from a study we conducted using cigarette smoke condensate. The beeswax pellet is clearly visible directly adjacent to the left lobar bronchus; the fibrous capsule can be seen on the other side of the cut surface of the lung.

The next slide, please. Histologically, the fibrous capsule is often seen near to a main bronchus. As can be seen in the present example taken from a benzo-(a)pyrene treated animal, the bronchial epithelia are not affected in most cases.

The next slide, please.

However, in a few cases as is demonstrated here, slight proliferations can be detected as early as after 20 weeks following implantation. It must also be mentioned here that such alterations have been observed in control animals treated with only beeswax pellets, as well as in the benzo(a)pyrene treated animals. This would indicate, therefore, that such alterations are dependent upon the pellet implantation itself. Nevertheless, in order to examine the effect of benzo(a)pyrene when administered by implantation and to compare these results with those obtained in instillation and inhalation experiments, we decided to conduct an experiment whereby different doses of benzo(a)pyrene were implanted into the lungs of Syrian golden hamsters.

This slide demonstrates the experimental design used. In this way we hoped to establish whether a single dose of benzo(a)pyrene was sufficient to exert a carcinogenic effect and if so whether a dose-dependent relationship for such could be established.

The next slide, please. As this table illustrates, very small doses, such as 0.05 or 0.1 mg benzo(a)pyrene resulted in sarcomas approximately 55 weeks after implantation. These tumors were very malignant, destroyed the lung parenchyma, and infiltrated the vessels and bronchi. The bronchus illustrated in this picture is surrounded by tumor tissue.

The next slide, please. As demonstrated here, tumor tissue that infiltrated the veins exhibited mitoses, as well as variously sized nuclei and nucleoli.

The next slide, please. With 1.0 mg benzo(a)pyrene, a high percentage of the induced tumors were sarcomas, while only a few neoplasms were of epithelial origin. This is in contrast to the results of Stanton, who reported initial metaplastic lesions and their subsequent development to squamous cell carcinomas after implantation of pellets containing cigarette smoke condensate in rats.

Hirano et al. also described similar findings in rats after implantation of different doses of methylcholanthrene. Sarcomas as diagnosed in the present experiment have not been reported by other authors using this technique.

The next slide, please. When pellets containing 1.0 mg of benzo(a)pyrene were implanted in Syrian golden hamsters, macroscopically visible tumors were observed as early as 30 weeks after implantation. Sometimes, as exemplified here, tumor tissue was only seen in the left lung. On other occasions, as illustrated in this slide, the tumor infiltrated all parts of the left and right lung, as well as the heart and diaphragm.

Histologically, as you can see in this slide, the tumors demonstrated mainly sarcomatous tissue with infiltration into the adjacent tissue, although sometimes, as in this case, they also exhibited epithelial parts with fibrous structures. These tumors were induced between 30 and 45 weeks after implantation of benzo(a)pyrene.

INHALATION

The third method to be discussed is that of inhalation. Such investigations have rarely been conducted in the past and the techniques and procedures for this are still very much in their infancy. It is, of course, the ideal method for providing a valid comparison with human experience, since the defense mechanisms of the lung are not disturbed in any way, nor is there any necessity for such external influences such as anesthetic surgical treatment, instillation via a hyperdermic syringe, or the use of vehicle solutions. Although ciliary clearance and macrophages remove particles from the respiratory tract, the dispersion of such benzo(a)pyrene particles to all areas of the lung is good, and more importantly they are of a good absorbable form so that sufficient amounts remain in the alveoli and small bronchi. Nevertheless, inhalation experiments with chronic exposure of laboratory animals to potentially carcinogenic compounds pose their own particular problems. For example, quite extensive legislation for the safety of such experiments means that special precautions must be taken to avoid contamination of the laboratory, the environment and the investigators. In addition, total body exposure of the animal must be avoided, since the contamination of skin could lead to neoplasms that might interfere with the actual inhalation evaluations. In order to try to meet such needs, a new inhalation chamber has been built.

In this slide you can see an inhalation chamber recently developed by Dr. Kimmerle. Using this equipment for the exposure of the Syrian golden hamster to different benzo(a)pyrene aerosol concentrations has demonstrated that the animal's behavior does not alter during long-lasting exposures, nor does its weight curves differ from those of the controls.

After 30 exposures with 40 mgs of benzo(a)pyrene per cubic meter of air, the concentration of benzo(a)pyrene in the respiratory tract is about 0.6 micrograms. Some of these pilot studies have now been running for more than 9 months. It has been possible to establish during this period that the distribution of particles is remarkably constant and also that the majority of particles are smaller than 0.5 microns. Animals that have been examined to date have shown no histological evidence of tumors.

In a further experiment, we exposed Syrian golden hamsters to chronic inhalation of 50 mg of benzo(a)pyrene per cubic meter of air for four and half hours daily over a total period of 120-240 days. In that time, hamsters inhaled more than 178 or 360 mg of benzo(a)pyrene. We were not able to detect any neoplastic alterations of the nasal, tracheal, or bronchial epithelium.

SUMMARY

Having now described a few of our studies that utilized these methods of instillation, implantation, and inhalation, I would like to summarize what I feel are the principal factors involved in an evaluation of their individual effectiveness.

As can be seen from this table, intratracheal instillation requires both minor surgical treatment and a vehicle solution or suspension medium. As we have demonstrated from our studies, the vehicle solution can influence the frequency of tumors induced in the respiratory tract. Moreover, intratracheal instillation does not permit the determination of the final location of deposition of the substance. This can be seen from the development of tumors not only in the lung, but also in the trachea and larynx. As with inhalation studies, the substance is also cleared by the normal pulmonary defense mechanisms, while the presence of forestomach tumors in such experiments also demonstrates that quantities of the substance are swallowed by the animals and hence cleared from the respiratory system. However, of the three methods this is probably the most tried and tested and is relatively simple to perform without the burden of high costs engendered by expensive equipment. The effectiveness is relatively good, with tumor induction being quite high, although again as our studies have shown, it is not particularly suitable for establishing a dose-response relationship.

In comparison to human exposure, the implantation method is highly unnatural and would, on first sight, seem to be of little relevance. Nevertheless, it can be highly effective. Neither instillation nor inhalation of as small a dose as 0.05 mg of benzo(a)pyrene is capable of producing tumors as seen after implantation of this amount. By means of this method it is also possible to establish a dose-dependency, with the largest dose producing high percentages of tumors. As yet it is not clear why hamsters develop mainly sarcomas, in contrast to rats that develop mainly carcinomas. Nor is the exact origin of tumor development known. Such factors could well be investigated in future studies using this technique. Again, however, certain major disadvantages exist, these being the relatively high temperature at the time of implantation, which can result in circumscribed necroses. And the introduction of a foreign body such as a beeswax pellet, which as previously described, could well induce epithelial alterations. Nevertheless, it would still seem to be a very sensitive method for the screening of various polycyclic hydrocarbons, since in such bioassay programs the major criterion is simply that of tumor development.

Despite the fact that the tracheobronchial system of the Syrian golden hamster is somewhat different from that of man, the inhalation method would still seem to offer a real comparison to the human situation. However, as was illustrated by my short description of some experiments with this method, it is not particularly suited to the testing of substances for their carcinogenicity. Very high dosages and first-class inhalation chambers are needed if any positive results are to be obtained. The use of such of first-class equipment also requires intensive cleaning and highly technical surveillance. For such reasons, the costs of such experimentation are prohibitive for most laboratories. The limited amount of experience with this type of technique does not really permit a final evaluation of its effectiveness.

In conclusion, it would seem appropriate to say that all three methods should be regarded as suitable instruments for the investigation of the carcinogenicity of polycyclic hydrocarbons on the respiratory tract. Each would appear to offer particular individual advantages and, therefore, it would perhaps now be an idea to turn our attention to the possibility of correlating them for a final overall estimation of the carcinogenic hazard to man posed by this group of substances.

DR. COULSTON: I will share in the leadership of our discussion with our good friend, Dr. Cranmer. He will take the major role in the discussion, but I would recommend if I may that we deal first with questions relating to Dr. Mohr's paper.

DR. TRUHAUT: Dr. Mohr, you are famous in lung carcinogenicity experimentation. You must know about the experiments of our Soviet colleagues, especially Shabad and Ianysheva, and my question is the following: I remember that they published at least a summary or data, based on experimentation in rats with the intratracheal instillation method, and they claimed not only to have been able to establish a dose-effect relationship but also to establish a threshold. And from this threshold they went ahead and applied a safety factor. I don't remember the value, but they established a proposed threshold for polycyclic aromatic hydrocarbons and especially for some of them, particularly benzo(a)-pyrene. If I remember correctly the value given for the permissible limit in rats was 15 mcg/kg. I was impressed at this time because certainly all who are here and who have knowledge in occupational hygiene know that as between values proposed for permissible limits, either MAC values or threshold-limit values, the values proposed by the Soviet expert are much lower. Surprisingly enough, when the majority of the Americans were of the opinion that there was no possibility of establishing a threshold for such carcinogenic chemicals, the Soviets claimed that they were able to establish a threshold and even recommended it. What is your opinion about that?

DR. MOHR: Well, it's very difficult for me to comment on their papers. I have to be very careful to say anything about that, because I'm on a committee in my country where we are looking for some permissible doses, and I don't like to comment on that, but we have done our work in hamsters and with a single administration we were unable to find a dose-relationship. If we gave the compound twice a week, however, we could find a very nice dose-relation curve. All these studies by the Russian people were done in rats, and I don't think that the rat is a good model for the intratracheal instillation procedure. You can use this animal for the implanation technique, but I think for the intratracheal studies you are using the wrong animal. But I cannot really answer your question.

DR. KENSLER: I seem to remember that Cuyler Hammond, among others, reported that people who inhaled milligrams, or at least a milligram or so per day, of benzo(a)pyrene (roofers, etc.) did not show any increase in lung cancer, isn't that so?

DR. HAMMOND: We followed roofers over a period over 30 years. After 15 years we couldn't show any increase in lung cancer at all. By 20-25 years, you got a slight increase. At 30 years it may have doubled in rate as compared with the general U.S. population. It is not very different from what Doll and his co-workers found with roofing workers. Of course, these roofers were not just exposed to benzo(a)pyrene. They were exposed to everything that is present in pitch. Pat Mosler's laboratory made chemical analyses for everything in that material. Now whether the benzo(a)pyrene (which was the strongest known carcinogen in the pitch) did it, or whether it was a combination of other agents, is uncertain, because we didn't know the smoking habits of these people, but it appears on inhalation to be a very weak carcinogen.

I am afraid that, based on the values we got from collected material in rats and that Dr. Wynder found in cigarette smoke, if benzo(a)pyrene in cigarette smoke were causing cancer, all these people should have died of cancer in no time flat. They were exposed thousands of times to an awful lot of things.

DR. CONNEY: I'd like to ask Dr. Hammond about the amount of material actually ingested that gets into the lung in people exposed in this manner, as compared to cigarette smoking.

DR. HAMMOND: We tested the material in several ways. We got the material molten as in the kettles and had the molten material analyzed. Then we had some gas samples analyzed, and then we had men wear masks during their whole working day. At least a good part of what was collected on the mask presumably would have fallen into the lung. Now the masks were not very good masks for the simple reason that you couldn't get men to wear them; they weren't effective masks. Probably, it took out between one quarter to one half of the fine particulate matter. However you look at it, these doses were simply enormous as compared with what Dr. Wynder and other people found. I think they were undoubtedly inhaling an enormous amount, even if it's a fraction of what was in the mask. This was collecting air samples.

DR. WYNDER: Well, for some reason we're getting involved here in tobacco carcinogenesis, which I thought was not intended this evening, but as long as it has been mentioned by some people I would like to comment first of all on the point of passive inhalation that Dr. Mohr referred to also.

We've got to recognize that man is unique among the two- and four-legged beings in that he inhales smoke directly into the mouth, and the amount of dose he gets is something immeasurably higher than anything he ever inhaled passively.

The clearance mechanism in our lungs is given by our good Lord to be very efficient, and we can probably handle much of the material that we inhale passively. Small animals particularly, as all of us know, have expecially well-developed nasal passages, and it is precisely for that reason that passive inhalation experiments in these small animals are so difficult.

After all, we need to recognize they've been walking on the ground for a few million years, and if they would succumb to the amount of dust on the ground they would have never made it over all these years. But we have walked erect for some time, so our nasal passages have become relatively defunct, even though they are still giving us a better defense system than our mouths, which were never really designed to catch inhaled particles. So we've got to make certain that we distinguish between passive and active inhalation.

Now. Dr. Hoffman and I, and others, have never claimed that benzo(a)-pyrene was the agent responsible for tobacco carcinogenesis. All we claim is that the polycyclic hydrocarbon fraction altogether is a key factor, and that's the only evidence we have for experimental tobacco carcinogenesis.

But the point that I think relates to Dr. Mohr's presentation, which I thought was a very fine one and very logically presented, was that it is very difficult to mimic man in this aspect, namely, the way in which he inhales. And through this conference we must be very clear that as much as we try as biologists to mimic man, there is unfortunately another problem where we find it increasingly difficult to duplicate man's behavior, and it's for that reason that Peter Greenwald and I said earlier that we've got to bring in the epidemiologists to help us make the final evaluation.

DR. HAMMOND: My impression from everything you have done on the action and other facts of various ingredients of cigarette smoke, is that we are dealing with a very complex situation, not just an agent. You have amply demonstrated that, and if we're going to duplicate man it should be under the conditions to which man is exposed, I think, and not just with one isolated substance. I very much doubt that one isolated substance is a key to any appreciable amount of comparison in man under conditions of very heavy occupational exposure.

DR. CRANMER: Could I ask each speaker to identify himself for the tape?

DR. KENSLER: I thought I was going to establish this Friday and I feel impinged upon, but I'm grateful for all the help all of you have given me. I agree with Cuyler and the reason I asked him the question about what the level of exposure was, is that they are horrendous in these groups, to at least one potent agent in the atmosphere. I think a point that Dr. Wynder has been raising for 15 years about the infiltration in the nasal passages has some merit. But Nettesheim at Oak Ridge, for example, has produced squamous carcinomas in the pulmonary bed of particular strain of rat with methylcholanthrene, etc., and he has shown by radioautographic procedures that cigarette smoke delivered at a dose which arrives there, going past the filter, at 3 mg per rat per day—which is one hell of a dose—didn't do it.

DR. CONNEY: I'm wondering if it's just possible with cigarette smoke that maybe it has to be absorbed, because Dr. Wynder has suggested large amounts are ingested orally, and maybe it's metabolism by the liver and then subsequent delivery to the lung that plays a role. Has anyone thought of this possibility? We've been working with a newborn mouse model where we inject benzo(a)pyrene interperitoneally, as others have done as well, and find pulmonary adenomas in a quite high yield and with some of the metabolites of benzo(a)pyrene I'll be talking about tomorrow, one can get down to as low as 28 in animals administered over a period of two weeks and get an appreciable incidence of lung adenomas, giving it interperitoneally in the newborn mouse.

DR. KENSLER: Well, my answer is that I think the adenoma story is different from the squamous carcinoma story, and I'd like to ask Dr. Mohr this: He's quoted Dr. Stanton and I think I remember the same thing—that he had mostly squamous carcinomas—and I think you've got one, perhaps, of mostly sarcomas. And I was just wondering, did you use the same beeswax, or did he have something that had something else in it, or what is beeswax, anyway?

DR. MOHR: Yes, Dr. Stanton gets only squamous carcinoma in his rats, and we had only a few squamous cell tumors. Most of our tumors were sarcomas going in the direction of mesotheliomas. But this story is not yet finished. We have to do some more work on it. We used the same beeswax as Stanton so we could show that only with beeswax you get nothing.

DR. CLAYSON: Can I now pass on to the general discussion? I'd like to take up three points which have been worrying me quite a bit during the day.

The first point is, that we heard from Dr. Wynder this morning a very interesting suggestion indeed for the creation of environmental cancer centers. The question which I'd like to put into people's minds is: Do we intend these to be in addition to our present effort, or extra to our present effort? The reason I ask this question is, that I think at the level of people who actually do the work, the skilled labor which we require with toxic substances coming in at this time, and with other interest in the environmental field over the whole of toxicology expanding, that we are rapidly approaching a critical situation.

This was even more clearly brought home to me before, talking to a colleague in industry, who was complaining bitterly that his histopathology was being held up, because the National Cancer Institute in their attempts to clear their backlog had, in fact, hired practically all of the pathological expertise available for this purpose, in this nation as a whole.

I think that this is going, in the very near future, to trouble us over a lot of toxicology. Maybe we have started training programs almost too late to remedy this deficiency; I don't know. As far as creative labor is concerned, the people who are going to conceive the new general ideas are even in shorter supply, and I wonder very much whether we should create additional environmental cancer centers? Are we are going to find ourselves in a position, which I think has happened before and has happened to a certain extent with the National Cancer Program, in which people are doing the same sort of thing over and over again? We're accumulating a vast number of facts, but we are making very little progress in broad concepts.

I put this out for discussion rather than direct criticism of what Dr. Wynder was saying, because I can see the great advantages in what he is suggesting: to get the people who are interested in development of mechanisms in doing the toxicological research. These are the people who will tell us whether this is reasonable from the point of view of man, as epidemiologists, working together either under one roof or under one pattern. I think is a first-rate concept, but I am very worried about the mechanics of it.

The second area, and I think it's similar, and that is that we're told from time to time that there are somewhere between 24 and 30,000 man-made chemicals in this country which, from time to time, penetrate into the environment. I can believe this, having just been shown from the outside the three volumes which the EPA has brought out on potentially controllable substances. They don't describe the substances, they just give them their names, and the three volumes were perhaps altogether nine inches to one foot high.

So many chemicals! How are we going to select which are the important chemicals among these?

The National Clearing House through the chemical selection group has begun to grapple with this problem as far as the national bioassay program is concerned, and I think I can put it to you that, perhaps, on a worldwide basis, we can now adequately test 100 environmental chemicals in any one year over a four-year period. That means that 24,000 chemicals or thereabouts will take approximately 250 years. That's inconceivable, but when you remember that the number of new compounds introduced every year is somewhere between 500 and 800, I think there would be something like another 250,000 chemicals of some concern at the end of that time. We very clearly have got to think of some means of deciding which chemicals should be tested, and we have a number of ideas of how this should be done using the annual output or the annual environmental escape for these chemicals, looking at chemical structure, perhaps, looking at other toxic properties, looking at the result of prescreens and animal tests and trying to accumulate this data to decide which are the important chemicals.

On the more general level, perhaps, we want to break down the 24,000 into smaller categories. We could look at these chemicals from the point of view of their structure, their analogy to known carcinogens—which I think is a very good approach until one realizes that, in fact, we have no knowledge at all of what we're speaking about, of what perhaps another 80-90% of the total chemicals are likely to do simply because they've never been through a proper carcinogenic screen.

The alternative approach I might personally favor is to consider the environment in terms of what one might call exposure categories containing measurable numbers of chemicals and then to start to look at these in turn, but that is going to be a terribly long process and I think this question of what we should look at is going to be of extreme importance if we're going to go into environmental cancer and environmental toxicological centers. It is of extreme importance to think about a national bioassay program to any form of toxicological approach, such as that which EPA is now mandated to look at, and I think we need a lot of input into that area.

The third point which I want to make is, perhaps, one of disappointment. Again we said that this afternoon we were going to look at Problem Area Number One, "Pesticides and Environmental Chemicals." I came to the conclusion, having listened to our conversations this afternoon, that perhaps the major problems with our chlorinated pesticides are that (a) we don't really know anything particularly about their metabolism, and (b) we don't know why they don't work in the Ames test. We had very little discussion of the pathology of the lesions, although I know we have at least one person in this audience who feels very strongly on this.

I was sorry that Dr. Ito's Japanese experiment wasn't mentioned. What Dr. Ito did was to give hexachlorobenzene in the diet at a reasonable level for 12, 24, and 36 weeks. He found that after being treated—for I think it was for 20-24 weeks, or something like that—the nodules which had already formed went away. But being a patient worker, he didn't say "I'll go to the end of the experiment," but kept his animals alive and kept on the serial killing. Near the end of the two-year period, different lesions, but nevertheless lesions concerning the liver, came back again. He described these as tumors, and I'm not enough of a pathologist to say that they were, and this doesn't sound to me like a promoting agent or a cofactor.

It does sound to me as if there is something more with these compounds and that maybe our attempts to dismiss them out of hand are wrong. Some of us still feel unhappy about them. It may be untrue, and I'll ask another question: Would we feel happier if we knew that these compounds were electrophilically activated by other carcinogens? Would we feel happier if we had some proper epidemiological evidence to show whether or not this type of compound produces tumors in man? I think that's really what I wanted to say.

DR. GREENWALD: I wanted to comment on a couple of things that Dr. Clayson referred to. One was the myriad of chemicals, and what do we do? We have a similar problem in epidemiology with all the different occupations, and so forth, and we have working with us in Albany (N.Y.) some engineers in operations research, and the question is, how can we add efficiency to this area? Really, what we're considering is a concept that we're calling epidemiological screening.

It has the same basic principle as disease screening. Can we, in a short study of a couple of months, by designing the study aimed at the group most likely to be positive, come up with an estimate of the probability of there being a problem there—if we went into it in much greater depth—and use this as a method of deciding where to focus down? I think there may be something in examining how each of us does this, toxicologists and epidemiologists, that may be worthwhile, because it's going to be essential to be able to think through where to focus that attention.

There was a second point—I'll come back to it later. Oh, I also wanted to ask the toxicologists about multiple thresholds. We were mentioning thresholds in terms of what is the lowest safe dose, but I mean thresholds in a very different sense. If you look at the literature, at the interface of genetics and epidemiology or the genetic literature, the geneticists tend to do their analysis by having mathematical models of the probability of genetic transmission, and then they compare their observations of disease incidence in first-degree relatives, and so forth, in order to make their inferences. There seems to be a great deal of extra power that can be gained statistically, if you have more than one threshold. Perhaps one of our weaknesses statistically in epidemiology and toxicology is having a dichotomy of either you have the disease or you don't.

One thing the geneticists tend to use is whether or not a disease is bilateral. Another one is that if there's a younger age of onset, or perhaps, the question is the grading of the tumor.

What I really wondered is whether the toxicologists can tell us anything from their animal studies to enable us to use some spectrum of disease where we can examine different thresholds, rather than just saying a person has cancer or not, and whether based on their work there may be a plausibility of using human studies.

DR. WYNDER: I would like to answer a couple of questions asked by David Clayson. The first one I will show, I guess on Friday morning, is what I visualize an environmental cancer center looks like. Clearly it can be built up in existing institutions and have at least two to three other categories, which I think ought to be included or are already at hand.

The next point you talked about was priorities. I like to think priorities ought to relate first to those cancers from which most of us die. I'm always amazed that as I travel around the world—and I suppose if I were a man from Mars and I came down to earth and the first medical journal I picked up as *Cancer Research*—I would certainly think that we would all die from liver cancer.

That is obviously not the case, but it happens to be a mighty experimental tool, like the blind man who looks for the key under the light, because that light is not necessarily where he lost the key. Many cancers are clearly for man—tobacco-related cancers—and sometimes I feel about those of us like Kensler and Hoffman and myself, and three or four others who labored in the vineyards of tobacco carcinogenesis for so many years, that they're still the same six or twelve people who have worked on this for 20 years. You can learn really marvelous chemistry and marvelous toxicology on tobacco smoke, and you really don't have to go to court about all those other things that we can more cheaply and easily buy in a drugstore.

It seems to me the first priority relates to the major cancers from which we die—cancer of the lung in man, cancer of the breast in women—and these are the kinds of cancer that we do not quite deal with. The same, of course, relates to the major agents which we know we are exposed to; I referred earlier to alcoholism, known for decades as a major tumor promoter in man, but we are not examining this either because we do not have a satisfactory animal model. Another great element arises because we have never gone into what I call metabolic epidemiology. I think one of the key priorities we neglect is using man as the experimental tool. After all, we drink the whiskey perhaps better than the mouse or the hamster. And third, there was the point you raised about DDT, and again it relates to priorities. If the epidemiology indicates that DDT—in spite of the fact that we have stored it in our fat pads for a long period of time—has not been demonstrated to relate to cancer in man, I would much rather see the great genius that I've heard here today (in terms of mechanism of potential toxic agents as related to liver cancer, or whatever), really concentrate on agents that we *know* produce cancer in man, instead of spending so much of our intellectual capabilities on agents which, in terms of epidemiology, were really shown for years not to cause cancer in man.

DR. CRANMER: Let me make one statement before I forget, and that is regarding the Toxic Substances Control Act and mechanisms by which the hierarchy approaches decisions on what's going to be tested: there will be a meeting the third week in August at NCTR, a full day's meeting at which the selection of chemicals and tests to be used regarding high-volume, suspect chemicals will be discussed. It will be announced in *Science* magazine and the *Federal Register*. For those of you who would like to submit papers or comments, please contact us at the laboratory, and Mrs. Magee will be happy to have that input.

DR. HAMMOND: I would say I thoroughly agree with what Dr. Wynder said in the general priority. There's one thing, however: We simply have to use animal models on substances to which people have been exposed but for which there are no animal data. I have in mind, for example, the enzyme detergents, soaps, and soap powders that were put around. The horrible thing about that was that close to half the total population was exposed to these by the huge promotion that went on, and this was in a matter of about two years; and with no human experience whatsoever. Now I'm not suggesting any evidence about these enzymes, I'm only talking about the testing for them. It seems to me, before you expose most of the human population to something under these conditions, I would give as high a priority as you're speaking about, Ernie (Wynder). I would say that they should be subjected to the most extreme test, much more elaborate than is ordinarily done in any of our animal screening tests. I think several methods that can be used for it, several different methods of exposure, and many more animals, and certainly in-utero exposure.

I just can't see any excuse whatsoever to expose such large numbers of people to considerable amounts of agents without knowing what they're all about, and I don't see how epidemiologists are going to help with that one little bit.

DR. WYNDER: I certainly agree with Cuyler (Hammond) that the new substances (which Weisburger and I have just written about) have got to be tested, not only for mutagenicity but in long-term tests, and just as you indicated, because clearly on anything that comes out new we do not have any prior information.

DR. HAMMOND: I was particularly speaking of those things where very, very large numbers of people are going to be exposed. In the chemical plant you may have 500 or 1,000 people exposed. If it gives them cancer, that's very sad. We want to prevent that. But when we're exposing a whole population to something, this can be an utter catastrophe; these are the materials I'd give a very, very high priority to before allowing their widespread use.

DR. CRANMER: I wonder if we could ask Dr. Kolbye to discuss some of the activities of the Bureau of Foods with respect to the potential need for testing additional compounds with the cyclic review of food additives. I know when we were in Omaha recently, John Kirschman made a comment about a multi-million dollar bioassay program for a series of colors. I asked Dr. Kolbye to discuss this because of the comments that were made with respect to saturation of capabilities that we have, and whether that saturation is being accomplished with the compounds which might have a higher societal need.

DR. KOLBYE: I'll take a few cracks at the general problem. In terms of the priorities that we face, much depends really upon which segment of society is grinding which axe. I was listening to Dr. Wynder's comments and Dr. Hammond's comments, and yes, you know, we can have a variety of viewpoints about what our priorities should be. But I think the fact of the matter is, that in part, the tail is wagging the dog.

If you deal with a cancerophobic phenomenon that occurs in the political arenas in this country, and if you deal with, if you will, the brainwashing that many people have about all the "carcinogens" in the food supply, if you deal with the pressures on FDA with respect to food additives and the GRAS review, and now the cyclical review of food additives, and if you deal with the consideration of whether or not the government has preclearance testing authority or authority to require testing *before* a product comes on the market (and that authority was lacking in the case of the detergents), you're dealing with a very complex matrix that you can turn in one direction and say, "Okay, we will assign scientific priority, and we'll attempt to do so on the basis of our index of suspicion about which agents are more important than others regarding the potential carcinogenic expression in humans." You can deal with a magnitude of exposures. But, in reality, if we're going to set priorities on a sensible basis, I think we've got a major job to educate the American public, and we have to deprogram them regarding some of the nonsense they've been stuck with.

But, as I view it right now, we have rapidly reached the point of saturation of our testing facilities, according to some of my colleagues on the industrial side. They're having problems locating contract laboratories to perform these tests. Ames and other mutageneticists come along and say, "Lo and behold, we have the instantaneous answers for you," and perhaps they have some relevant information. I don't know that I'm ready, and I've so stated, to start making decisions merely on the basis of some of the mutagenicity screening tests.

So, I have the feeling that I'm a flea on the tail of a dog and the tail is driving the dog. I'm afraid I'm just going along for the ride, and it really bothers me. In our societal desire to achieve an instant utopia, instant chaos is developing, and I think sooner or later we have the responsibility not just to talk among ourselves, but to talk in a meaningful forum with some of the people that really control both the destiny of science and carcinogenesis research. I would like one way or another to get the message across to Congress that what is important is the toxicology of carcinogens and the epidemiology of the expression of carcinogenic factors in human population. I don't think we can get to the point where magically we can wave our wand blindly and say, "There shall be no carcinogens on the face of the earth."

I'll end my comment by saying that in the area of indirect additives, we face a real societal problem. Whether or not you've thought about it, in the United States we've got many food additives because we regulate many indirect additives and packaging additives, which in some other countries are classified as processing aids and not regulated at all.

We face a problem when an intermediate solvent may be present in a final product in very low parts per billion range, and yet like chloroform or some other solvent, it has been demonstrated under certain test circumstances to be carcinogenic.

If we apply a Delaney philosophy right across the board blindly, we're going to run out of solvents. Even though it's my responsibility to work within the constraints and the strengths of the Food and Drug Act, as a private individual I sometimes wonder when we are unknowingly going to take the next step and start heading into the dark ages of technology. Thank you.

DR. BUTLER or DR. THORPE: Fred Coulston has remarked that the term food additive used in a rather loose sense, and I must concur entirely with what he said. As far as I know, there is only one situation in which one can clearly demonstrate two stages in chemical carcinogenesis in animals, and that is on the skin of the mouse and on the skin of the rabbit, and, in fact, I think none of the other species really demonstrates this particular phenomenon very well. Dr. Berenblum has said that he can do this with lymphoma induction and using phorbol. I'm not sure about those experiments. They bother me a little bit. There are obvious cases in which that kind of two-stage situation seems to extrapolate very nicely to other situations, but I do not really believe that there is any rigid proof to satisfy most people in other experimental situations that one can really say that two stages of carcinogenesis do indeed occur. I think that, as a matter of fact, this is one of the situations that perhaps we should try and subject to more rigid proof, both between the experimentalists in the laboratory and those who did experimental epidemiology, and see if we can find better reasons for believing that there are indeed two stages.

There is much talk about tobacco carcinogenesis involving promoting agents. I must say that in reviewing the experimental data on the promoters in tobacco, I am not too terribly convinced that they are clearly and demonstrably there, and that there are the two clear-cut stages one has seen in the mouse skin experiments that started this whole situation.

There are a series of features in those mouse experiments that make it unequivocal, I think, that one has a two-stage situation. The other situation, I think, that is quite clearcut is one that was mentioned today by Dr. Kraybill in the old and very elegant experiment by Dr. Tannenbaum where he restricted caloric intake at different stages in skin carcinogenesis and showed there was undoubtedly a situation that occurred that was quite similar to the two-stage skin carcinogenesis experiments with croton oil; as you all know phorbol esters are singularly specific agents. Originally croton oil was produced by Dr. Berenblum to follow some of his old ideas on irritation and carcinogenesis. And he finished up with the irritation phase being the much more specific of the two stages. This has bothered me ever since I got involved in these experiments. I don't know exactly how to sort it out. Numerous experiments that people have done with hepatectomy and liver carcinogenesis are in no instance, as far as I know, terribly convincing. They're borderline situations.

The idea that some of these things, like the chlorinated hydrocarbons, are different is obvious. They *are* different. But I think it would be an error to start out by saying that these are possibly promoting factors, that there are two stages involved that are analogous to these other situations, and use the same words that describe specific and clearly defined situations. The same applies to much of the lung work. What we obviously need is a vast burst of experimental work to put this sort of concept on a sound footing and see whether or not it is real.

DR. KENSLER: I would like to compliment Al Kolbye for both his spunk, his common sense, and his stamina. And I wish him well in biting the tail of the dog, flea, or whatever it is. But now I'd like to get back to science as we tend to recognize it, and talk about promotion from a nutritional point of view, or something which might be considered promotional.

Years ago, working with the azo dyes, it was found that if you fed them with a deficient diet, tumors were developed. However, if you feed them with a sufficient diet for about 45 days and then stop feeding them carcinogens and put the animals on a protective diet, the animals do not get tumors, and the lesions reverse. If you put them on a sufficient diet without any more carcinogen, there's very little carcinogen in the liver at that point. You find that the majority of the animals go on to develop the tumors.

In other words, you have a nutritional situation which parallels a promotion situation which you have initiated, but you don't get the effect unless you stress the animal one way or another. And I submit that nutritional stress is one of those possible stresses. Dr. Wynder doesn't like phorbol esters (I don't know why, because I do think you have to study things that some people don't think are important in order to find out important things). Therefore, I support the phorbol ester group because I think they are learning things, and I also support both Ernst Wynder's environmental center and Shubik's environmental center where they combine epidemiology and carcinogenesis, and molecular this and that and immunology. We've got to take a broad perspective here and we've got to support Al Kolbye's idea of educating the public to approach our problem and their problem intelligently with the limited resources we have, both in dollars and more particularly, in skilled personnel.

DR. KOLBYE: I just wanted to ask Dr. Shubik if he would clarify his semantic use of the word "promoter." As you were using the word "promoter," I got the impression you were really talking about what I denote as a carcinogen. I use the term "promoter" more broadly. I may be using the term "promoter" somewhat inappropriately.

DR. SHUBIK: If you want to have it in historical context, the term "cocarcinogen" was coined by Dr. Murray Shear at the National Cancer Institute, who discovered that there were some fractions of creosote that had no carcinogenic activity, but which when combined with a weak solution of benzo(a)pyrene succeeded in producing tumors when the two things were combined together.

The term "promoting agent" was, in fact, produced by some experiments in which Shear showed that if you tied the ear of a rabbit, or subsequently painted it with a chemical carcinogen, tumors developed, but if you stopped painting, the tumors would go away. And if you then punched a hole through the ear (or, in fact, he used an irritant—turpentine—which was rather peculiar because it was kind of specific), after the tumor had gone away it would come back again.

The term "promoter" was used subsequently by *Berenblum* and myself in our first experiments to denote the action of a substance which made a tumor appear in a tissue previously treated with a subeffective dose of a carcinogen.

The term "cocarcinogen" was used to denote the effect of the substances given together. To try and separate out the two things and make it easier to do experimental analyses—that's all the terms were used for by a relatively small group of people who played games with mouse skin and rabbit ears.

DR. MOFIDI(?): I wanted to endorse what Dr. Shubik and also Dr. Kensler mentioned about the question of the mutation in the background and the promoter of the two-stage aspect in many of these studies. As Dr. Greenwald said, he had to take the immunological approach in some of these experiments, although the psychologists hadn't found their thinking.

The reproduction of human exposure may be difficult, but I think one may look at the analytical approach. For instance, we know about the effect of asbestos as related to the size and shape of the particle. I assume that in many of these cases, maybe the irritation phase before the experiment with the proposed carcinogen would be of great interest. In other words, stress the tissue and then study it experimentally.

In connection with the epidemiology of cancer, there is a great need for retrospective studies of exposed people during a year. In many of these places, there is a great need for record linkers which is not much permitted in many parts of the world. I assume now that this has been discussed in many of the committees, it may be again emphasized that it is important for the epidemiologist to correlate the data of various types. I assume you know that in the study of asbestos cases, it has been always difficult to go back and study the case of the workers in years past for the information on these points.

One more point. I want to stress the fact that in many cases in the developing countries, some of the industrial carbon compounds you have we don't have. In other words, I'm thinking of the epidemiology of nonexisting disease, or the epidemiology of, let's say, occupational stress. For these data are not available, and many of the data are from areas where there are too many carcinogens in the environment; the information about the background is not available, and such projects as are devised may be extended beyond the area like that.

Unfortunately, of course it's clear that the scientists, toxicologists, and epidemiologists are not available in those areas to do the jobs. That one may take the question not from a local point of view but from the individual or international point of view was already mentioned this morning.

DR. GREENWALD: First, I appreciate the concern that Dr. Mofidi and Dr. Clemmesen have for the need for record linkage. We do have a concern in this country relating to extensions of the Privacy Act and our ability in the future to do these large-scale types of studies.

Another question I wanted to raise was, if we accept that it will take many years to look into these many problems that have been raised, I wonder what we might recommend as prudent policy decisions that could be made today? If we look at the history of public health, I think we can see that there may be certain things which could be done, and which although we may not understand their mechanisms, might still lessen risks.

For example, general industrial standards. Much as we have something like a coliform count relating to water supplies and water standards for clean restaurants, I wonder if some sort of general standards to minimize exposure might be prudent? Another possible example might be the stepwise introduction of selected new products or drugs, perhaps with voluntary registration of a certain number of the first ones, and I just wonder if we might not consider what would be prudent policy decisions given the current state of knowledge?

DR. NEWILL: We've talked a little bit about the scarcity of the toxicity resource, but nobody has talked about the scarcity of the epidemiology resource. It seems to me that there are far fewer epidemiologists, probably not many over a couple of hundred in the whole world, engaged in chronic disease epidemiology at the present time. I don't know how we're going to carry this out, unless we do get on with some kind of training in this particular area.

DR. KOLBYE: I just wanted to come back for a moment, not necessarily to prolong the discussion, but I would hope during the course of this meeting I would at least get a clearer distinction between where one draws the line between a promoting agent and a modifying factor; I think some of these semantical distinctions may be very, very important in the not too distant future in determining how society will treat "carcinogens," classify them, and decide the degree of control to be exerted over the different classes of "carcinogens." Thank you.

DR. UPHOLT: (EPA.) There are three comments I would like to make. The first is in regard to resources: I represent the EPA on the statutory committee set up by the Toxic Disease Control Act on selecting up to 50 chemicals for priority and testing. That act requires that we consider the availability of resources to do the testing. We will be considering this matter sometime between the 23rd of this month and probably some time in late August (1977), and I noted with interest Dr. Clayson's suggestion that we could possibly do 100 tests for carcinogenicity (that is, testing 100 substances for carcinogenicity each year). If he or any of you have information of this sort that can be reasonably well documented, at least the basis for it, it would be extremely helpful to our committee.

The second thing is that I am quite concerned about what I think I heard regarding the epidemiology on DDT. If I understood correctly, I think Phil Shubik said something about the large number of people who had been exposed to DDT, some of them with heavy exposures and many of them with much less. I believe he said he knew of no one who had really looked at this population, and invited anybody who did know to contribute such information. I haven't heard anybody contribute such information, but I believe I heard somebody say that since we had this exposure to DDT for so many years and have found no epidemiological evidence, therefore DDT must not be causing cancer. If I heard correctly, I think this is about the most unscientific type of conclusion that could be reached, and I hope the epidemiologists did not come to such conclusions, or if they did, we have a better basis for it than I have heard.

Third, I raised some questions earlier about a definition of threshold. A few minutes ago Fred (Coulston) asked me if I wanted to bring this up again. My answer is no. I really think the question of threshold is not particularly important. The reason I raised it is because I think too much concern for thresholds gets the attention of scientists and the public away from the really critical issue, not only with carcinogenicity but with other toxicants; namely, as a recent speakers commented, what we should be looking for are methods to reduce exposure, not simply classifying and trying to give the public the impression that we, as regulatory agencies, can guarantee safety from any group of chemicals.

The concept of threshold implies zero risk, and I think most scientists have pretty well refused the concept that through regulatory mechanisms for chemicals in the environment, it is possible for us to guarantee anything approaching zero risk. Our problem, rather, is to reduce the risk as far as is consistent with the cost to society of that reduction in risk.

If we can get the help of groups such as this toward encouraging the enforcement agencies, the regulatory agencies, to express clearly how they have estimated the risk, how much reduction in risk they can reasonably expect to accomplish through the regulation, and what considerations they have given of the cost to society of such regulations, we'll be doing a whole lot more for society than just worrying about whether or not there is a threshold. Thank you.

DR. WYNDER: I talked to Dr. Frederickson some weeks ago about a suggestion that we got when we pointed out that we thought it was unlikely that we could have full training of an M. D. epidemiologist, which would require an additional three years. Rather I suggested that we could take people who are going to take the examinations in preventive medicine to see whether, by training them for one year in epidemiology, we could give them credit for this toward the examinations.

Even better, I suggested, would be if physicians specializing in internal medicine would take one year out of the three, for which the Board of Internal Medicine would give them full credit, to study clinical epidemiology. It's my belief that if I'm a good physician who can treat well in internal medicine, I should also be a physician who knows something about etiology. Call them etiologists.

"Well," I was asked, "where would the money come from?" Well, I don't know where the money would come from, but clearly if this nation needs epidemiologists, we ought to make the money available. My suggestion is, therefore, that as a part of preventive medicine and internal medicine we might get more physicians interested in this.

A talk was given about record linkage. The one record that we think we can study throughout the nation is liver cancer registries. At the American Health Foundation, in 20 hospitals where we interview we take detailed histories of all patients (including the occupations) with hepatic diseases and all liver cancer patients; I think by having set this kind of registry, we can be more alert to a new agent that may affect a particular liver cancer.

One of my best friends, Charlie (Kensler), canceled my best friend's work with phorbol ester. I did not say I'm against phorbol ester, I just put it in perspective. I said at a meeting in Gatlinburg that I saw 250 people work on phorbol ester, and I thought at least a couple of them should have worked on alcohol carcinogenesis.

I certainly feel that the excellent work that Dr. Kensler did with riboflavin years ago may well be the basis whereby alcoholism promotes tobacco carcinogenesis.

In our view alcohol is not a carcinogen to man, since it does not produce cancer by itself. But it certainly does in tobacco carcinogenesis act as a promoter. And, finally, we all applauded Al Kolbye: I must say I was equally impressed with the vigor and elegance with which he presented his point of view, but it's actually we, the scientists, who put the FDA in the position in which it is today, and not only we as scientists, but obviously as a society.

The other day, I was going in one of those lousy taxicabs in New York City, and the driver was talking away. I always learn from field studies, so I asked this fellow: "How come you're still smoking?" He used a nonfilter brand, said he smoked about 40 a day, and commented, "Listen, you've got to have something. After all, with saccharin, air pollution, etc., we live in a 'sea of carcinogens.'"

Well, we have put this taxicab driver thinking in this area, because if he reads not even the *New York Times* but the *Daily News,* he really believes that everything that he eats and inhales is carcinogenic. And I very strongly believe that we as scientists have the obligation to warn the public when the public really ought to be warned, and really shut up until we have the scientific evidence before we warn the public not to use certain substances. The point I want to make is that we are very sympathetic to the position in which you are, and we as scientists have really put you there.

And, I believe I think it was Burke who stated: "The only way for evil to triumph is if good men say nothing." This is a kind of paraphrasing of what he said, but I think it's very important. Sometimes it's difficult, because there's rising in this country something that is certainly McCarthyism in science; sometimes when we take a stand and somebody says, "Well, don't you know that such and such produces cancer?" and we say, "No, it is my view as an epidemiologist or clinician that I do not regard this evidence as sufficient to really warn the public or take this product off the market," that oftentimes the question is "Are you being paid by this particular industry?"

I know that this is a great problem to many of us, and many of us have not taken industrial funds precisely for this reason. But I think these matters have to be discussed in here; in other words, we must not only discuss science, but we must discuss the politics of science.

DR. KRAYBILL: I'd like to extend Bill Upholt's remarks. I alluded to the work on DDT and epidemiology. Back in the 1960's men like Deichmann and

John Davies and Griffith Quinby and the people at California collected a lot of data, particularly down in Florida. To do a study on DDT where whole populations turn it around as a stress in their body fat (even the penguins in Antarctica have it in their body fat), is a difficult study. The only person I know that volunteered to do it (and I think it's long overdue) is the one I mentioned and that is Tom Mason, who said they were going to do it, and I hope they do it. They should start looking at formulators and people who get a high exposure, because to do anything otherwise you get a washout, so the statisticians told me, *in* the data. You've got to look at a very highly exposed group

I'd like to say something more about what Al Kolbye said, because I think it was germane. I read elsewhere on other subjects that scientists only talk to scientists. And that's a tragedy in this country. Here we are all gathered for these couple of days and we're talking to one another, but I think we need to get the message out in a missionary sort of way.

We get calls, at least the Cancer Institute does, I do, and our office repeatedly does from the outside, and they're not scientific people, they're lay public. My wife works for the American Cancer Society. She started in the information bureau, and she comes home at night and tells me all these questions she gets, and I'm dissatisfied with the kind of information she relays back. But they try, and the people are happy.

But the Cancer Institute has a speakers' bureau, and they ask people to go out and give talks, and I've done that on several occasions. The American Cancer Society also has this sort of thing, and they ask people to volunteer, to go out and talk. If we don't start talking to the lay public, and we just talk among ourselves, we're not going to get the message across. So I think it's about time to get on with it, because if we don't it's that other group out there that gets in the newspaper and causes all this emotion and all this folderol, and we're tearing our hair out. As I mentioned this morning, I went home one night and this woman on the TV spouted off a lot of "information" on the incidence of cancer from these compounds in water; I was horrified to hear it. So *somebody* is getting through to this woman. She gave a very emotional plea about these cancer wards filled with people getting cancer from these compounds in the water. I think we need to help and not just talk to one another, but get out and talk to other people.

DR. CRANMER: We have about five more minutes of discussion, and then we'll need to close it off. Dr. Hammond?

DR. HAMMOND: I'd like to comment on what Dr. Shubik said about promoters. Obviously, we want to know the mechanisms, but first I think we need to answer a very simple question. All other things being equal, does exposure to Agent X alter the risk of getting cancer? It might do so in dozens of different ways. Dr. Kensler showed one way: phenol, I believe inhibited ciliary action. Well, in this case by breaking down a defense mechanism, it could greatly increase the probability of getting cancer under exposure to something else.

I personally am a little cold to these words that are used for it: "promoters," "initiators," and what not. We want to know the mechanisms, but first we ask for the facts. Does something, or does it not, increase the risk of getting cancer?

DR. UPHOLT(?): That has absolutely nothing to do with what I said.

DR. HAMMOND: But somebody else asked the question of defining it. I wasn't contradicting anything.

DR. UPHOLT(?): It wasn't what I was talking about there.

DR. HAMMOND: I'm sorry, I misunderstood you.

DR. CRANMER: Do you want redirect there, Dr. Shubik?

DR. KENSLER: Actually I think phenol is for the birds, both in cigarette smoke and ciliary action. But I do think, whether you talk about promoters, co-carcinogens, or procarcinogens—which is a word we use for the effect of a compound that one adds to a diet which otherwise didn't induce cancer—there are all sorts of words, but when we have "initiation," I think of a clearly established event. Then we have a variety of factors which can make this event evolve into malignancy, and I hope Al (Kolbye) that you and the regulators don't get hung up on semantics here.

DR. CRANMER: One last question, or comment? Dr. Coulston is going to close the meeting.

DR. COULSTON: Thank you. I want to thank everyone around this table for what I think has been a very exciting and very painless and wonderful first day of our meeting. Tomorrow morning, as you know, we'll meet at 8:45, and Dr. Wynder will take the chair; I'll be very delighted to get back into the audience, so to speak. Thank you very much, one and all.

DR. WYNDER: I would like to say that I appreciate being here; to me one of the best parts of these meetings is that one meets old friends, over breakfast, over lunch, and this to me is the most enjoyable part of this type of get together. In addition, so many different groups can exchange views about their various specialties; hopefully, we'll all learn from one another.

The meeting this morning or this afternoon is divided into roughly two parts, one dealing with mechanistic studies and the other one with drugs as human carcinogens. We'll hear from Dr. Miller and Dr. Conney. For many years I've always felt as I read *Cancer Research* the articles on mechanism were so complex that I for one, really could not understand them. When I look at this in the historic perspective, I wonder whether perhaps both speakers could comment on whether they believe the particular mechanistic studies in which they are involved can really contribute not only to understanding carcinogenesis, but what really is important to prevention?

In other words, do these studies suggest preventive mechanisms? I'm reminded that in the history of infectious diseases, John Snow was able to tell us how to prevent cholera in 1849, but not until something like 1895 did Koch identified the causative agent. Similarly, in the late 1840s we knew how to prevent childbed fever, but it was not until 1895 that Pasteur identified the streptococcus. So there were some 40-odd years between identifying a way to prevent a disease and determining the causative agent. I like to believe that the probable identification of an infectious agent would be easier than identifying the mechanism whereby different carcinogens produce cancer, an identification that would lead to preventive measures.

Now we will talk about drugs as carcinogens to man. It's important here, and we have stressed this throughout, that we become better epidemiologists; for one thing we must have better records. I've never been able to understand how it is that our hospitals are technologically so advanced today—we have all kinds of extremely expensive equipment—but if you look at the average hospital and the patient histories taken by interns, residents, or medical students, you are amazed at how poor these records are in terms of etiological factors. In fact, particularly today, a young intern or resident feels that history-taking is a thing of the past and should be done by some allied health professional. I would hope that this could improve, and that indeed not only would hospital records be better, but that they would be put on computers for us to retrieve this data at a later time.

There's another problem in taking records that I would like to share with you. It so happens that in our Division of Epidemiology we have young interviewers all over the country and, recently, they have developed a problem in terms of the privacy act. It used to be that once we had permission from the hospital to interview a patient, we could go to the patient's bed and ask our questions. Today, in most hospitals, we need permission from every division. We need to have signed permission from the patient, and we then need the document signed by a witness. By this time I want to ask the patient how much he smokes. He thinks: "My God, they probably want to know what my bank number is in Switzerland," and he feels very worried. Not only could this lead to possible interview bias, but it doubles or triples the amount of time it takes us to get one patient interviewed. It is a significant problem which I'm sure Dr. Hammond and others are aware of. I think you can really take this privacy act too far, particularly since all we are interested in is identifying questions that relate to a patient's case.

Now today we will hear about drugs, about how these drugs could relate to cancer. Drug history happens to be a very difficult history to acquire. One is amazed how many people do not know what drugs they are taking. They say: "Well my doctor gave me that, and I didn't ask him really what it was." We also know that a high percentage of people who are given prescriptions don't take them. The drugs remain in the medicine cabinet. We also know that the drug users are not necessarily the same as the controls. For instance, you could do a special study on the epidemiology of Premarin use. Our studies have indicated—and I'm sure that Peter will show you—that a correlation exists between the use of Premarin and cancer of the endometrium, although we have not found it for cancer of the breast. Clearly, the Premarin user is different. In other words, the lady who reaches menopause and is given Premarin by a doctor may have a different socioeconomic background from one who does not take it. You'd better believe that in New York if you go on Park Avenue, you'll find more Premarin users than you'll find in our ghetto population.

So these things are important. Important also are animal studies in which a drug is given during pregnancy in very high concentration. Can we draw a correlation of that in women to a drug being present in the liver of cattle? Sometimes we say "Well, obviously, we know that DES, for instance, causes cancer in the offspring of women who have taken it during pregnancy at very high doses," which leads the average person to believe that the presence of this drug in beef liver will equally produce cancer in human offspring. Nowhere do we relate this problem in terms of dose-response.

Finally, I'd like you to consider, as we review these various aspects this morning, something that I referred to yesterday pertinent to societal action. It is important that when we take a societal action, (a) we do something that is useful for the population; and (b) if we do, future generations will thank us for having taken this measure. Let me take as an example the saccharin story. In this case, we have had this agent with us for some 80 years. What I have always said is that it is indeed true that the epidemiological evidence doesn't indicate there is an increase of bladder cancer, but perhaps there could be an increase of bladder cancer, nevertheless.

I've heard a debate about the data presented by Richard Doll regarding the frequency of bladder cancer and other cancer in diabetic populations. Diabetic populations, as all of us know, use significantly more sweeteners than control people. I can only report that, after reviewing the retrospective studies on all cancers that we have done over the last 20 years (and with one possible exception of female cancer of the pancreas) I have found no difference in diabetes frequence between study and control populations. But most important are case control studies. There are several case control studies (including those that we have just presented) that show the patients with bladder cancer do not take more sweeteners in their coffee than controls. To me a case control study is really the final proof in this area, particularly since it already relates to the data available on diabetes.

What are the case control studies doing? We take patients with cancer of the bladder and match them against 130 patient controls. We find the bladder cancer patients by frequency and duration did not take more sweeteners than the controls, even before standardizing for coffee and cigarette smoking. Somebody said, "Well how do you know the next 100 cases will show the same?" All I can report is that our data show a relative risk for all of these variables of strictly 1.0, and having had some experience with case control studies, I can tell you that if you do a case control study on cigarette smoking you pick up the first statistical significance in the first 20 cases.

So this is where we are, and yet as a society we obviously make a tremendous noise about the sweetener story. I think it's about time that we think about modifying existing federal statutes, including the Delaney Clause relative to food additives and other environmental carcinogens. In an editorial that appears in the June issue of *Preventive Medicine,* we are recommending a modification of the Delaney Clause. This modification includes two facets that I'd like you to consider. Number one is that the National Clearing House on Environmental Carcinogenesis, and perhaps similar groups in other federal agencies, should carefully consider the medical risk assessment relative to this agent. In other words, we have our tests of mutagenicity, we have our long-term test in animals, and they should carefully consider the medical risk that applies or does not apply when we're dealing with a new drug. I should think that in the case of saccharin, in the case of DDT, and in the case of certain hair dyes we have many years of experience; then, if a group of experts should decide that there is a significant risk for man, we are calling for a special panel to be set up by the President or by the Secretary of HEW to review the societal risk and benefits of this decision. I think it is very important that we do this because you and I take risks all the time. If we have an agent that gives us a certain risk and the alternative will give us a greater risk, then clearly this is the decision of society, which should evaluate the risk-benefit.

Finally, it is just not a scientific decision, but it is rather a societal decision, as well. Clearly, we have made the decision as a society that we want to smoke cigarettes. Clearly, we are prepared to take the consequences. Clearly, as a society we are making the decision that we want to drink alcohol, and we are prepared to take 28,000 deaths on our highways. Clearly, we are prepared to take the risk! We have many instances in which we have taken such decisions, and we are suggesting in the *Preventive Medicine* editorial that we take a similar societal view regarding decisions that we make in respect to environmental carcinogens.

With this as a background, let us then proceed to two aspects of our discussion this morning and this afternoon, one dealing with mechanistic studies and the other one dealing with drugs. I would therefore like first to call on Dr. Miller, who has for many years been one of the outstanding investigators in our country concerned with investigating, together with his wife, various aspects of carcinogenic activation and inactivation as key to species and tissue differences in response.

7. Carcinogen Activation and Inactivation as Keys to Species and Tissue Differences in Response*

James A. Miller
McArdle Laboratory for Cancer Research
University of Wisconsin Medical Center
Madison, Wisconsin

It is an honor to have this opportunity to speak on chemical carcinogenesis before this critical international audience, which includes many of my colleagues in experimental chemical carcinogenesis.

When one considers the complexities of carcinogenesis by chemicals it is evident why we experience difficulty in extrapolating data from chemical carcinogenesis in experimental animals to our own species. To show these complexities, I have listed in Table 1 some of the characteristics which are common to carcinogenesis by many chemicals.

You will note in point 2 that I differ with my good friend, Phil Shubik, on the generality of the stages of initiation and promotion in chemical carcinogenesis. I feel that recent data have provided fairly convincing evidence that these stages occur in carcinogenesis in a variety of tissues.

In this brief overview I will deal primarily with point 4 on the structural variety and activation and inactivation of chemical carcinogens. Today, it is a central fact in chemical carcinogenesis that organic and inorganic carcinogens exhibit great structural heterogeneity. This was not the case in 1939 when I began graduate study in biochemistry at Madison and started to work with these chemicals. At that time only aromatic compounds were known to be carcinogenic. The carcinogenicity of certain polycyclic aromatic hydrocarbons had been found in England, workers in Japan had discovered the aromatic aminoazo dyes, and in France the great pioneer Lacassagne had found that the aromatic steroid estrogen estrone could induce tumors in the mouse mammary gland. This dis-

*This study was supported by Grants CA-07175 and CA-15785 of the National Cancer Institute, USPHS.

TABLE 1
CHARACTERISTICS OF CARCINOGENESIS BY CHEMICALS

1. Long induction times (often large fraction of life span)

2. Multistep process: *initiation* (rapid, irreversible?) followed by *promotion* (protracted, reversible?). Tumors undergo *progression* to more malignant states.

3. Noncarcinogenic dose of carcinogen can initiate and noncarcinogenic promoters can complete process.

4. Wide range of carcinogenic structures (synthetic and natural). Majority require metabolic activation. All subject to inactivation in vivo.

5. Tumor response depends on:
   a. Activity of carcinogen, degree of activation and inactivation of carcinogen.
   b. Total dose and dose frequency.
   c. Susceptibility factors: species, strain, sex, diet, hormonal and immunologic status, previous exposures to carcinogens, subsequent exposures to promoters, age at exposure, etc.

tinction disappeared soon thereafter and research in the last 40 years has revealed chemical carcinogens among over a dozen different classes of aromatic and aliphatic organic structures. In addition, inorganic chemical carcinogens were discovered. So today one cannot find any common chemical structure among these agents which have the common property of inducing tumors.

For example, let's look at just a very small sampling of synthetic chemical carcinogens in Fig. 1. The majority of the chemical carcinogens we now know are synthetic compounds and the majority of these agents are nonreactive *per se*. That is, these carcinogens do not react directly in a covalent manner with cellular macromolecules such as nucleic acids and proteins.

However, some synthetic chemical carcinogens are reactive *per se* in this manner; these chemicals include the alkylating agents, of which there are now at least 8 different classes, and a few acylating agents. These agents cover a very wide range of structures, but they have a common chemical property that will soon be evident.

This great structural heterogeneity of chemical carcinogens is also evident for those agents which occur naturally as metabolites of certain fungi, bacteria, and green plants. About twenty of these nonreactive naturally-occurring carcinogens are now known, and examples are shown in Fig. 2. I think it is inevitable that many more of these naturally-occurring chemical carcinogens will be discovered among the thousands of uncharacterized and untested, nonpolar, low molecular weight, minor non-nutritive constituents of fungi, bacteria, plants, and animal cells that humans use as food.

To complete the roster of chemical carcinogens I will mention, but not discuss further, the small number of carcinogenic metal ions that are now known. Likewise, I will exclude from this discussion those polymeric chemicals where surface characteristics or fiber size seem to determine their carcinogenic activity, primarily in mesenchymal tissues.

134

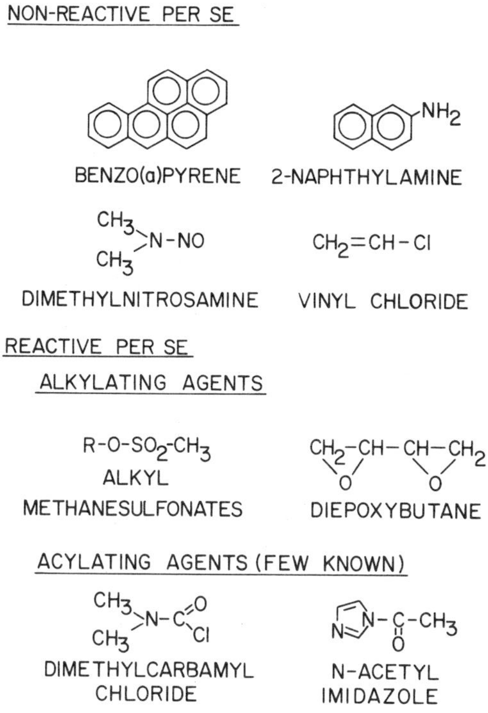

NON-REACTIVE PER SE

BENZO(a)PYRENE   2-NAPHTHYLAMINE

DIMETHYLNITROSAMINE   VINYL CHLORIDE

REACTIVE PER SE

ALKYLATING AGENTS

$R-O-SO_2-CH_3$

ALKYL
METHANESULFONATES   DIEPOXYBUTANE

ACYLATING AGENTS (FEW KNOWN)

DIMETHYLCARBAMYL   N-ACETYL
CHLORIDE   IMIDAZOLE

FIGURE 1
Examples of Synthetic Chemical Carcinogens.

A great deal of work on tumor induction and metabolism has been carried out with these synthetic and naturally-occurring chemical carcinogens in various experimental systems. Most of these studies have used intact animals, usually rodents, but more recent studies have also shown it is possible to induce malignant transformation of mammalian cells in culture with chemicals.

Many of these studies have involved the metabolism of these chemical agents, in an effort to understand how they initiate the malignant transformation of cells both in whole animals and in cell culture. This work has revealed an important aspect of carcinogenesis by the majority of synthetic and naturally occurring carcinogens. That is, studies on their mechanisms of action strongly indicate that these compounds are not carcinogenic as such, but are really *precarcinogens* that require metabolic conversion into reactive and carcinogenic forms which we call the *ultimate carcinogens* (Fig. 3). Sometimes intermediate metabolites, the *proximate carcinogens,* are formed. At every level, metabolic inactivation occurs. This is the general situation for the great majority of chemical carcinogens. The balance between the amounts of inactivation and activation is a primary factor in determining the rate and level of tumor formation.

It is axiomatic that chemical carcinogens must induce tumors through interaction(s), direct or indirect, with critical cell components. Since the malig-

135

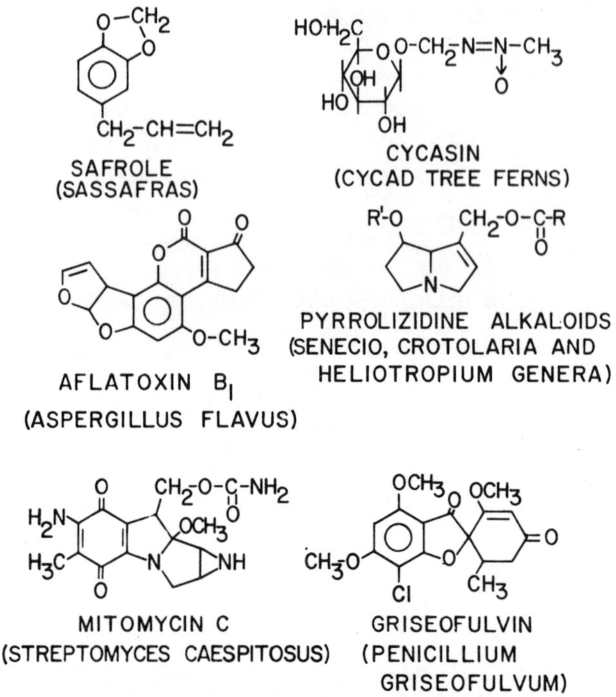

FIGURE 2

Examples of Naturally Occurring Carcinogens.

nant phenotype is heritable, it would appear that among the critical cellular molecules involved in chemical carcinogenesis must be informational macromolecules such as nucleic acids or proteins or both that are involved in the control of growth. Interactions in vivo between chemical carcinogens and cellular macromolecules have been known for quite some time. Indeed, in 1947 my wife and I were fortunate enough to find the first example of this. In all cases that have been adequately studied, covalent binding of a part of the chemical carcinogen occurs with nucleic acids and protein of the target tissues. Today we know a wide variety of chemical carcinogens that interact in vivo in this manner.

This statement is contrary to the impression that Dr. Klein gave in his talk. In addition to the carcinogenic alkylating agents that he mentioned, chemical determinations of the structures of macromolecular covalent adducts formed in vivo have been reported for several structurally different precarcinogens. They include 2-acetylaminofluorene, N-methyl-4-aminoazobenzene, benzo(a)pyrene, dimethylnitrosamine, ethionine, and aflatoxin B_1. This is a significant list, considering the difficulty in elucidating the structures of the small amounts of these covalently bound forms present in vivo.

I agree with Dr. Klein that the finding of apparently bound carcinogen in macromolecules after physical extraction of the free carcinogen and its metabo-

136

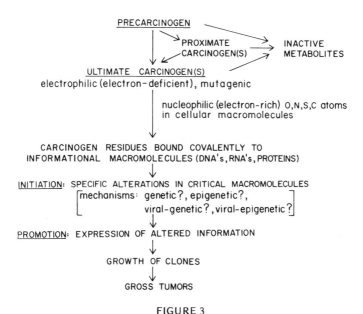

FIGURE 3

Overall Metabolism of the Majority of Synthetic and Naturally Occurring Chemical Carcinogens.

lites by solvent is not enough. The chemical characterization of the bound carcinogen must be carried out in each case. We have never excluded the possibility that some chemical carcinogens might bind to macromolecules in vivo through multiple weak noncovalent bonds. For example, we have hypothesized that this might be the mechanism of binding of the carcinogen actinomycin D to DNA in vivo. Furthermore, at this year's meeting of the American Association for Cancer Research, Dr. Hans Marquardt of New York City gave rather convincing evidence that in cell cultures the rat kidney carcinogen and mutagen adriamycin binds strongly to DNA only by noncovalent bonds.

In a number of cases, good correlations exist between the gross amounts of macromolecular binding and the carcinogenicities of a series of like structures of high, medium, low, or no carcinogenicity. Taken as a whole we believe the data indicate that macromolecular binding of many carcinogens is necessary, but not sufficient, for the induction of tumors.

Numerous sites of covalent binding of the carcinogen residues in cellular macromolecules have been found. Furthermore, some of the more complex chemical carcinogens form more than one reactive metabolite in vivo. So it seems probable that only one or a few of the found forms will be found to be critical in the initiation of chemical carcinogenesis.

The nature of these covalent interactions in vivo has become very much clearer in recent years, particularly as covalent bound forms have been characterized. It is now evident that the ultimate reactive forms of most, if not all,

137

chemical carcinogens are strongly electrophilic in nature. Thus despite the great structural variety of the precarcinogens, these compounds appear to be metabolized to a common electronic form—an electrophile—in which carbon or, sometimes, a nitrogen atom is relatively electron deficient.

Inside cells these reactive species seek out relatively electron-rich or nucleophilic sulfur, nitrogen, oxygen, or occasionally, carbon atoms in macromolecules to form the covalently bound carcinogen residues which have been recognized for so many years. This occurs nonenzymatically. The alkylating and acylating agents (Fig. 1) are electrophiles *per se.*

It has also become quite evident in the last few years that, wherever it has been possible to bring these reactive electrophilic forms of chemical carcinogens into contact with DNA in mutagenicity test systems, usually bacterial systems, these reactive forms exhibit mutagenicity. It is this observation that has revived interest in what now appears to be a strong formal relationship between chemical carcinogenesis and chemical mutagenesis. This relationship not only has important mechanistic implications but points to methods for detection of potentially carcinogenic substances in our environment.

The actual mechanisms involved in the initiation step are not known unequivocally and may be genetic, epigenetic, viral-genetic, or viral-epigenetic in nature. I believe it is very likely that many chemical carcinogens induce one or more critical mutations in the initiation step. However, the evidence for this is equivocal and we must continue to consider possible epigenetic mechanisms.

Numerous nucleophilic sites in proteins and nucleic acids are attacked by ultimate carcinogens or ultimate reactive metabolites of chemical carcinogens in vivo (Fig. 4). In proteins the sulfur atoms of methionine and cysteine, the ring nitrogens of histidine, and the 3-position of tyrosine can be involved. Guanine is the most nucleophilic base in the nucleic acids and is attacked at least at the N-3, N-7, C-8, and O-6 atoms and the 2-amino group. The nucleic acid phosphate-sugar backbones are also attacked.

Most of the known ultimate carcinogens are built around an electrophilic carbon atom; a few contain an electrophilic nitrogen atom. I think it is probable that eventually some electrophiles based on sulfur and oxygen atoms in the proper structures will be recognized. An important part of the electrophilic reaactant is the so-called "leaving" group, and a variety of these groups exist. Thus, despite the fact that we already know many hundreds of chemical carcinogens within more than a dozen different chemical classes, many more of these agents will probably be found. Therefore, the metabolic activation of structures to give electrophiles can apparently be achieved in many different ways.

The principles discussed above can be illustrated by specific examples of the metabolic activation of chemical carcinogens to reactive mutagenic electrophiles. Dr. Conney will present the beautiful work that he and others have done recently on the metabolic activation of polycyclic aromatic hydrocarbons. Accordingly, I will comment on four other classes of chemical carcinogens with

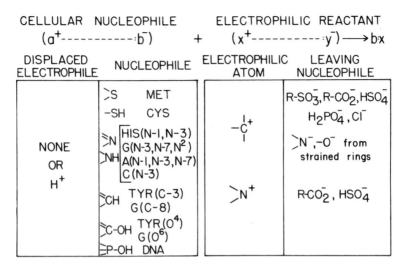

CELLULAR NUCLEOPHILE $(a^+ \text{----------} :b^-)$		ELECTROPHILIC REACTANT $(x^+ \text{----------} :y^-) \longrightarrow b{\cdot}x$	
DISPLACED ELECTROPHILE	NUCLEOPHILE	ELECTROPHILIC ATOM	LEAVING NUCLEOPHILE
NONE OR H^+	$>$S MET	$-\overset{\mid}{\underset{\mid}{C}}{}^+$	$R\text{-}SO_3^-, R\text{-}CO_2^-, HSO_4^-$ $H_2PO_4^-, Cl^-$ $>$N$^-$,$-O^-$ from strained rings
	$-$SH CYS		
	$\equiv$N$\begin{bmatrix}$HIS(N-I,N-3)$\\$G(N-3,N-7,N^2)$\\\end{bmatrix}$		
	$>$NH$\begin{bmatrix}$A(N-I,N-3,N-7)$\\$C(N-3)$\end{bmatrix}$		
	$>$CH TYR(C-3) G(C-8)	$>$N$^+$	$R\text{-}CO_2^-, HSO_4^-$
	$>$C-OH TYR(O^4) G(O^6)		
	$\equiv$P-OH DNA		

FIGURE 4

Nucleophilic Targets of Chemical Carcinogens *In Vivo.*

representatives of two classes of synthetic carcinogens and two classes of naturally occurring carcinogens. These are compounds that my colleagues and I have worked with in recent years.

Figure 5 shows the structure of the relatively well-studied aromatic amide 2-acetylaminofluorene (AAF). This compound is inactivated by ring or C-hydroxylation at seven positions. N-hydroxylation, however, leads to the proximate carcinogen N-hydroxy-AAF, which is more carcinogenic than the parent amide and is active in a wider variety of tissues and species. N-hydroxy AAF is nucleophilic, but its further metabolism can lead to several electrophilic forms that can react nonenzymatically to yield macromolecular-bound, 2-acetylaminofluorene and 2-aminofluorene residues.

The major activation route in the male rat liver is shown in Fig. 6. N-hydroxy-AAF is sulfonated by PAPS (3'-phosphoadenosyl-5'-phosphosulfate) by a cytosolic sulfotransferase to yield the extremely reactive electrophile and mutagen AAF-N-sulfate. This electrophile forms the principal nucleic acid- and protein-bound forms of AAF found in the liver.

It is of interest to note that PAPS is also a potential electrophile. However, PAPS is not electrophilic *per se* at physiological pH; it requires an enzyme to make it electrophilic for specific substrates. The same is true for S-adenosyl methionine and acetyl CoA; these coenzymes are electrophilic in cells only in the presence of the proper enzymes.

There is considerable biochemical evidence that AAF-N-sulfate is a major ultimate carcinogen in the male rat liver. As noted in Table 2, the levels of hepatic sulfotransferase activity in male and female Sprague-Dawley rats cor-

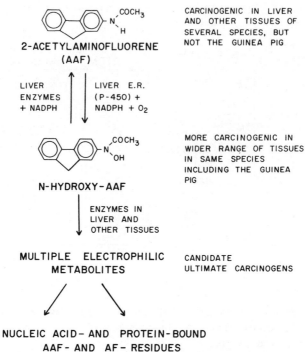

2-ACETYLAMINOFLUORENE
(AAF)

CARCINOGENIC IN LIVER
AND OTHER TISSUES OF
SEVERAL SPECIES, BUT
NOT THE GUINEA PIG

LIVER
ENZYMES
+ NADPH

LIVER E.R.
(P-450) +
NADPH + O_2

N-HYDROXY-AAF

MORE CARCINOGENIC IN
WIDER RANGE OF TISSUES
IN SAME SPECIES
INCLUDING THE GUINEA
PIG

ENZYMES IN
LIVER AND
OTHER TISSUES

MULTIPLE ELECTROPHILIC
METABOLITES

CANDIDATE
ULTIMATE CARCINOGENS

NUCLEIC ACID- AND PROTEIN-BOUND
AAF- AND AF- RESIDUES

FIGURE 5

Initial Steps in the Metabolic Activation of 2-Acetylaminofluorene (AAF).

relate very well with the carcinogenic activities of AAF and N-hydroxy-AAF in these livers (Debaun, Miller, & Miller, 1970). The male and female rats of this strain N-hydroxylate AAF to about the same extent, but they differ very much in their ability to carry out this important second step of activation. Likewise, there is a good correlation between sulfotransferase activity and carcinogenicity for the livers of males of the other species listed. The level of binding of AAF residues to the sulfur atoms of methionyl residues in the liver protein also parallels the observed carcinogenicity.

Further crucial evidence that the N-sulfate is an ultimate carcinogen in the liver was provided by the Weisburgers and their associates (1972) at the National Cancer Institute. They lowered the level of PAPS in the rat liver in vivo by feeding the rats acetanilide. This amide is metabolized and excreted as a stable ring sulfate. Feeding acetanilide with N-hydroxy-AAF also lowered the carcinogenicity of N-hydroxy AAF in the male rat liver. Recovery of about two thirds of the loss in carcinogenicity was accomplished by supplementing the diet with sodium sulfate. The level of PAPS is limiting in the rat liver because of the slow

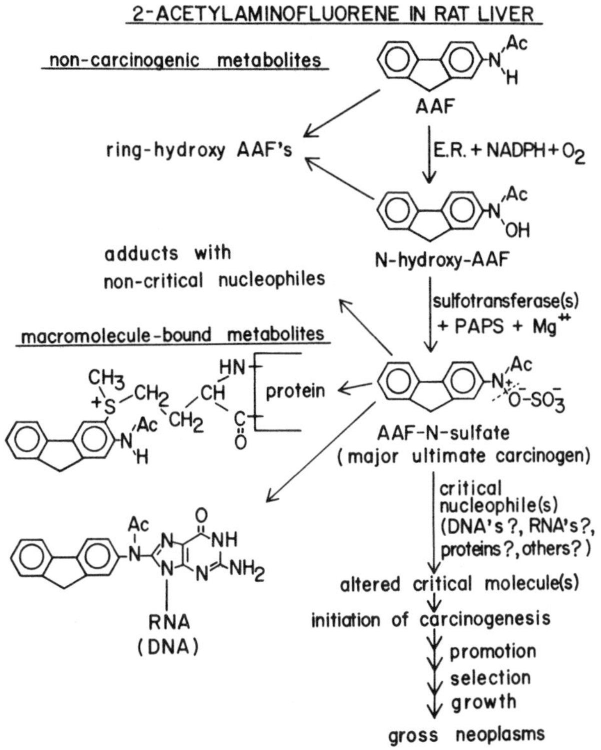

FIGURE 6

The Metabolic Activation and Inactivation of 2-Acetylaminofluo-
rene in the Rat Liver.

terminal oxidation of the sulfur of cysteine and can be increased simply by providing more sulfate ion to the animal.

However, no sulfotransferase activity for N-hydroxy AAF has been found
in other tissues such as the mammary gland, ear duct gland, and the subcutaneous
tissue in the rat where this proximate carcinogen also produces tumors. Subsequent work showed other enzymatic pathways can form several electrophiles
from N-hydroxy AAF as noted in Fig. 7. The peroxidatic pathway was first
shown by Bartsch and Hecker (1971) in Heidelberg. It involves a one-electron
oxidation to a free nitroxide radical which spontaneously dismutates to form
two carcinogenic, electrophilic and mutagenic compounds. N-acetoxy-AAF is
entirely analogous in its reactivity to the metabolically formed AAF-N-sulfate.
So far this pathway has not been demonstrated in mammalian tissues. Another
pathway is the formation of the 0-glucuronide of N-hydroxy AAF. This glucuronide is the principal circulatory and excretory form of N-hydroxy-AAF in

TABLE 2
COMPARISON OF HEPATIC N-HYDROXY-AAF
SULFOTRANSFERASE ACTIVITY AND THE *IN VIVO*
FORMATION OF HEPATIC PROTEIN-BOUND METHIONYL-AAF
DERIVATIVES IN ANIMALS SUSCEPTIBLE AND RESISTANT
TO HEPATOCARCINOGENESIS BY N-HYDROXY-AAF
(DEBAUN, MILLER, AND MILLER, 1970)

	o-CH$_3$S-AAF from		
Species	*Liver sulfotransferase in vitro* ug/mg prot./30 min	*Liver protein in vivo* ug/5 g liver	*Hepatocar. of* N-HO-AAF
Rat (M)	21 ± 2	37 ± 7	++++
Rat (F)	4 ± 1	5 ± 1	+
Mouse (M)	0.7	<1.5	+
Hamster (M)	<0.5	<0.3	+
Guinea Pig (M)	0.5	<0.3	−
Rabbit (M)	2 ± 0.5^a	<0.5	−

^{a}Figures for rabbit are o-CH$_3$S-AAF + o-CH$_3$S-AF.

the rat. In collaboration with Charles Irving at Memphis we found this metabolite to have weak electrophilic activity (Miller et al., 1968). At pH 7, it will insert both AAF and AF residues into nucleic acids. This candidate ultimate carcinogen has not received much further study.

More recently, Helmut Bartsch (Bartsch et al., 1972, 1973) in our laboratory found a soluble acetyl transferase activity for N-hydroxy-AAF in a variety of rat tissues including some where AAF and N-hydroxy-AAF produce tumors. This system has also received extensive study by King and his associates (King, 1974; King & Olive, 1975). This enzyme transfers the acetyl group of N-hydroxy-AAF from the nitrogen to the oxygen atom and generates the extremely powerful electrophile N-acetoxy-AF. This reactive metabolite could give rise to the macromolecular bound AF residues noted in vivo. Considerable acetyl transferase activity was found in several nonhepatic rat tissues including the mammary gland and small intestine where AAF induces tumors (Bartsch et al., 1973, King, 1974; King & Olive, 1975). However, no adequate study of this enzyme activity in relation to tumor formation is available at present.

There has been much comment at this meeting on inducers of cytochrome P-450, such as phenobarbital. This compound has been found to have two effects on the hepatocarcinogenicity of AAF. As shown by the data of Peraino and his associates (1971; see also Table 3), phenobarbital fed with a low level of AAF greatly reduces the incidence of hepatomas. This presumably results from overall loss of carcinogen from an increased level of ring-hydroxylation relative to that of N-hydroxylation, but this has not been fully demonstrated by analysis.

A more striking fact, perhaps, is the effect of phenobarbital given sub-

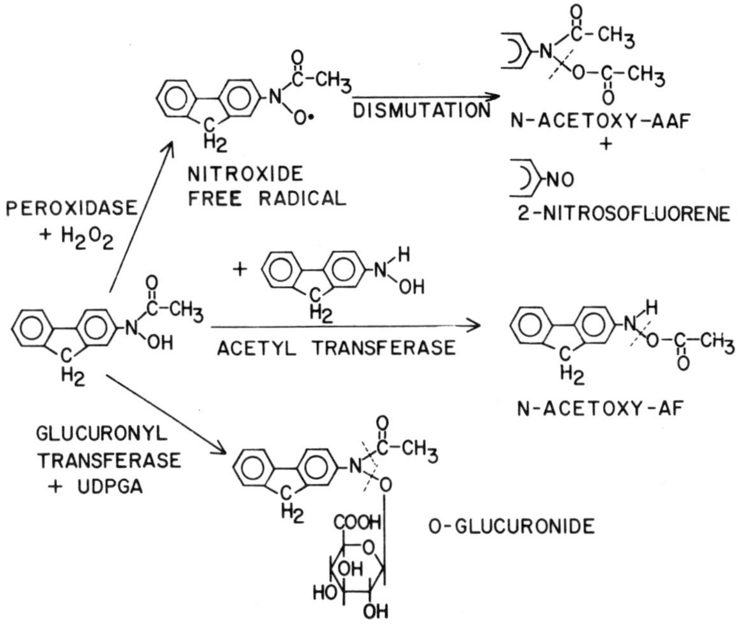

FIGURE 7

Other Enzymatic Pathways in the Metabolic Activation of N-Hydroxy-2-acetyl-aminofluorene.

sequent to a very short period of AAF administration. In this situation this barbiturate enhances tumor formation considerably. Interestingly, the tumors obtained in this way are generally much more highly differentiated than those produced by the long-term administration of AAF alone. Thus it appears that in this situation the short period of administration of AAF initiates hepatic tumors

TABLE 3
REDUCTION AND ENHANCEMENT BY
PHENOBARBITAL ADMINISTRATION OF
HEPATOMA INDUCTION BY AAF IN THE
MALE SPRAGUE-DAWLEY RAT
(PERAINO, FRY, AND STAFFELDT, 1971)

Dietary regimen		% rats with Hepatomas
Control diet	180 days	0
0.05% PB	180 days	0
0.02% AAF	180 days	83
0.02% AAF + 0.05% PB	180 days	22
0.02% AAF, 26 days; control,	234 days	26
0.02% AAF, 26 days; 0.05% PB,	234 days	84

and the long subsequent period of phenobarbital administration promotes tumor development in the rat liver. Tumor formation elsewhere in the rat by AAF is not affected by the subsequent period of phenobarbital administration. Several laboratory groups are now studying this interesting model system of liver tumor formation.

Other aromatic amine derivatives are metabolically activated in ways which are similar to those discussed above for AAF but with interesting differences. Figure 8 shows the pathway that Dr. Kadlubar (Kadlubar, Miller, & Miller, 1976a, 1976b) has found in our laboratory for the rat liver carcinogen N-methyl-4-aminoazobenzene (MAB). N-Hydroxylation of MAB also occurs in rat liver, but, unlike the oxidation of AAF, this is catalyzed by a noncytochrome-P-450, mixed-function amine oxidase. This enzyme appears to be the microsomal flavoprotein amine oxidase that was first found in pig liver by Ziegler and his group (Ziegler & Mitchell, 1972; Ziegler, McKee, & Poulsen, 1973) in Austin, Texas. It is of considerable interest that Ziegler and his associates found high levels of this enzyme in human liver and that many synthetic drugs containing N-methyl and N-dimethyl groups are substrates for this oxidase.

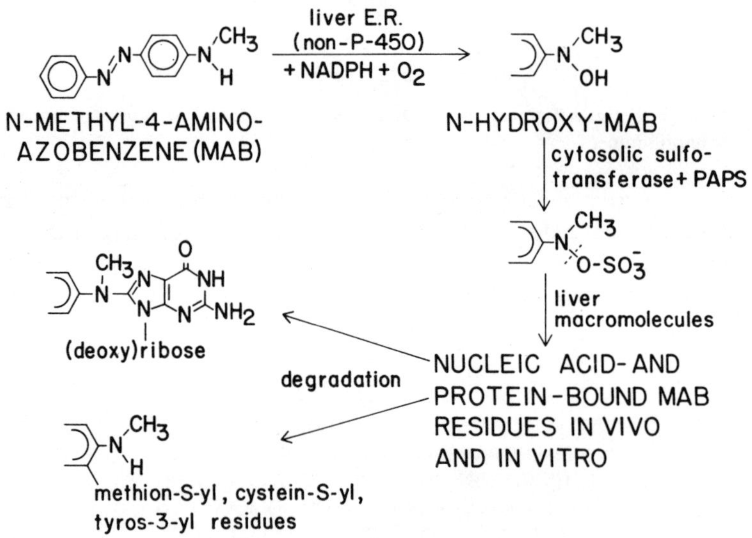

FIGURE 8

The Metabolic Activation of N-Methyl-4-aminoazobenzene (MAB) in the Rat Liver.

As with the activation of AAF, the second step in the activation of MAB involves a cytosolic sulfotransferase, but it appears to be a different enzyme from that found for N-hydroxy-AAF. Table 4 shows levels of the two activation enzymes in various rat tissues in relation to the susceptibilities of these tissues

TABLE 4

METABOLISM OF N-METHYL-4-AMINOAZOBENZENE
BY RAT TISSUES IN RELATION TO ITS
CARCINOGENIC ACTIVITY
(KADLUBAR, MILLER, & MILLER, 1976a, 1976b)

	Microsomal N-hydroxlation of MAB (nmoles/min/mg of protein)	Cytosolic sulfonation of N-HO-MAB	Tumor induction by MAB
Liver	2.1	3.6	+++
Kidney	<0.2	0.5	0
Small intenstie Mucosa	<0.2	0.5	0
Muscle	—	<0.2	0
Lung	<0.2	<0.2	0
Spleen	<0.2	—	0

to carcinogenesis by MAB. MAB is primarily a liver carcinogen, and we found very much lower levels of the two enzyme activities in the extrahepatic tissues where tumors are not found. Likewise, Table 5 indicates that there is a good correlation of hepatic enzyme level with species susceptibility to liver tumor induction.

Similar and different mechanisms of activation have been found with the naturally occurring carcinogen, safrole (Fig. 9). Safrole is a major component of oil of sassafras and a minor constituent of many spices that we use. It was once used in the United States as a flavor in soft drinks until it was banned under the Delaney Amendment when it was found to be a weak hepatocarcinogen in the rat. A metabolite of safrole, 1'-hydroxysafrole (5), is a proximate carcinogen for it has considerably stronger hepatocarcinogenic activity in both

TABLE 5

HEPATIC METABOLISM OF N-METHYL-4-AMINOAZOBENZENE
IN RELATION TO ITS HEPATOCARCINOGENIC ACTIVITY
(KADLUBAR, MILLER, & MILLER, 1976a, 1976b)

	Microsomal N-hydroxylation of MAB (nmoles/min/mg of protein)	Cytosolic sulfonation of N-HO-MAB	Hepatic tumor induction by DAB
Rat	2.1	3.6	+++
Mouse	0.3	1.1	+
Hamster	0.8	0.2	0
Guinea Pig	0.6	1.3	0
Rabbit	0.1	1.9	0

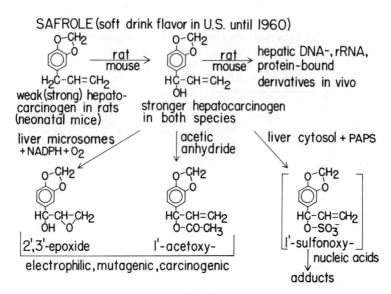

SAFROLE (soft drink flavor in U.S. until 1960)

FIGURE 9
The Metabolic Activation of Safrole in Rat and Mouse Liver.

the rat and mouse than safrole (4). It yields hepatic macromolecular-bound forms in vivo.

Wislocki et al. (1976) demonstrated that 1'-hydroxysafrole can be activated by two enzymatic pathways (Fig. 9). Liver microsomes contain a mixed-function oxidase which epoxidizes the vinyl group to form 1'-hydroxysafrole-2',3'-epoxide. This metabolite was isolated from the enzyme reaction mixture and also synthesized chemically. It is electrophilic, mutagenic, and active as an initiator of skin carcinogenesis in the mouse (Wislocki et al., 1977).

1'-Hydroxysafrole can also be activated by acetylation to form the synthetic ester 1'-acetoxysafrole (Borchert, Wislocki, Miller, & Miller, 1973). This derivative is electrophilic, mutagenic and carcinogenic (Borchert, Miller, Miller, & Shires, 1973; Wislocki et al., 1976, 1977). Subsequently, Wislocki et al. (1976) found that liver cytosol generates the analogous sulfuric acid ester in the presence of PAPS. As expected, this metabolite reacted readily with nucleic acids.

Only limited data have been obtained so far relating these epoxy and sulfonoxy metabolites to liver tumor formation (Table 6). The very low level of formation of these electrophiles may account for the weak hepatocarcinogenecity of safrole (Wislocki et al., 1976). It may account also for the failure of safrole and its 1'-hydroxy metabolite to exhibit mutagenic activity in the *S. typhimurium*-microsome test (McCann et al., 1975; Wislocki et al., 1977).

As noted above, phenobarbital decreased the carcinogenicity of AAF when it was fed with this carcinogen. However, recent work in our laboratory (Wislocki et al., 1977) showed that concurrent administration of phenobarbital increases

146

TABLE 6

THE METABOLIC ACTIVATION OF 1'-HYDROXYSAFROLE
IN RELATION TO ITS HEPATOCARCINOGENICITY
(WISLOCKI et al., 1976)

		Sulfonation	Epoxidation	Liver tumors
		(pmoles/40 mg liver/10 min)		
Rat	M	920	380	+++
(CR)	F	680	130	(no data)
Mouse	M	200	1100	+
(CD-1)	F	600	900	++

the carcinogenicity of safrole (see Table 7). Rats pretreated with phenobarbital and given safrole excrete more of the proximate carcinogen 1'-hydroxysafrole than do rats given safrole alone (Borchert, Wislocki, Miller, & Miller, 1973).

My last example of carcinogen activation concerns the mycotoxin aflatoxin B_1 (Fig. 10). This difuranocoumarin derivative is at least one million times more active than safrole in producing liver tumors in the rat. Considerable epidemiological evidence exists that this mycotoxin is hepatocarcinogenic in man (Peers & Linsell, 1973; Shank et al., 1972; Van Rensberg et al., 1974).

Aflatoxin B_1 appears to be metabolically inactivated in several ways by ring-hydroxylation and by demethylation of the methoxy group to give products which have less or far less toxicity than the parent mycotoxin (Campbell & Hayes, 1976). One of these metabolites, aflatoxin M_1, is less carcinogenic than aflatoxin B_1. While the other metabolites have not been tested for carcinogenicity, their low degrees of hepatotoxicity (Campbell & Hayes, 1976) and mutagenicity (Wong & Hsieh, 1976) suggest that they would be far less active as hepatocarcinogens than aflatoxin B_1.

The metabolic activation of aflatoxin B_1 appears to proceed via epoxida-

TABLE 7

EFFECT OF PHENOBARBITAL ADMINISTRATION
ON THE CARCINOGENICITY OF SAFROLE IN
MALE CHARLES RIVER CR RANDOM—BRED RATS
(WISLOCKI ET AL., 1977)

	% with hepatic ca. by	
Diet additives	12 mo.	22 mo.
0.5% safrole	0	17
0.55% 1'-hydroxysafrole	61	89
0.5% safrole + 0.1%		
phenobarbital (water)	0	67
0.1% phenobarbital (water)	0	6
None	0	0

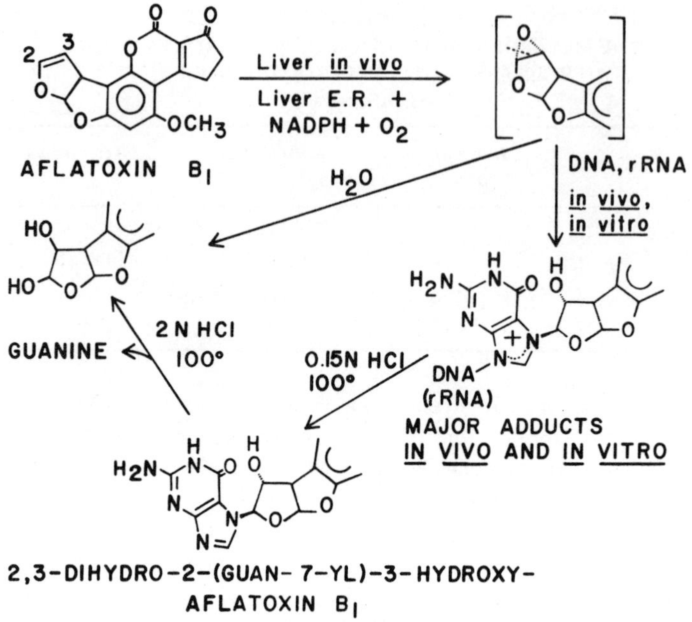

AFLATOXIN B_1

2,3-DIHYDRO-2-(GUAN-7-YL)-3-HYDROXY-AFLATOXIN B_1

FIGURE 10

The Metabolic Activation of Aflatoxin B_1 in the Rat Liver

tion at the 2,3-double bond (Garner, 1973; Garner, Miller, & Miller, 1972; Swenson et al., 1973, 1974, 1977) to form a highly reactive electrophile (Fig. 10). This figure also shows the structure of the major nucleic acid adducts formed in vitro and in vivo (Essigmann et al., 1977; Lin, Miller, & Miller, 1977). The levels of such adducts in the nucleic acids of several rat tissues are shown in

TABLE 8

LEVELS OF NUCLEIC-ACID–BOUND DERIVATIVES
OF AFLATOXIN B_1 IN VARIOUS RAT TISSUES
IN RELATION TO ITS CARCINOGENICITY
(SWENSON ET AL., 1977)

	DNA-AFB$_1$ adducts[a]	rRNA-AFB$_1$ adducts[a]	% tumors[b] 20 mo.
	pmoles/mg		
Liver	130	260	100
Kidney	10	30	0
Spleen	1	2	0
Small intestine	1	1	0

[a]18 hour. after one I.P. dose (520 µg/kg body weight).

[b]0.3 ppm in diet for 15 months.

Table 8; aflatoxin B_1 is primarily a liver carcinogen and binds very much less to the other tissues studies.

Table 9 shows the inhibitory effect of phenobarbital on the carcinogenicity of aflatoxin B_1 when fed concurrently with this carcinogen (Swenson et al., 1977). The lower levels of the nucleic acid-bound aflatoxin residues presumably reflect an altered balance of activation and inactivation of aflatoxin B_1 in these rats.

Table 9 also presents the low level of binding and carcinogenicity of aflatoxin B_2 (2,3-dihydro-aflatoxin B_1). Swenson and Lin (1977) in our laboratory have shown that these activities result from a limited desaturation of aflatoxin B_2 to aflatoxin B_1. The nucleic acid adducts derived from aflatoxin B_2 are identical to those formed from aflatoxin B_1. These results again emphasize the role of the 2,3-double bond in the activation and carcinogenicity of aflatoxin B_1.

While the data presented for these four carcinogens are limited in scope, it is evident that the degrees of activation and inactivation of the chemical carcinogens are important parameters in determining tissue and species selectivity. It is also clear that there are other important keys to species and tissue selectivities of carcinogens. For example, work in several laboratories, such as that of Dr. Magee, suggests very strongly that the rate of repair of DNA-containing carcinogen residues in target tissues may also be a strong determinant of tissue response. Likewise, promotion by a carcinogenic or noncarcinogenic promoter following initiation by a carcinogen can have profound effects on the magnitude of the tumor response.

While progress in understanding the mechanism of action of chemical carcinogens has been encouraging, I believe we have farther to go than we have already come on the road to full understanding in this difficult but intriguing field of research.

TABLE 9
FORMATION OF NUCLEIC ACID-BOUND DERIVATIVES
FROM TUMORS IN THE LIVERS OF MALE RATS
GIVEN AFLATOXIN B_1 OR AFLATOXIN B_2
(SWENSON ET AL., 1977)

	DNA-AFB_1 adducts[a]	rRNA-AFB_1 adducts[a]	% tumors[b]	
	pmoles/mg		15 mo.	20 mo.
AFB_1	130	260	60	100
AFB_1 + phenobarbital	15	35	11	67
None or phenobarbital	—	—	0	0
AFB_2	1.4	2		(6)[c]

[a]18 hr after one I.P. dose (520 μg/kg body weight).

[b]0.3 ppm in diet for 15 months.

[c]Wogan et al., (1971).

REFERENCES

Bartsch, H., Dworkin, C., Miller, E. C., & Miller, J. A. Formation of electrophilic N-acetoxy-arylamines in cytosols from rat mammary gland and other tissues by transacetylation from the carcinogen N-hydroxy-4-acetylaminobiphenyl. *Biochem. Biophys. Acta*, 1973, *304*, 42-55.

Bartsch, H., Dworkin, M., Miller, J. A., & Miller, E. C. Electrophilic N-acetoxy-aminoarenes derived from carcinogenic N-hydroxy-N-acetylaminoarenes by enzymatic deacetylation and transacetylation in liver. *Biochim. Biophys. Acta*, 1972, *286*, 272-298.

Bartsch, H., & Hecker, E. On the metabolic activation of the carcinogen N-hydroxy-2-acetylaminofluorene. III. Oxidation with horseradish peroxidase to yield 2-nitroso-fluorene and N-acetoxy-N-2-acetylaminofluorene. *Biochim. Biophys. Acta*, 1971, *237*, 567-578.

Becker, F. F. (Ed.). Cancer. Vol. 1, Etiology: Chemical and Physical Carcinogenesis. New York: Plenum Press, 1975.

Borchert, P., Miller, J. A., Miller E. C., & Shires, T. K. 1'-Hydroxysafrole, a proximate carcinogenic metabolite of safrole in the rat and mouse. *Cancer Res.*, 1973, *33*, 590-600.

Borchert, P., Wislocki, P. G. Miller, J. A., & Miller, E. C. The metabolism of the naturally occurring hepatocarcinogen safrole to 1'-hydroxysafrole and the electrophilic reactivity of 1'-acetoxysafrole. *Cancer Res.*, 1973, *33*, 575-589.

Campbell, T. C., & Hayes, J. R. The role of aflatoxin metabolism in its toxic lesion. *Toxicol. Appl. Pharmacol.*, 1976, *35*, 199-222.

DeBaun, J. R., Miller, E. C., & Miller, J. A. N-Hydroxy-2-acetylaminofluorene sulfotransferase: Its probable role in carcinogenesis and in protein-(methion-S-yl) binding in rat liver. *Cancer Res.*, 1970, *30*, 577-595.

Essigmann, J. M., Croy, R. G., Nadzan, A. M., Busby, W. F., Jr., Reinhold. V. N., Buchi, G., & Wogan, G. N. Structural identification of the major DNA adduct formed by aflatoxin B_1 in vitro. *Proc. Natl. Acad. Sci., U.S.*, 1977, *74*, 1870-1874.

Garner, R. C. Chemical evidence for the formation of a reactive aflatoxin B_1 metabolite by hamster liver microsomes. *Federation European Biochem. Soc. Letters*, 1973, *36*, 261-264.

Garner, R. C., Miller, E. C., & Miller, J. A. Liver microsomal metabolism of aflatoxin B_1 to a reactive derivative toxic to *Salmonella typhimurium* TA1530. *Cancer Res.*, 1972, *32*, 2058-2066.

Kadlubar, F. F., Miller, J. A., & Miller, E. C. Microsomal N-oxidation of the hepatocarcinogen N-methyl-4-aminozobenzene and the reactivity of N-hydroxy-N-methyl-4-aminoazobenzene. *Cancer Res.*, 1976(a), *36*, 1196-1206.

Kadlubar, F. F., Miller, J. A., & Miller, E. C. Hepatic metabolism of N-hydroxy-N-methyl-4-aminoazobenzene and other N-hydroxy arylamines to reactive sulfuric acid esters. *Cancer Res.*, 1976(b), *36*, 2350-2359.

King, C. M. Mechanism of reaction, tissue distribution, and inhibition of arylhydroxamic acid acyltransferase. *Cancer Res.*, 1974, *34*, 1503-1515.

King, C. M., & Olive, C. W. Comparative effects of strain, species and sex on the acyltransferase- and sulfotransferase-catalyzed activations of N-hydroxy-N-2-fluorenylacetamide. *Cancer Res.*, 1975, *35*, 906-912.

Lin, J.-K., Miller, J. A., & Miller, E. C. 2,3-dihydro-2-(guan-7-yl)-3-hydroxyaflatoxin B_1, a major acid hydrolysis product of aflatoxin B_1-DNA or -rRNA adducts formed in hepatic microsome-mediated reactions and in rat liver in vivo. *Cancer Res.*, 1977, *37*, 4430-4438.

McCann, J., Choi, E., Yamasaki, E., & Ames, B. N. The detection of carcinogens as mutagens in the *Salmonella*/microsome test: Assay of 300 chemicals. *Proc. Natl. Acad. Sci., U.S.,* 1975, *72,* 5135-5139.

Miller, E. C., Lotlikar, P. D., Miller, J. A., Butler, B. W., Irving, C. C., & Hill, J. T. Reactions in vitro of some tissue nucleophiles with glucuronide of the carcinogen N-hydroxy-2-acetylaminofluorene. *Mol. Pharmacol.,* 1968, *4,* 147-154.

Miller, E. C., & Miller, J. A. The metabolism of chemical carcinogens to reactive electrophiles and their possible mechanisms of action in carcinogenesis. In: *Chemical carcinogens,* Searle, C. E. (Ed.), ACS Monograph 173. Washington, D.C.: American Chemical Society, 1976, pp. 737-762.

Peers, F. G., & Linsell, C. A. Dietary aflatoxins and liver cancer–A population based study in Kenya. *Br. J. Cancer,* 1973, *27,* 473-484.

Peraino, C., Fry, R. J. M., & Staffeldt, E. Reduction and enhancement by phenobarbital of hepatocarcinogenesis induced in the rat by dietary phenobarbital. *Cancer Res.,* 1971, *31,* 1506-1512.

Searle, C. E. (Ed.). *Chemical carcinogens.* ACS Monograph 173. Washington, D.C.: American Chemical Society, 1976.

Shank, R. C., Bhamarapravati, N., Gordon, J. E., & Wogan, G. N. Dietary aflatoxins and human liver cancer. IV. Incidence of primary liver cancer in two municipal populations of Thailand. *Food Cosmet. Toxicol.,* 1972, *10,* 171-179.

Swenson, D. H., Lin, J.-K., Miller, E. C., & Miller, J. A. Aflatoxin B_1-2,3-oxide as a probable intermediate in the covalent binding of aflatoxins B_1 and B_2 to rat liver DNA and ribosomal RNA in vivo. *Cancer Res.,* 1977, *37,* 172-181.

Swenson, D. H., Miller, E. C., & Miller, J. A. Aflatoxin B_1-2,3-oxide: Evidence for its formation in rat liver in vivo and by human liver microsomes in vitro. *Biochem. Biophys. Res. Commun.,* 1974, *60,* 1036-1043.

Swenson, D. H., Miller, J. A., & Miller, E. C. 2,3-dihydro-2,3,-dihydroxyaflatoxin B_1: An acid hydrolysis product of an RNA-aflatoxin B_1 adduct formed by hamster and rat liver microsomes in vitro. *Biochem. Biophys. Res. Commun.,* 1973, *53,* 1260-1267.

Van Rensberg, S. J., Van Der Watt, J. J., Purchase, I. F. H., Pereira Coutinho, L., & Markham, R. Primary liver cancer rate and aflatoxin intake in a high cancer area. *S. Afr. Med. J.,* 1974, *48,* 250a-d.

Weisburger, J. H., & Williams, G. M. Metabolism of Chemical Carcinogens. In: Cancer Vol. 1 (Becker, F. F., Ed.), pp. 185-234. Plenum Press, New York, 1975.

Weisburger, J. H., Yamamoto, R. S., Williams, G. M., Grantham, P. H., & Weisburger, E. K. On the sulfate ester of N-hydroxy-N-2-fluorenylacetamide As a key ultimate hepatocarcinogen in the rat. *Cancer Res.,* 1972, *32,* 491-500.

Wislocki, P. G., Borchert, P., Miller, J. A., & Miller, E. C. The metabolic activation of the carcinogen 1'-hydroxysafrole in vivo and in vitro and the electrophilic reactivities of possible ultimate carcinogens. *Cancer Res.,* 1976, *36,* 1686-1695.

Wislocki, P. G., Miller, E. C., Miller, J. A., McCoy, E. C., & Rosenkranz, H. S. Carcinogenic and mutagenic activities of safrole, 1'-hydroxysafrole, and some known or possible metabolites. *Cancer Res.,* 1977, *37,* 1883-1891.

Wong, J. J., & Hsieh, D. P. H. Mutagenicity of aflatoxins related to their metabolism and carcinogenic potential. *Proc. Natl. Acad. Sci., U.S.,* 1976, *73,* 2241-2244.

Ziegler, D. M., McKee, E. M., & Poulsen, L. O. Microsomal flavoprotein-catalyzed N-oxidation of arylamines. *Drug. Metab. Disposition,* 1973, *1,* 314-321.

Ziegler, D. M., & Mitchell, C. H. Microsomal oxidase IV: Properties of a mixed-function amine oxidase isolated from pig liver microsomes. *Arch. Biochem. Biophys.,* 1973, *150,* 116-125.

8. Metabolism of Polycyclic Aromatic Hydrocarbons to Reactive Intermediates with High Biological Activity

A. H. Conney, W. Levin, A. W. Wood
Hoffmann-La Roche, Inc., Nutley, New Jersey

H. Yagi, D. R. Thakker, R. E. Lehr and D. M. Jerina
*National Institute of Arthritis, Metabolism
and Digestive Diseases
National Institute of Health, Bethesda, Maryland*

The pioneering research of Drs. J. A. Miller and E. C. Miller demonstrated that many chemical carcinogens undergo metabolism to highly reactive electrophiles that covalently bind with cellular constituents to initiate the carcinogenic event (Miller & Miller, 1947, 1974; Miller, 1970, 1978). Since thousands of tons of a mixture of benzo[a]pyrene (BP[1]) and other carcinogenic polycyclic aromatic hydrocarbons are released into the environment of the United States each year as unwanted by-products of combustion (Committee on the Biologic Effects of Atmospheric Pollutants, 1972), it is of considerable importance to determine how these chemicals are metabolized. Evidence for the metabolic activation of a polycyclic aromatic hydrocarbon to reactive intermediates was first obtained in 1951 from a key study by E. C. Miller. She applied BP to mouse skin and found that metabolites of this hydrocarbon were covalently bound to skin protein (Miller, 1951). Subsequent studies by many other investigators demonstrated that application of BP or other carcinogenic polycyclic hydrocarbons to mouse skin resulted in the covalent binding of metabolites to DNA, RNA and protein. In 1957, the liver microsomal metabolism of BP to several hydroxylated products and quinones by an inducible monooxygenase system was described (Conney et al., 1957), and several years later the microsomal-mediated metabolism of BP to DNA-bound metabolites was demonstrated (Grover & Sims, 1968; Gelboin, 1969). More recently, Borgen et al. (1973) found that metabolism of BP 7,8-dihydrodiol by liver microsomes resulted in significantly higher binding of metabolites. Shortly thereafter, Sims et al. (1974) provided evidence that a BP 7,8-diol-9,10-epoxide was involved in the binding of BP 7,8-dihydrodiol to DNA,

153

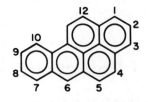

BP

BP 4,5 – OXIDE

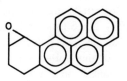

BP 7,8 – DIOL – 9,10 – EPOXIDE 1

BP 7,8 – DIOL – 9,10 – EPOXIDE 2

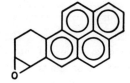

9,10 – EPOXY – 7,8,9,10 –
TETRAHYDRO BP

7,8 – EPOXY – 7,8,9,10 –
TETRAHYDRO BP

FIGURE 1
Structures of BP and some mutagenic BP derivatives.

and the possibility of diastereomeric diol epoxides of BP (Fig. 1) was pointed out by Yagi et al. (1975).

Several years ago, our laboratories in Bethesda and Nutley initiated collaborative studies on the synthesis and testing for biological activity of as many of the known and potential metabolites of BP as were possible, and we have also investigated the metabolism of BP and certain of its metabolites (Conney et al., 1977; Jerina et al., 1976c; Levin et al., 1977a). The results of our studies on the metabolism, mutagenicity, and carcinogenicity of BP and its metabolites are summarized below, and a generalized theory (Jerina et al., 1977) of polycyclic hydrocarbon carcinogenesis that has evolved from this research is also described.

154

MUTAGENIC ACTIVITY OF POTENTIAL BP METABOLITES[1]

We chose to study the mutagenic activity of BP derivatives as an initial test of biological activity, because the mutagenic activity of these compounds under physiological conditions provides an index of their ability to interact with genetic material in a way that results in an altered and heritable phenotype. Since somatic cell mutation may be involved in the chemical initiation of cancer, studies on the mutagenicity of BP derivatives should help in our efforts to determine how BP is activated to its ultimately reactive forms. Inherent mutagenic activity of BP derivatives was examined in *Salmonella typhimurium* strains TA 98, 100, and 1538 developed by Ames et al. (1973a, 1973b) and in the Chinese hamster V-79 cell line of Chu and Malling (1968). Both the bacterial and mammalian cells selected for testing the mutagenic activity of the BP derivatives lack detectable levels of polycyclic hydrocarbon-metabolizing enzymes (Ames et al., 1973a; Huberman and Sachs, 1974), and thus the parent hydrocarbon, BP, is inactive in these test systems.

In 1975 we reported that BP 4,5-oxide was a potent mutagen in *S. typhimurium* and in V-79 cells, that BP 7,8-oxide and BP 9,10-oxide were very weakly mutagenic, and that 4-, 5-, 7-, 8-, 9-, and 10-HOBP had little or no mutagenic activity (Wood et al., 1975). We also reported, at a symposium on reactive metabolites during the summer of 1975, on the mutagenic activity of more than

[1]The abbreviations used are: BP, benzo[a]pyrene; 1-HOBP, 1-hydroxybenzo[a]-pyrene; 2- to 12-HOBP, other benzo[a]pyrene phenols; BP 4,5-oxide, benzo[a]pyrene 4,5-oxide; BP 7,8-, 9,10-, and 11,12-oxide, other benzo[a]pyrene oxides; BP 4,5-dihydrociol, *trans*-4,5-dihydroxy-4,5-dihydrobenzo[a]pyrene; BP 7,8-, 9,10-, and 11,12-dihydrodiol, other *trans* dihydrodiols of benzo[a]pyrene; BP 7,8-diol-9,10-epoxide-*1*, (±)-7β,8α-dihydroxy-9β,10β-epoxy-7,8,9,10-tetrahydrobenzo[a]pyrene; BP 7,8-diol-9,10-epoxide-*2*, (±)-7β,8α-dihydroxy-9α,10α-epoxy-7,8,9,10-tetrahydrobenzo[a]pyrene; BP, 9,10-diol-7,8-epoxide-*1*, (±)-9α,10β-dihydroxy-7β,8β-epoxy-7,8,9,10-tetrahydrobenzo[a]pyrene; BP 9,10-diol-7,8-epoxide-2, (±)-9α,10β-dihydroxy-7α,8α-epoxy-7,8,9,10-tetrahydrobenzo[a]pyrene; BP 7,10-diol-8,9-epoxide, (±)-7α,10β-dihydroxy-8α,9α-epoxy-7,8,9,10-tetrahydrobenzo[a]-pyrene; BA, benzo[a]anthracene; BA 3,4-diol-1,2-epoxide-*1*, (±)-3α,4β-dihydroxy-1β,2β-epoxy-1,2,3,4-tetrahydrobenzo[a]anthracene; BA 3,4-diol-1,2-epoxide-2, (±)-3α,4β-dihydroxy-1α,2α-epoxy-1,2,3,4-tetrahydrobenzo[a]anthracene, BA 8,9-diol-10,11-epoxides *1* and *2*, and BA 10,11-diol-8,9-epoxides *1* and *2*, other diol epoxides of benzo[a]anthracene with analogous stereochemistry; BA 5,6-oxide, benzo[a]anthracene 5,6-oxide; BA 3,4-dihydrodiol, *trans*-3,4-dihydroxy-3,4-dihydrobenzo[a]anthracene; BA 1,2-, 5,6-, 8,9-, and 10,11-dihydrodiol, other BA dihydrodiols; DMSO, dimethylsulfoxide. The above compounds are racemic mixtures wherever optical enantiomers are possible.

The abbreviations used for the optically pure enantiomers of BP 7,8-diol-9,10-epoxide are: (−)-BP 7,8-diol-9,10-epoxide-*1*, (−)-7β,8α-dihydroxy-9β,10β-epoxy-7,8,9,10-tetrahydrobenzo[a]pyrene; (+)-BP 7,8-diol-9,10-epoxide-*1*, (+)-7α,8β-dihydroxy-9α,10α-epoxy-7,8,9,10-tetrahydrobenzo[a]pyrene; (−)-BP 7,8-diol-9,10-epoxide-2, (−)-7α,8β-dihydroxy-9β,10β-epoxy-7,8,9,10-tetrahydrobenzo[a]pyrene; (+)-BP 7,8-diol-9,10-epoxide-2, (+)-7β,8α-dihydroxy-9α,10α-epoxy-7,8,9,10-tetrahydrobenzo[a]pyrene.

30 BP derivatives, and we indicated that a BP 7,8-diol-9,10-epoxide was one of the most potent mutagens ever tested (Conney et al., 1977). We indicated that BP 7,8-diol-9,10-epoxide-*1* (Fig. 1) was at least four- to fivefold more mutagenic than BP 4,5-oxide in the bacterial *S. typhimurium* strains TA 98 and TA 100, and that this diol epoxide was about 40-fold more mutagenic than the highly mutagenic BP 4,5-oxide in mammalian V-79 cells. We described additional studies on the mutagenic activities of the BP 7,8-diol-9,10-epoxides and other BP derivatives the following year (Wislocki et al., 1976a, 1976b; Wood et al., 1976c). Studies on the high mutagenic activities of the BP 7,8-diol-9,10-epoxides were also reported by Huberman et al. (1976) and by Newbold and Brookes (1976).

Table 1 summarizes the mutagenic activities of 19 BP derivatives in bacterial and mammalian cells. Structures of the most potent mutagens are given in Fig. 1. A comparison of the inherent mutagenic activity of the BP derivatives was made from the linear portions of the dose-response curves for mutations whenever the particular BP derivative had sufficient mutagenic activity to determine a dose-response relationship. The most mutagenic compound in each test

TABLE 1

COMPARISON OF THE INHERENT MUTAGENIC ACTIVITY OF
BENZO(A)PYRENE DERIVATIVES IN SALMONELLA
TYPHIMURIUM AND IN CHINESE HAMSTER V79 CELLS

Compound	Relative % activity[a]			
	TA 1538	TA 98	TA 100	V-79
BP 7,8-diol-9,10-epoxide-*1*	40	100	100	40
BP 7,8-dio-9,10-epoxide-*2*	15	35	65	100
BP 9,10-diol-7,8-epoxide-*1*	—	2	0.4	<0.1
BP 9,10-diol-7,8-epoxide-*2*	—	11	1	0.2
BP 7,10-diol-8,9-epoxide	—	<0.1	0.4	<0.1
9,10-Epoxy-7,8,9,10-tetrahydro BP	100	95	90	40
7,8-Epoxy-7,8,9,10-tetrahydro BP	20	10	2	0.2
BP 4,5-oxide	60	20	6	1
BP 7,8-oxide	2	1	0.6	<0.1
BP 9,10-oxide	1	1	0.6	<0.1
BP 11,12-oxide	1	0.5	0.2	0.3
6-HOBP	5	5	0.6	0.3
12-HOBP	2	1.5	≤0.1	<0.1
1-HOBP	1.5	0.5	<0.1	0.1
3-HOBP	1	0.5	<0.1	<0.1
2-, 4-, 5-, 7-, 8-, 9-, 10-, 11-HOBP	<1	<0.1	<0.1	<0.1
BP 1,6-, 3,6-, 6,12-, 4,5-, 7,8-, 11,12-quinone	<0.1	<0.1	<0.1	<0.1
BP 4,5-, 7,8-, 9,10-, 11,12-dihydrodiol	<0.1	<0.1	<0.1	<0.1
BP	<0.1	<0.1	<0.1	<0.1

[a]The comparisons are derived from data obtained in several different experiments. In each experiment, BP 4,5-oxide or one of the diastereomeric BP 7,8-diol-9,10-epoxides was used as a positive control for comparative purposes.

system was assigned 100% activity. The importance of comparing mutagenic potency of a series of compounds at several doses cannot be overemphasized. At low concentrations, where cytotoxicity is very low, mutagenicity increases proportionately with dose (Wislocki et al., 1976b; Wood et al., 1976c). The comparative mutagenic activities of the 19 BP derivatives given in Table 1 indicate that 9,10-epoxy-7,8,9,10-tetrahydro BP and the diastereomeric BP 7,8-diol-9,10-epoxides were the most potent mutagens tested in *S. typhimurium* strains TA 98 and TA 100 and in V-79 cells. In strain TA 1538 of *S. typhimurium,* BP 4,5-oxide was a more potent mutagen than the diastereomeric BP 7,8-diol-9,10-epoxides but was less active than 9,10-epoxy-7,8,9,10-tetrahydro BP. In all three bacterial strains, BP 7,8-diol-9,10-epoxide-*1* was a more potent mutagen than BP 7,8-diol-9,10-epoxide-*2,* while the reverse was true in V-79 cells. We found that BP 7,8-diol-9,10-epoxides-*1* and *2* were, respectively, about 40- and 100-fold more mutagenic toward the mammalian V-79 cells than was BP 4,5-oxide (Wislocki et al., 1976b; Wood et al., 1976c). High mutagenic activities for both BP 7,8-diol-9,10 epoxides-*1* and *2* were also reported in V-79 cells by Newbold and Brookes (1976). Although Huberman et al. (1976) found exceptionally high mutagenic activity for BP 7,8-diol-9,10-epoxide-*2* in V-79 cells, they reported that BP 7,8-diol-9,10-epoxide-*1* was only as active as BP 4,5-oxide in these cultured cells. Malaveille et al. (1975) found relatively low mutagenic activity for a BP 7,8-diol-9,10-epoxide of unstated stereochemistry in *S. typhimurium* strain TA 100, but a later study by this group (Malaveille et al., 1977a) found high mutagenic activities for BP 7,8-diol-9,10-epoxides-*1* and *2* that were similar to those reported from our laboratories in strain TA 100 (Wood et al., 1976c). The high mutagenic potency of the BP 7,8-diol-9,10-epoxides and 9,10-epoxy-7,8,9,10-tetrahydro BP relative to the other BP derivatives shown in Table 1 is undoubtedly an underestimation of biological activity because these compounds are extremely unstable in aqueous solution (Whalen et al., 1977; Wood et al., 1976c). Although BP 4,5-oxide is stable in aqueous solution for many hours (Levin et al., 1976a; Wood et al., 1975), the biologically measured half-lives of BP 7,8-diol-9,10-epoxide-*1,* BP 7,8-diol-9,10-epoxide-*2,* and 9,10-epoxy-7,8,9,10-tetrahydro BP in phosphate-buffered saline are about 30, 120, and 30 seconds, respectively (Wood et al., 1976c).

Since the chemically synthesized BP 7,8-diol-9,10-epoxides-*1* and *2* described in Table 1 are each racemic mixtures, we have prepared the optically pure (+)- and (−)-enantiomer of each diasteriomer (Yagi et al., 1977), and we have determined their mutagenic activities (Wood et al., 1977b). Substantial differences were observed in the mutagenic activities of the optically pure (+)- and (−)-enantiomers of the BP 7,8-diol-9,10-epoxides-*1* and *2* in bacterial and mammalian cells (Table 2). In strains TA 98 and TA 100 of *S. typhimurium,* the (−)-enantiomer of BP 7,8-diol-9,10-epoxide-*1* was 1.3 to 9.5 times more mutagenic than the three other optically active stereoisomers. In Chinese hamster V-79 cells, the (+)-enantiomer of BP 7,8-diol-9,10-epoxide-*2* was 6 to 18 times more

Table 2

MUTAGENICITY OF OPTICALLY PURE ENANTIOMERS OF THE

BENZO [a] PYRENE 7,8-DIOL-9,10-EPOXIDES

Compound tested	S. typhimurium strain		V-79 cells
	TA 98	TA 100	(8-AG resistant
	(revertants / nmole / plate)		colonies/nmole/10⁵ survivors)
(−)-diol epoxide 1	5200	9500	60
(+)-diol epoxide 1	3900	5200	34
(−)-diol epoxide 2	1800	1000	22
(+)-diol epoxide 2	2500	6000	400

mutagenic than the other three isomers. This study, which is the first example of differences in the mutagenicity of optically pure enantiomers, suggests the presence of highly stereospecific receptors, detoxification mechanisms and/or transport systems.

Since an ultimate carcinogenic metabolite of a compound such as BP need not be a primary (or even a secondary) oxidative metabolite, we have tested the mutagenic activity of many of the BP derivatives listed in Table 1 in the presence of a reconstituted monooxygenase system that metabolizes polycyclic hydrocarbons. Of the BP derivatives tested in strains TA 1538 and TA 98 of *S. typhimurium,* only BP 7,8-dihydrodiol was metabolically activated to mutagenic metabolites to a greater extent than was BP (Wood et al., 1976b, 1977e). Studies by Malaveille et al. (1975) and by Huberman et al. (1976) also revealed that BP 7,8-dihydrodiol was metabolized to a potent mutagen(s) to a greater extent than BP or the 4,5- and 9,10-dihydrodiols of BP. In our study with a reconstituted monooxygenase system, 1-, 2-, 3-, 6-, 9-, and 12-HOBP were metabolically activated to mutagenic metabolites, but to a lesser extent than BP. BP 7,8-oxide was metabolized to mutagenic metabolites by a combination of a purified monooxygenase system and purified epoxide hydrase, but metabolism to a mutagen did not occur by either enzyme alone (Wood et al., 1976b). The active metabolites generated from BP 7,8-oxide and BP 7,8-dihydrodiol were presumably one or more of the four optically active enantiomers of the diastereomeric BP 7,8-diol-9,10-epoxides. Although earlier studies had indicated that epoxide hydrase was primarily involved in the detoxification of arene oxides and epoxides, the present study with purified monooxygenase and epoxide hydrase is the first to demonstrate that epoxide hydrase can participate in the metabolism of a chemical to a more toxic and mutagenic compound.

STEREOSELECTIVE METABOLISM AND COVALENT BINDING OF BP AND ITS METABOLITES

Metabolism

Since the stereospecificity of metabolism of BP by monooxygenase systems and by epoxide hydrase may play a critical role in the expression of biological activity, the stereochemical course of BP metabolism has been the subject of intensive investigation. Liver microsomal enzymes from 3-methylcholanthrene-pretreated rats metabolize BP to the (−)-enantiomers of BP 4,5-dihydrodiol, BP 7,8-dihydrodiol, and BP 9,10-dihydrodiol to a greater than tenfold excess relative to the (+)-enantiomers (Thakker et al., 1976, 1977a, 1977b; Yang & Gelboin, 1976). This high degree of stereoselective metabolism of BP is shown in Table 3 (Thakker et al., 1977a).

TABLE 3
OPTICAL PURITY OF DIHYDRODIOLS OBTAINED DURING
INCUBATION OF BP OR BP 7,8-OXIDE WITH LIVER
MICROSOMES FROM 3-METHYLCHOLANTHRENE-
TREATED RATS

$[C^{14}]$-substrate incubated	Dihydrodiol formed	% Each enantiomer		% Optical purity[a]
		%(+)	%(−)	
BP	BP 4,5-dihydrodiol	4	96	92
BP	BP 9,10-dihydrodiol	4	96	92
BP	BP 7,8-dihydrodiol	4	96	92
Racemic BP 7,8-oxide[b]	BP 7,8-dihydrodiol	46	54	8

[a]Percent optical purity is defined as the specific rotation of the enantiomeric mixture divided by the specific rotation of one pure enantiomer × 100.

[b]Racemic $[C^{14}]$-BP 7,8-oxide was incubated with liver microsomes or purified epoxide hydrase.

Interestingly, racemic BP 4,5-oxide is metabolized by liver microsomal or by purified epoxide hydrase predominantly to the (−)-enantiomer of BP 4,5-dihydrodiol, whereas racemic BP 7,8-oxide and BP 9,10-oxide are each hydrated to appreciable amounts of both the (+) and (−)-enantiomers of the *trans*-dihydrodiols (Thakker et al., 1977b). These results indicate a high degree of stereospecificity in the formation of BP 7,8-oxide and BP 9,10-oxide by the monooxygenase system and epoxide hydrase depends on the substrate studied. It can be seen in Table 4 that liver microsomes from 3-methylcholanthrene-treated rats metabolize (−)-BP 7,8-dihydrodiol to (+)-BP 7,8-diol-9,10-epoxide-*2* and (−)-BP 7,8-diol-9,10-epoxide-*1* in a 6:1 ratio, while (+)-BP 7,8-dihydrodiol is converted to (+)-BP 7,8-diol-9,10-epoxide-*1* and (−)-BP 7,8-diol-9,10-epoxide-*2* in a 22:1 ratio (Thakker et al., 1977a). Interestingly, liver microsomes from untreated or phenobarbital-pretreated rats are less stereospecific in the metabolism of the optically active BP 7,8-dihydrodiol enantiomers than are liver microsomes from 3-methylcholanthrene-treated rats (Thakker et al., 1977a). Additional studies on the stereoselective metabolism of BP in tissues sensitive to BP carcinogenesis are needed. Studies by Huberman et al. (1976) suggested that BP was metabolized almost exclusively to BP 7,8-diol-9,10-epoxide-*2* relative to BP 7,8-diol-9,10-epoxide-*1,* but in a subsequent study, the same investigators (Yang et al., 1976) recognized that BP 7,8-diol-9,10-epoxide-*1* was also formed. The large differences in biological activity of the optically active enantiomers of the BP 7,8-diol-9,10-epoxides (Table 2) indicate that stereospecificity of the monooxygenase and epoxide hydrase systems described above could play a highly important role in determining the susceptibility of a particular tissue, organ, or species toward the carcinogenicity and toxicity of polycyclic aromatic hydrocarbons.

Covalent Binding

Although only BP 7,8-diol-9,10-epoxide-*2* was found bound to RNA when BP was metabolized by bovine bronchial explants (Jeffrey et al., 1976; Weinstein et al., 1976), studies with cultured BHK 21/C13 cells (King et al., 1976), cultured hamster embryo cells (Baird & Diamond, 1977) and BHK 21/C13 as well as secondary mouse embryo fibroblast cells (Remsen et al., 1977) provided chromatographic evidence for the binding of both BP 7,8-diol-9,10-epoxides-*1* and *2* to DNA after exposure of the cells to BP. In the studies where bovine explants were exposed to BP, evidence for the binding of (+)-BP 7,8-diol-9,10-epoxide-*2* to RNA was provided (Nakanishi et al., 1977). Both (+)-BP 7,8-diol-9,10-epoxide-*2* and (+)-BP 7,8-diol-9,10-epoxide-*1* were found bound to DNA, RNA, and protein of skin after topical application of BP to the backs of C57BL/6J mice (Koreeda et al., in press; More et al., 1977; Yagi et al., 1977). The relative amounts of the two diol epoxides bound depended on whether binding to DNA, RNA, or protein was measured, but in all cases the amount of (+)-BP 7,8-diol-9,10-epoxide-2 that was bound was greater than the amount of (+)-BP

Table 4

METABOLISM OF OPTICALLY PURE ENANTIOMERS OF BP-7,8-DIHYDRODIOL

SUBSTRATE	PRODUCTS FORMED	% OF TOTAL METABOLITES FORMED		
		CONTROL MICROSOMES	PHENOBARBITAL MICROSOMES	3-METHYLCHOLANTHRENE MICROSOMES
(−)-BP 7,8-dihydrodiol	(−)-diol epoxide 1	24	20	13
	(+)-diol epoxide 2	53	51	83
(+)-BP 7,8-dihydrodiol	(+)-diol epoxide 1	58	54	90
	(−)-diol epoxide 2	10	12	4

7,8-diol-9,10-epoxide-*1*. Although the above studies demonstrated that most of the binding of the BP diol epoxides to nucleic acid occurred at the exocyclic 2-amino group of guanine, some occurred at the backbone phosphate oxygen (Koreeda et al., 1976), and this binding may be of high biological significance (Gamper et al., 1977). The metabolism of BP to diol epoxides and the structures of the two major guanine adducts of the BP diol epoxides that were isolated from mouse skin DNA and RNA after application of BP are shown in Fig. 2.

CARCINOGENICITY OF BENZO[A]PYRENE METABOLITES

Since not all mutagens are carcinogens, and since covalent binding of chemicals need not be accompanied by tumor formation, the identification of proximate and ultimate carcinogenic metabolites of BP can only come from carcinogenicity studies. These studies have been ongoing in our laboratories for the past several years. We have investigated the carcinogenic activities of four arene oxides of BP, all 12 possible isomeric phenols of BP, BP 7,8-dihydrodiol, BP 9,10-dihydrodiol, and the diastereomeric BP 7,8-diol-9,10-epoxides-*1* and *2*. In addition to our

161

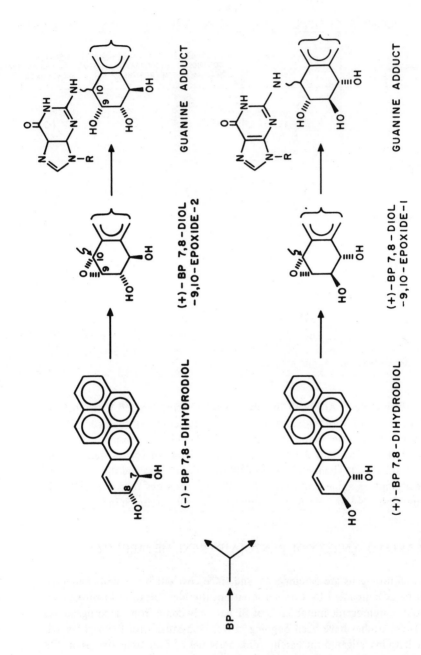

FIGURE 2

Metabolism of BP to diol-epoxides and their covalent binding to guanine in DNA and RNA. R = ribose in RNA and deoxyribose in DNA.

162

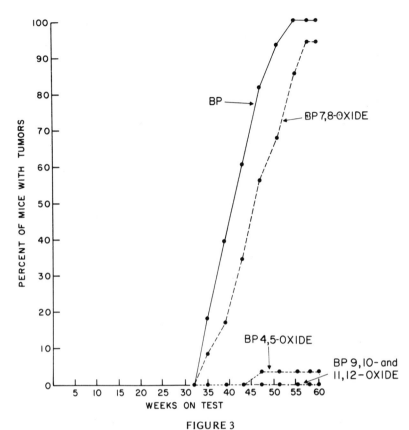

FIGURE 3

Carcinogenicity of BP arene oxides on the skin of female C57BL/6J mice. Compounds (0.4 μmole per application) were applied in 20 μl of acetone; NH₄OH 1000:1 once every two weeks for 60 weeks. Thirty mice were used in each experimental group. The percent of animals with tumors was calculated from surviving nontumor and tumor-bearing mice and from tumor-bearing mice that died during the 60 weeks of treatment.

studies with the above racemic compounds, we have also studied the carcinogenic activities of the optically pure (+)- and (−)-enantiomers of BP 7,8-dihydrodiol.

Carcinogenicity of BP Arene Oxides on Mouse Skin

Application of 0.4 μmole of BP every two weeks to the skin of C57BL/6J mice for 60 weeks resulted in a 100% tumor incidence after 55 weeks of treatment (Fig. 3) (Levin et al., 1976a). The first tumors were observed after 35 weeks of treatment. At equimolar doses, BP 9,10- and 11,12-oxide were inactive as carcinogens, and BP 4,5-oxide produced only one skin tumor among the 30 mice that were treated with the hydrocarbon for 60 weeks (Levin et al., 1976a;

163

Wislocki et al., 1977). BP 7,8-oxide was the most potent carcinogen of the four BP arene oxides and was only slightly less active than BP as a complete carcinogen at this dose (Fig. 3). As will be shown later, however, BP 7,8-oxide was significantly less carcinogenic than BP when a lower dose was used.

Histological examination revealed that most of the tumors in the treated animals were squamous-cell carcinomas. Since the stability of the arene oxides could be a determining factor in their ability to reach critical receptor sites within the cell, we have determined the stability of the BP arene oxides in 100 mM potassium phosphate buffer (pH 7.4) at 37°. BP 7,8-, 9,10-, and 11,12-oxides had half-lives of 30, 2, and 15 minutes, respectively, and BP 4,5-oxide showed less than 10% decomposition after incubation for 24 hr at 37° (Levin et al., 1976a; Wislocki et al., 1977). Thus, the very poor carcinogenic activity of BP 4,5-oxide and the relatively high carcinogenic activity of BP 7,8-oxide do not appear related to the stability of these arene oxides in aqueous solution.

Carcinogenicity of BP 7,8-Dihydrodiol on Mouse Skin

Although BP 7,8-oxide is a potent carcinogen on mouse skin, this compound only has very weak intrinsic mutagenicity in *S. typhimurium* and Chinese hamster V-79 cells (Table 1). It should be noted, however, that BP 7,8-oxide can be metabolically activated to potent mutagens by a combination of both epoxide hydrase and a monooxygenase system (Wood et al., 1976b). Presumably, the mutagenic products produced are BP 7,8-diol-9,10-epoxides which could be formed via hydration of BP 7,8-oxide to BP 7,8-dihydrodiol and subsequent oxidation of this dihydrodiol at the 9,10-position by the monooxygenase system. If this is the case, BP 7,8-dihydrodiol should be a more potent carcinogen than BP 7,8-oxide.

Figure 4 shows that application of 0.15 μmole of BP or BP 7,8-dihydrodiol to C57BL/6J mice once every two weeks for 60 weeks resulted in a tumor incidence of 100%, whereas only 20% of the mice treated with an equimolar amount of BP 7,8-oxide had skin tumors (Levin et al., 1976b). BP 7,8-dihydrodiol was at least equipotent to BP as a complete carcinogen at the dose tested, and other studies have shown that BP 7,8-dihydrodiol is a potent tumor initiator on mouse skin (Chouroulinkov et al., 1976; Slaga et al., 1976).

Results of other studies in our laboratories (Levin et al., 1977c) indicate that BP 7,8-dihydrodiol is slightly more active than BP as a complete carcinogen on mouse skin when tested at lower doses than shown in Figure 4. Seven,8-Epoxy-7,8,9,10-tetrahydro BP and 7,8-dihydroxy-7,8,9,10-tetrahydro BP, compounds related to BP 7,8-oxide and BP 7,8-dihydrodiol but with the double bond removed from the 9,10-position of the molecule, were completely inactive in eliciting tumors (Fig. 4). Seven,8-Epoxy-7,8,9,10-tetrahydro BP can be metabolized to 7,8-dihydroxy-7,8,9,10-tetrahydro BP by epoxide hydrase (Wood et al., 1976c), but this compound cannot be converted to the BP 7,8-diol-9,10-

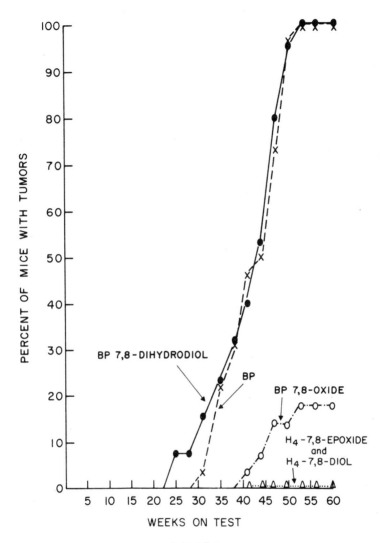

FIGURE 4

Skin tumors produced in C57BL/6J female mice treated topically with BP or benzo-ring derivatives of BP. The compounds (0.15 μmole per application) were applied once every two weeks for 60 weeks in 25 μl of acetone: NH$_4$OH (1000:1). Each treatment group originally consisted of 30 mice. H$_4$-7,8-epoxide and H$_4$-7,8-diol are 7,8-epoxy-7,8,9,10-tetrahydro BP and *trans*-7,8-dihydroxy-7,8,9,10-tetrahydro BP, respectively.

epoxides (Fig. 5). The lack of carcinogenicity of BP 7,8-oxide and BP 7,8-dihydrodiol when the 9,10-double bond has been saturated (i.e., 7,8-epoxy-and 7,8-dihydroxy-7,8,9,10-tetrahydro BP) suggests that the carcinogenicity of BP

165

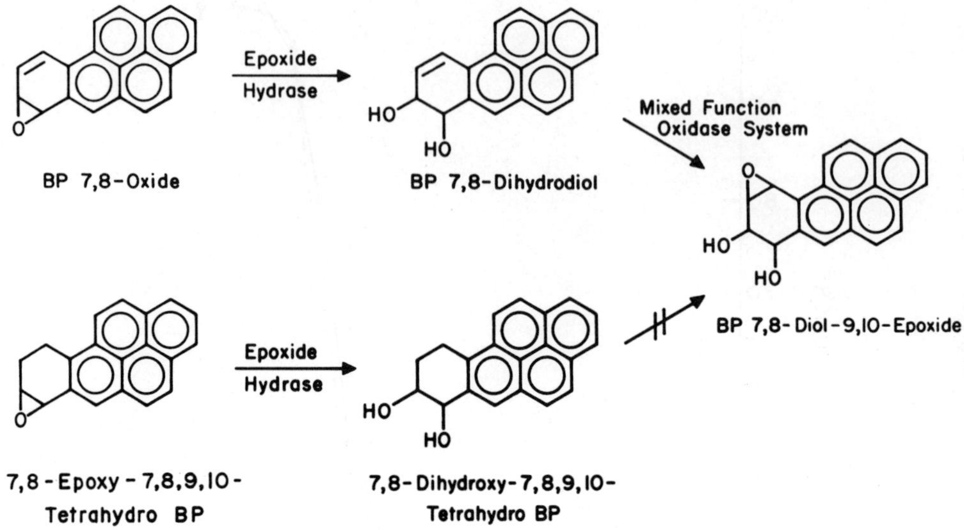

FIGURE 5

Metabolism of BP 7,8-oxide and 7,8-epoxy-7,8,9,10-tetrahydro BP by the microsomal monooxygenase system and epoxide hydrase.

7,8-oxide and BP 7,8-dihydrodiol is due to metabolic conversion of these compounds to one or more of the BP 7,8-diol-9,10-epoxides.

Differences in the Carcinogenicity of the Optically Pure (+)- and (−)-Enantiomers of BP 7,8-Dihydrodiol

Although considerable stereoselectivity exists in the metabolism of BP to the (+)- and (−)-enantiomers of BP 7,8-dihydrodiol (Table 3) and in the further metabolism of these compounds to the (+)- and (−)-enantiomers of BP 7,8-diol-9,10-epoxides-*1* and -*2* (Table 4), all of the above carcinogenicity studies, as well as those done in other laboratories, have been done with racemic derivatives or derivatives of unknown stereochemistry. Since the mutagenic activities of the (+)- and (−)-enantiomers of the BP 7,8-diol-9,10-epoxides were markedly different (Table 2), it seemed possible that the carcinogenic activities of the optically active enantiomers of the diol epoxides and the carcinogenic activities of the optically pure (+)- and (−)-enantiomers of BP 7,8-dihydrodiol might differ from one another. The ability of optically pure (+)- and (−)-BP 7,8-dihydrodiol to initiate skin tumors in a two-stage tumorigenesis model in mice was evaluated (Levin et al., 1977b), and the results are shown in Fig. 6. A single application of 100 nmole of BP, (+)-BP 7,8-dihydrodiol, or (−)-BP 7,8-dihydrodiol to the backs of mice, followed by twice weekly applications of 12-0-tetradecanoylphorbol-13-acetate, revealed that the (−)-enantiomer of BP 7,8-dihydrodiol was 5- to 10-fold more potent than the (+)-enantiomer as a tumor initiator. The (−)-enan-

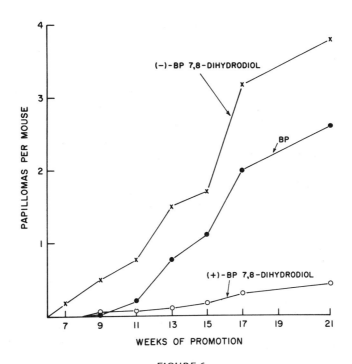

FIGURE 6

Papillomas produced on the skin of female CD-1 mice after a single initiating dose of 0.1 μmole of BP or (+)- and (−)-BP 7,8-dihydrodiol followed by twice weekly application of 16 nmole of 12-0 tetrade-canoylphorbol-13-acetate as a promoting agent. Each treatment group originally consisted of 30 mice.

tiomer was more potent than BP, whereas the (+)-enantiomer was considerably less active. Similar marked differences in the carcinogenicity of the (+)- and (−)-enantiomers of BP 7,8-dihydrodiol have been observed in newborn mice when pulmonary adenomas and malignant lymphomas were determined, (Kapitulnik et al., in prep.). These results are the first examples of differences in the carcinogenic activities of optically active enantiomers.

Carcinogenicity of the Diastereomeric
BP 7,8-Diol-9,10-Epoxides on Mouse Skin

The carcinogenic activities of the racemic BP 7,8-diol-9,10-epoxides-*1* and *2* on mouse skin are shown in Table 5. We found that BP 7,8-diol-9,10-epoxide-*1* was inactive as a complete carcinogen at all doses tested, while BP 7,8-diol-9,10-epoxide-*2* had weak activity compared to BP (Levin et al., 1977c). Slaga et al. (1976, 1977) recently reported that the diastereomeric BP 7,8-diol-9,10-epoxides are considerably less active than BP and BP 7,8-dihydrodiol as tumor initiators in

167

initiation-promotion experiments on mouse skin. Since the BP 7,8-diol-9,10-epoxides are extremely unstable compounds, their poor carcinogenic activity on mouse skin may be related to their short biological half-lives and/or their high reactivity. It is of considerable interest that racemic BP 7,8-diol-9,10-epoxides-*1* and *2* have strong activity for causing hypertrophy and hyperplasia in mouse skin when these compounds are applied topically (Table 6) (Bresnick et al., 1977).

Among the 12 phenolic BP derivatives tested, 2-HOBP and 9-HOBP also possessed strong hypertrophic and hyperplastic activity (Table 6). The strong hyperplastic activity and low carcinogenicity of the BP 7,8-diol-9,10-epoxides on mouse skin may mean that the compounds are not stable enough to reach critical cellular receptors for tumor initiation within the cell, but that they can interact with receptors on the cell surface that are important for cellular hyperplasia and hypertrophy. It is possible that other BP derivatives—perhaps in combination with the BP 7,8-diol-9,10-epoxides—may be ultimate carcinogenic metabolites of BP on mouse skin.

High Carcinogenicity of BP 7,8-Dihydrodiol and BP 7,8-diol-9,10-Epoxide-2 in Newborn Mice

Whenever possible, it is desirable to use several different tumor models to evaluate the carcinogenic potential of a series of compounds, since many factors—including

TABLE 5
CARCINOGENICITY OF BP AND BP 7,8-DIOL-9,10-EPOXIDES
ON MOUSE SKIN[a]

Compound	Dose every two weeks (μmole)	% of mice with tumors
Benzo[a]pyrene	0.40	100
	0.10	50
	0.02	4
BP 7,8-diol-9,10-epoxide-*1*	0.40	0
	0.10	0
	0.02	0
BP 7,8-diol-9,10-epoxide-2	0.40	13
	0.10	7
	0.02	0

[a]Thirty C57BL/6J female mice were painted with BP or the BP 7,8-diol-9,10-epoxides once every two weeks for 60 weeks. Compounds were dissolved in acetone:DMSO (3:1), and 50 μl was applied to the backs of the mice.

TABLE 6
EPIDERMAL HYPERPLASIA IN MOUSE SKIN AFTER TOPICAL
APPLICATION OF BENZO[A]PYRENE DERIVATIVES[a]

Compound	No. of nuclei per 61μ length	No. of layers (% increase)	Epidermal thickness (μ)
Benzo[a]pyrene	37	30	53
BP 7,8-diol-9,10-epoxide-1	128	160	402
BP 7,8-diol-9,10-epoxide-2	140	130	440
BP 7,8-dihydrodiol	29	0	38
BP 7,8-oxide	17	0	12
7,8-Epoxy-7,8,9,10-tetrahydro BP	18	0	45
2-HOBP	86	90	174
9-HOBP	142	100	282

[a]Female C57BL/6J mice were painted with BP derivatives (1.2 μmole) in 200 μl of solvent. The mice were killed four days later, and the skin was removed and processed for morphometric analysis. For each skin specimen, 50 evenly spaced, separate vision fields were analyzed. The values represent the average percent increase for four mice.

the age of the animal, the route of administration, absorption, distribution, and metabolism of the test chemical, and the susceptibility of a particular tissue to the carcinogen—all influence the carcinogenicity of the compound.

The newborn mouse is a useful model for carcinogenicity studies because of its high susceptibility to the effects of many chemical carcinogens (Della Porta & Terracini, 1969; Toth, 1968; Toth & Shubik, 1967). We found that 1400 nmole of racemic BP 7,8-dihydrodiol administered intraperitoneally to newborn mice during a two-week interval was more than 10 times as potent as an equimolar dose of BP in causing malignant lymphomas and pulmonary adenomas (Experiment 1, Table 7) (Kapitulnik et al., 1977). The two racemic BP 7,8-diol-9,10-epoxides-1 and 2 were highly toxic, and survival of the animals could be achieved only when 1/50 of the above dose of the diol epoxides was administered. Even with this low dose, the survival of animals treated with BP 7,8-diol-9,10-epoxide-1 was poor, whereas the low dose of BP 7,8-diol-9,10-epoxide-2 resulted in good survival. A quantitative comparison of pulmonary adenomas after a 1400-nmole dose of BP, a 1400-nmole dose of BP 7,8-dihydrodiol, and a 28-nmole dose of BP 7,8-diol-9,10-epoxide-2 suggested that BP 7,8-dihydrodiol and BP 7,8-diol-9,10-epoxide-2 were, respectively, approximately 12- and 40-fold more tumorigenic than BP (Experiment 1, Table 7). Because unequal doses of BP and BP 7,8-diol-9,10-epoxide-2 were tested in experiment 1, we compared the tumorigenicity of low equimolar doses (28 nmole) of BP, BP 7,8-dihydrodiol, BP 7,8-diol-9,10-epoxide-1, BP 7,8-diol-9,10-epoxide-2, and the tetraols which result from the spontaneous hydrolysis of BP 7,8-diol-9,10-epoxide-2 in aqueous medium (Experiment 2, Table 7).

TABLE 7
TUMORIGENICITY OF BENZO[A]PYRENE, BENZO[A]PYRENE
7,8-DIHYDRODIOL AND THE BENZO[A]PYRENE
7,8-DIOL-9,10-EPOXIDES IN NEWBORN MICE[a]

Experiment	Treatment	Total dose (nmole)	No. of animals autopsied	% of mice with malignant lymphomas	Lung adenomas per animal
1	Control	0	48	0	<0.1
	Benzo[a]pyrene	1400	45	0	6.3
	BP 7,8-dihydrodiol	1400	50	70	75.0
	BP 7,8-diol-9,10-epoxide-2	28	37	0	4.9
2	Control	0	67	0	0.13
	Benzo[a]pyrene	28	63	0	0.24
	BP 7,8-dihydrodiol	28	62	0	1.77
	BP 7,8-diol-9,10-epoxide-1	28	21	0	0.14
	BP 7,8-diol-9,10-epoxide-2	28	64	2	4.42
	Tetraols (from BP 7,8-diol-9,10-epoxide-2)	28	61	2	0.05

[a]Swiss-Webster mice were injected i.p. with one-seventh of the indicated total dose of the hydrocarbon on the first day of life, two-sevenths on the eight day, and four-sevenths on the fifteenth day. The study was terminated when the animals were 21-24 weeks old in Exp. 1 and at 28 weeks in Exp. 2

Animals treated with the very low dose of 28 nmole of BP had about twice as many pulmonary adenomas per mouse as animals treated with DMSO alone (Experiment 2, Table 7). BP 7,8-diol-9,10-epoxide-1 and the BP tetraols derived from BP 7,8-diol-9,10-epoxide-2 did not cause lung tumors, whereas BP 7,8-diol-9,10-epoxide-2 and BP 7,8-dihydrodiol were highly tumorigenic at the dose tested. After correcting for the small number of lung adenomas in control mice, the data in experiment 2 indicate that BP 7,8-dihydrodiol and BP 7,8-diol-9,10-epoxide-2 were, respectively, 15- and 39-fold more active than BP in causing pulmonary adenomas in newborn mice (Kapitulnik et al., 1978). One mouse treated with BP 7,8-diol-9,10-epoxide-2, and another mouse treated with the BP tetraols derived from BP 7,8-diol-9,10-epoxide-2, developed malignant lymphoma. The significance of this low incidence of malignant lymphoma in the hydrocarbon-treated animals is uncertain. The results described here indicate that BP 7,8-dihydrodiol is a proximate carcinogenic metabolite and that BP 7,8-diol-9,10-epoxide-2 is an ultimate carcinogenic metabolite of BP in the newborn mouse. Studies on the carcinogenic activities of the optically pure (+)- and (−)-enantiomers of BP 7,8-diol-9,10-epoxide-2 in the newborn mouse are in progress. The reason for the high carcinogenic activity of racemic BP 7,8-diol-9,10-epoxide-2 in newborn mice and the very weak activity of this compound on mouse skin is not known. These results dramatically illustrate the need for studies with several animal systems during the evaluation of the carcinogenic activity of chemicals.

Carcinogenicity of the Twelve Isomeric BP Phenols on Mouse Skin

A comparison of the carcinogenic potency of BP with that of its 12 possible isomeric phenols (Kapitulnik et al., 1976; Wislocki et al., 1977) revealed that only 2- and 11-HOBP were complete carcinogens on mouse skin (Fig. 7). 2-HOBP was equipotent to BP in causing skin tumors; 11-HOBP was weakly active, and 1-, 3-, 4-, 5-, 6-, 7-, 8-, 9-, 10- and 12-HOBP were inactive when 0.4 μmole of each compound was applied to mouse skin once every two weeks for 60 weeks. All of the mice treated with BP or 2-HOBP had tumors after 53 weeks of treatment. Further studies with lower doses of 2-HOBP and BP indicate that 2-HOBP is less

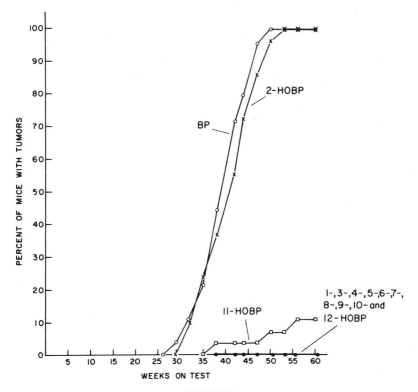

FIGURE 7

Skin tumors produced in C57BL/6J female mice treated topically with BP or BP phenols. Compounds (0.4 μmole per application) were applied once every two weeks for 60 weeks in 25 μl of acetone. Each treatment group originally consisted of 30 mice.

carcinogenic than BP on mouse skin, but that 2-HOBP is more active than BP in causing pulmonary adenomas in the newborn mouse (Chang et al., in prep.; Wislocki et al., in prep.). 2-HOBP is the first example of a phenolic polycyclic aromatic hydrocarbon with strong carcinogenic activity. Additional studies are needed to determine whether 2-HOBP is a metabolite of BP and whether or not this compound plays a role in BP carcinogenesis. The lack of carcinogenic activity of 7- and 8-HOBP indicates that the strong carcinogenic activity of BP 7,8-oxide is not due to either of its phenolic isomerization products. Recent studies with the twelve isomeric BP phenols have indicated that only 2-HOBP has strong tumor-initiating activity (Slaga et al., 1978).

THE BAY REGION THEORY OF POLYCYCLIC HYDROCARBON CARCINOGENESIS

In an attempt to correlate the structures of polycyclic hydrocarbons with their carcinogenic activities, the literature was surveyed to determine the effects of halogen or alkyl substituents on carcinogenic activity, and it was found that substituents on angular benzo rings of polycyclic hydrocarbons reduce carcinogenic activity, presumably through blocking metabolism at that portion of the molecule (Jerina & Daly, 1976a). Furthermore, perturbational molecular orbital calculations for a number of polycyclic hydrocarbons predicted that benzylic carbonium ions derived from epoxides on an angular tetrahydrobenzo ring of carcinogenic hydrocarbons would have an unusual ease of formation when the carbonium ion is located in the bay region of the hydrocarbon (Jerina et al., 1976b). The prototype of a bay region in a polycyclic hydrocarbon is the sterically hindered region between C_4 and C_5 of phenanthrene. Examples of bay regions and bay region diol epoxides of polycyclic hydrocarbons are given in Fig. 8. In accord with the bay region concept, 9,10-epoxy-7,8,9,10-tetrahydro BP, with the benzylic carbon atom of the oxirane ring in the bay region of the hydrocarbon, is far more mutagenic than the isomeric 7,8-epoxy-7,8,9,-10-tetrahydro BP (Wood et al., 1976c) (Table 1), in which the oxirane ring is remote from the bay region. In addition, the BP 7,8-diol-9,10-epoxides are much more mutagenic than BP 7,10-diol-8,9-epoxide or the BP 9,10-diol-7,8-epoxides (Thakker et al., 1978b) (Table 1).

Studies with the hydrocarbon benzo[a]anthracene (BA) were initiated as a test of the bay region theory. Even though BA is a weak carcinogen, perturbational molecular orbital calculations indicated an unusual ease of carbonium ion formation (at the bay region 1-position) for the BA 3,4-diol-1,2-epoxides, when compared with other BA diol epoxides (Jerina et al., 1976b, 1978). Wood et al. (1976a) evaluated the metabolic activation of the five metabolically possible *trans* dihydrodiols of BA to mutagens. The structures of these compounds are given in Fig. 9. Our prediction that among the several dihydrodiols of BA the BA 3,4-dihydrodiol should be metabolically activated to the most mutagenic

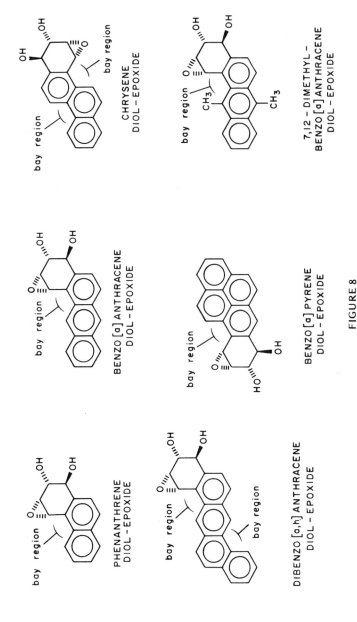

CHRYSENE
DIOL – EPOXIDE
bay region

7,12 – DIMETHYL –
BENZO [a] ANTHRACENE
DIOL – EPOXIDE
bay region
CH_3
CH_3

BENZO [a] ANTHRACENE
DIOL – EPOXIDE
bay region

BENZO [a] PYRENE
DIOL – EPOXIDE
bay region

PHENANTHRENE
DIOL – EPOXIDE
bay region

DIBENZO [a,h] ANTHRACENE
DIOL – EPOXIDE
bay region
bay region

FIGURE 8

Structures of bay region diol epoxides (isomer 2 series shown) of polycyclic hydrocarbons.

173

metabolite (presumably one or more of the BA 3,4-diol-1,2-epoxides) was confirmed. BA 3,4-dihydrodiol was metabolized by a highly purified monooxygenase system to products which are at least ten times more mutagenic to *Salmonella typhimurium* strain TA 100 than are the metabolites of BA or the other four metabolically possible *trans* dihydrodiols of BA (Fig. 10).

In addition, Wood et al. (1977a) examined the mutagenic and cytotoxic activities of several diol epoxides and tetrahydro-epoxides of BA. The structures of these compounds are indicated in Fig. 11. As anticipated, the bay region BA 3,4-diol-1,2-epoxides were manyfold more mutagenic than the BA 8,9-diol-10, 11-epoxides or the BA 10,11-diol-8,9-epoxides (Table 8). In addition, the bay region 1,2-epoxy-1,2,3,4-tetrahydro BA was considerably more mutagenic than the 3,4-epoxy-1,2,3,4-tetrahydro BA (Table 8). In accord with observations on the mutagenic activity of the BA derivatives, Wood et al. (1977c) found that BA 3,4-dihydrodiol was at least 10 times more tumorigenic than BA or the 1,2-, 5,6-, 8,9-, or 10,11-dihydrodiols of BA on mouse skin (Fig. 12). In addition, BA 3,4-dihydrodiol is at least 30-fold more active than BA or the other metabolically

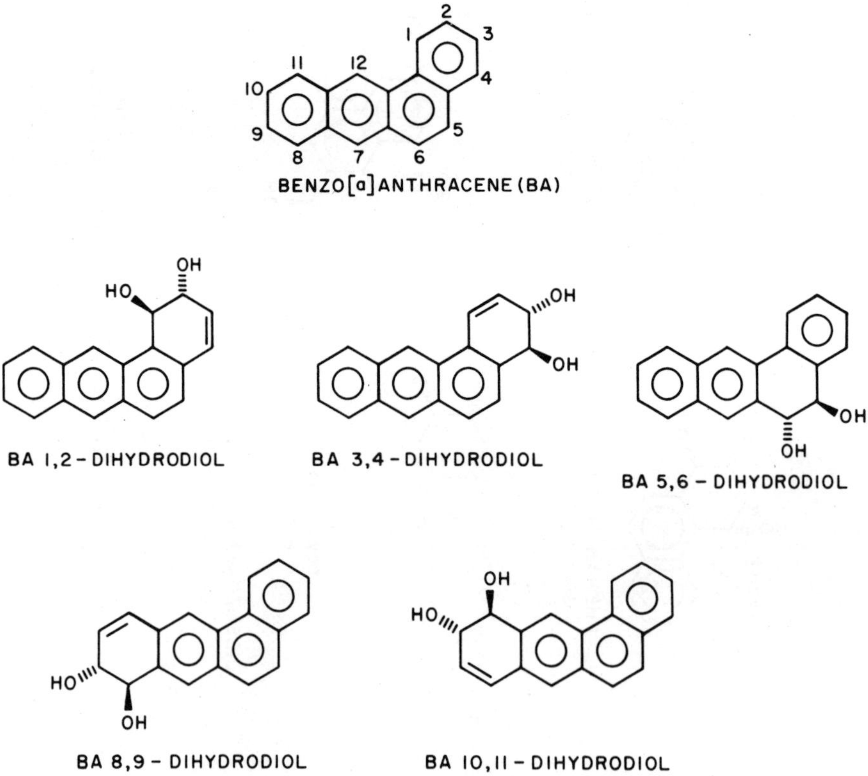

BENZO[a]ANTHRACENE (BA)

BA 1,2 – DIHYDRODIOL   BA 3,4 – DIHYDRODIOL

BA 5,6 – DIHYDRODIOL

BA 8,9 – DIHYDRODIOL   BA 10,11 – DIHYDRODIOL

FIGURE 9
Structures of metabolically possible dihydrodiols of benzo[a]anthracene.

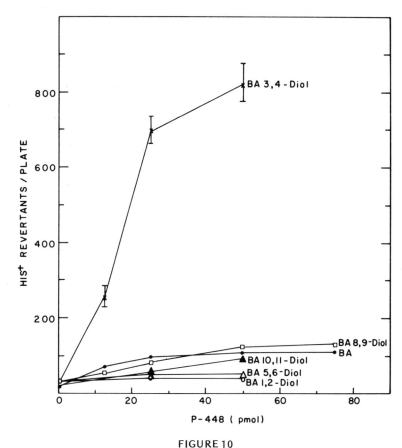

FIGURE 10

Ability of a purified and reconstituted monooxygenase system from rat liver microsomes to activate benzo[a]anthracene and dihydrodiols of benzo[a]anthracene to compounds which are mutagenic toward *S. typhimurium* strain TA 100.

possible BA dihydrodiols in causing pulmonary adenomas and malignant lymphomas in newborn mice (Wislocki et al., 1978).

Recent studies have indicated exceptionally high tumorigenic activity for the BA 3,4-diol-1,2-epoxides on mouse skin (Levin et al., ms. submitted for publ.). These studies indicate that the BA bay region diol-epoxides are ultimate carcinogens. Evidence was recently obtained indicating that 7-methyl-BA (Malaveille et al., 1977b; Marquardt et al., 1977), chrysene (Wood et al., 1977d), 7,12-dimethyl BA (Moschel et al., 1977), 3-methylcholanthrene (King et al., 1977; Thakker et al., 1978a; Vigny et al., 1977), and dibenzo[a,h]anthracene (Wood et al., ms. submitted for publ.) undergo metabolism to reactive intermediates at the bay region. Additional studies with other hydrocarbons are in progress to determine the general validity of the bay region theory of polycyclic hydrocarbon carcinogenesis.

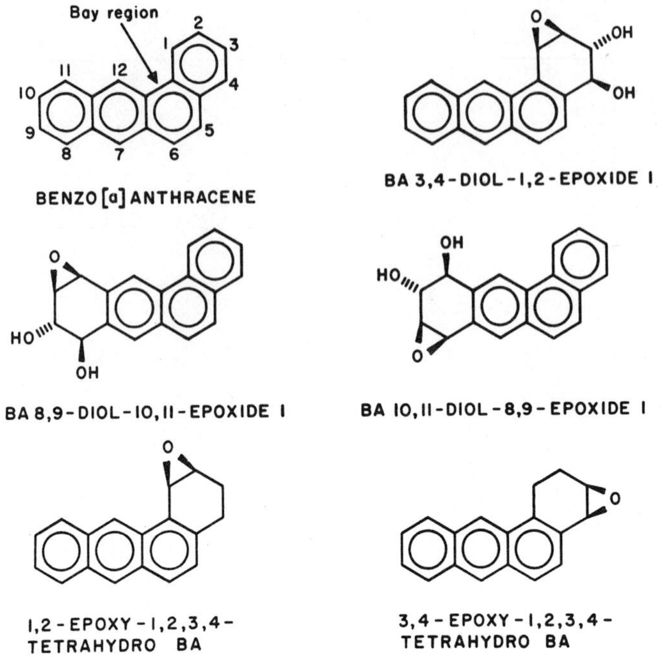

FIGURE 11

Structures of some diol epoxides and tetrahydroepoxides of benzo[a] anthracene.

TABLE 8

MUTAGENICITY OF BENZO[A] ANTHRACENE DIOL EPOXIDES AND
TETRAHYDRO EPOXIDES IN BACTERIAL AND MAMMALIAN CELLS

	Mutation frequency	
Compound[a]	S. typhimurium TA 100[b]	Chinese hamster V79 cells [c]
BA 3,4-diol-1,2-epoxide		
Isomer 1	1650	8.5
Isomer 2	850	10.9
BA 8,9-diol-10,11-epoxide		
Isomer 1	16	0.06
Isomer 2	50	0.10
BA 10,11-diol-8,9-epoxide		
Isomer 1	6	0.03
Isomer 2	55	0.21
1,2-Epoxy-1,2,3,4-tetrahydro BA	2300	26
3,4-Epoxy-1,2,3,4-tetrahydro BA	460	1.0
BA 5,6-oxide	100	0.2
BP 7,8-diol-9,10-epoxide		
Isomer 2	8800	120

[a] In isomer 1, the benzylic hydroxyl group is *cis* to the expoxide oxygen (Fig. 11). In isomer 2, the benzylic hydroxyl group is *trans* to the epoxide oxygen. All diol-epoxides used in this study were racemic.

[b] Histidine revertants/nmole/plate.

[c] 8-Azaguanine-resistant colonies/nmole/10^5 surviving cells.

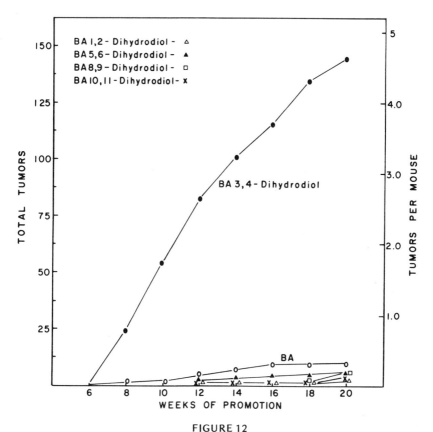

FIGURE 12

Papillomas produced on the skin of female CD-1 mice after a single initiating dose of 2 μmole of benzo[a]anthracene or the *trans*-dihydrodiols of benzo[a]anthracene followed by twice weekly application of 16 nmole of 12-0-tetradecanoylphorbol-13-acetate as a promoting agent. Each treatment group originally consisted of 30 mice.

CONCLUDING REMARKS

We have described how benzo[a]pyrene and other polycyclic aromatic hydrocarbons undergo metabolism to reactive intermediates that are highly mutagenic and carcinogenic. By knowing how polycyclic hydrocarbons and other environmental carcinogens are metabolized, it should be possible to devise ways of measuring the ability of different individuals in our population to detoxify and to activate these chemicals. Such studies would allow us to identify high risk individuals in our population. In addition, it may be possible to give suitable enzyme inducers or inhibitors that enhance the detoxification or block the activation of chemical carcinogens. Finally, the design of safe nucleophiles that

177

would react with and inactivate reactive ultimate carcinogenic metabolites is an important area for future research. Thus, it may some day be possible to prevent human cancer by administration of a suitable nucleophile or by modulating the metabolism of environmental carcinogens.

ACKNOWLEDGMENT

We thank Mrs. MaryAnn Augustin for her excellent help in the preparation of this manuscript.

REFERENCES

Ames, B. N., Durston, W. E., Yamasaki, E., & Lee, F. D. Carcinogens are mutagens: A simple test system combining liver homogenates for activation and bacteria for detection. *Proc. Natl. Acad. Sci. U.S.*, 1973(a), *70*, 2281-2285.

Ames, B. N., Lee, F. D., & Durston, W. E. An improved bacterial test system for the detection and classification of mutagens and carcinogens. *Proc. Natl. Acad. Sci. U.S.*, 1973(b), *70*, 782-786.

Baird, W. M., & Diamond, L. The nature of benzo(a)pyrene-DNA adducts formed in hamster embryo cells depends on the length of time of exposure to benzo(a)pyrene. *Biochem. Biophys. Res. Comm.*, 1977, *77*, 162-167.

Borgen, A., Darvey, H., Castagnoli, N., Crocker, T. T., Rasmussen, R. E., & Wang, I. Y. Metabolic conversion of benzo[a]pyrene by Syrian hamster liver microsomes and binding of metabolites to DNA. *J. Med. Chem.*, 1973, *16*, 502-506.

Bresnick, E., McDonald, F., Yagi, H., Jerina, D. M., Levin, W., Wood, A. W., & Conney, A. H. Epidermal hyperplasia after topical application of benzo[a]pyrene, benzo[a]-pyrene diol epoxides, and other metabolites. *Cancer Res.*, 1977, *37*, 984-990.

Chang, R. L., Wood, A. W., Levin, W., Yagi, H., Thakker, D. R., Mah, H. D., Jerina, D. M., and Conney, A. H., in preparation.

Chouroulinkov, I., Gentil, A., Grover, P. L., & Sims, P. Tumor-initiating activities on mouse skin of dihydrodiols derived from benzo[a]pyrene. *Brit. J. Cancer*, 1976, *34*, 523-532.

Chu, E. H. Y., & Malling, M. V. Mammalian cell genetics. II. Chemical induction of specific locus mutations in Chinese hamster cells in vitro. *Proc. Natl. Acad. Sci. U.S.*, 1968, *61*, 1306-1312.

Committee on the Biological Effects of Atmospheric Pollutants. *Particulate polycyclic organic matter*. Washington, D.C.: National Academy of Sciences, 1972.

Conney, A. H., Miller, E. C., & Miller, J. A. Substrate-induced synthesis and other properties of benzpyrene hydroxylase in rat liver. *J. Biol. Chem.*, 1957, *228*, 753-766.

Conney, A. H., Wood, A. W., Levin, W., Lu, A. Y. H., Chang, R. L., Wislocki, P. G., Holder, G. M., Dansette, P. M., Yagi, H., & Jerina, D. M. Metabolism and biological activity of benzo[a]pyrene and its metabolic products. In D. Jallow, J. Kocsis, R. Snyder, & H. Vainio (Eds.), *Reactive intermediates: Formation, toxicity and inactivation*. New York: Plenum Press, 1977, pp. 335-356.

Della Porta, G., & Terracini, B. Chemical carcinogenesis in infant animals. In F. Homburger (Ed.), *Progress in experimental tumor research*, Basel, Switzerland: S. Karger, 1969, pp. 334-363.

Gamper, H. B., Tung, A. C., Straub, K., Bartholomew, J. C., & Calvin, M. DNA strand scission by benzo[a]pyrene diol epoxides. *Science,* 1977, *197,* 671-674.

Gelboin, H. V. A microsome-dependent binding of benzo[a]pyrene to DNA. *Cancer Res.,* 1969, *29,* 1272-1276.

Gelboin, H. V., Kinoshita, N., & Wiebel, F. J. Microsomal hydroxylases: Induction and role in polycyclic hydrocarbon carcinogenesis and toxicity. *Fed. Proc.,* 1972, *31,* 1298-1309.

Grover, P. L., & Sims, P. Enzyme-catalysed reactions of polycyclic hydrocarbons with deoxyribonucleic acid and protein in vitro. *Biochem. J.,* 1968, *110,* 159-160.

Huberman, E., & Sachs, L. Cell-mediated mutagenesis of mammalian cells with chemical carcinogens. *Int. J. Cancer,* 1974, *13,* 326-333.

Huberman, E., Sachs, L., Yang, S. K., & Gelboin, H. V. Identification of mutagenic metabolites of benzo[a]pyrene in mammalian cells. *Proc. Natl. Acad. Sci. U.S.,* 1976, *73,* 607-611.

Jeffrey, A. M., Jennette, K. W., Blobstein, S. H., Weinstein, I. B., Beland, F. A., Harvey, R. G., Kasai, H., Miura, I., & Nakanishi, K. Benzo[a]pyrene-nucleic acid derivative found in vivo: Structure of a benzo[a]pyrenetetrahydrodiol epoxide-guanosine adduct. *J. Am. Chem. Soc.,* 1976, *98,* 5714-5715.

Jerina, D. M., & Daly, J. W. Oxidation at carbon. In D. V. Parke & R. L. Smith (Eds.), *Drug metabolism.* London: Taylor & Francis, 1976, Pp. 15-33.

Jerina, D. M., Lehr, R., Schaefer-Ridder, M., Yagi, H., Karle, J. M., Thakker, D. R., Wood, A. W., Lu, A. Y. H., Ryan, D., West, S., Levin, W., & Conney, A. H. Bay region epoxides of dihydrodiols: A concept which may explain the mutagenic and carcinogenic activity of benzo[a]pyrene and benzo[a]anthracene. In H. H. Hiatt, J. D. Watson, & J. A. Winsten (Eds.), *Origins of human cancer.* New York: Cold Spring Harbor, 1977. Pp. 638-658.

Jerina, D. M., Lehr, R. E., Yagi, H., Hernandez, O., Dansette, P.M., Wislocki, P. G., Wood, A. W., Chang, R. L., Levin, W., & Conney, A. H. Mutagenicity of benzo[a]pyrene derivatives and the description of a quantum mechanical model which predicts the ease of carbonium ion formation from diol epoxides. In F. J. deSerres, J. R. Fouts, J. R. Bend, & R. M. Philpot (Eds.), In vitro metabolic activation in mutagenesis testing. Amsterdam: Elsevier North-Holland Biomedical Press, 1976. Pp. 159-177.

Jerina, D. M., Thakker, D. H., Yagi, H., Levin, W., Wood, A. W., & Conney, A. H. Carcinogenicity of benzo[a]pyrene derivatives: The bay region theory. *Proc. 26th IUPAC Congress, Pure & Applied Chemistry,* Tokyo, 1978, in press.

Jerina, D. M., Yagi, H., Hernandez, O., Dansette, P. M., Wood, A. W., Levin, W., Chang, R. L., Wislocki, P. G., & Conney, A. H. Synthesis and biological activity of potential benzo[a]pyrene metabolites. In R. I. Freudenthal, & P. W. Jones (Eds.), *Polynuclear aromatic hydrocarbons: Chemistry, metabolism, and carcinogenicity (Volume 1).* New York: Raven Press, 1976(c). Pp. 91-113.

Kapitulnik, J., Levin, W., Conney, A. H., Yagi, H., & Jerina, D. M. Benzo[a]pyrene 7,8-dihydrodiol is more carcinogenic than benzo[a]pyrene in newborn mice. *Nature,* 1977, *266,* 378-380.

Kapitulnik, J., Levin, W., Yagi, H., Jerina, D. M., & Conney, A. H. Lack of carcinogenicity of 4-,5-,6-,7-,8-,9-, and 10-hydrobenzo[a]pyrene on mouse skin. *Cancer Res.,* 1976, *36,* 3625-3628.

Kapitulnik, J., Wislocki, P. G., Levin, W., Yagi, H., Jerina, D. M., & Conney, A. H. Tumorigenicity studies with diol-epoxides of benzo[a]pyrene which indicate that (±)-trans-7β,8α-dihydroxy-9α,10α-epoxy-7,8,9,10-tetrahydrobenzo[a]pyrene is an ·ultimate carcinogen in newborn mice. *Cancer Res.,* 1978, *38,* 354-358.

Kapitulnik, J., Wislocki, P., Levin, W., Yagi, H., Thakker, D. R., Akagi, H., Koreeda, M., Jerina, D. M., & Conney, A. H., in preparation.

King, H. W. S., Osborne, M. R., Beland, F. A., Harvey, R. G., & Brookes, P. (±)-7α,8β-Dihydroxy-9β,10β-epoxy-7,8,9,10-tetrahydrobenzo[a]pyrene is an intermediate in the metabolism and binding to DNA of benzo[a]pyrene. *Proc. Natl. Acad. Sci. U.S.A.*, 1976, *73*, 2679-2681.

King, H. W. S., Osborne, M. R., and Brookes, P. The metabolism and DNA binding of 3-methylcholanthrene. *Int. J. Cancer*, 1977, *20*, 564-571.

Koreeda, M., Moore, P. D., Wislocki, P. G., Levin, W., Conney, A. H., Yagi, H., & Jerina, D. M. Binding of benzo[a]pyrene 7,8-diol-9,10-epoxides to DNA, RNA and protein of mouse skin occurs with high stereoselectivity. *Science*, 1978, *199*, 778-781.

Koreeda, M., Moore, P. D., Yagi, H., Yeh, H. J. C., & Jerina, D. M. Alkylation of poly-guanylic acid at the 2-amino group and phosphate by the potent mutagen (±)-*trans*-7β,8α-dihydroxy-9β,10β-epoxy-7,8,9,10-tetrahydrobenzo[a]pyrene. *J. Am. Chem. Soc.*, 1976, *98*, 6720-6722.

Levin, W., Lu, A. Y. H., Ryan, D., Wood, A. W., Kapitulnik, J., West, S., Huang, M.-T., Conney, A. H. Properties of the liver microsomal monooxygenase system and epoxide hydrase: Factors influencing the metabolism and mutagenicity of benzo[a]pyrene. In H. H. Hiatt, J. D. Watson, & J. A. Winsten (Eds.), *Origins of human cancer.* Cold Spring Harbor, N.Y.: Cold Spring Harbor Laboratory, 1977(a). Pp. 659-682.

Levin, W., Thakker, D. R., Wood, A. W., Chang, R. L., Lehr, R. E., Jerina, D. M., & Conney, A. H., manuscript submitted for publication.

Levin, W., Wood, A. W., Chang, R. L., Slaga, T. J., Yagi, H., Jerina, D. M., & Conney, A. H. Marked differences in the tumor-initiating activity of optically pure (+)- and (−)-*trans*-7,8-dihydroxy-7,8-dihydrobenzo[a]pyrene on mouse skin. *Cancer Res.*, 1977(b), *37*, 2721-2725.

Levin, W., Wood, A. W., Wislocki, P. G., Kapitulnik, J., Yagi, H., Jerina, D. M., & Conney, A. H. Carcinogenicity of benzo-ring derivatives of benzo[a]pyrene on mouse skin. *Cancer Res.*, 1977(c), *37*, 3356-3361.

Levin, W., Wood, A. W., Yagi, H., Dansette, P. M., Jerina, D. M., & Conney, A. H. Carcinogenicity of benzo[a]pyrene 4,5-, 7,8-, and 9,10-oxides on mouse skin. *Proc. Natl. Acad. Sci. U.S.A.*, 1976(a), *73*, 243-247.

Levin, W., Wood, A. W., Yagi, H., Jerina, D. M., & Conney, A. H. (±)-*trans*-7,8-Dihydroxy-7,8-dihydrobenzo[a]pyrene: A potent skin carcinogen when applied topically to mice. *Proc. Natl. Acad. Sci. U.S.A.*, 1976(b), *73*, 3867-3871.

Malaveille, C., Bartsch, H., Grover, P. L., & Sims, P. Mutagenicity of non-K-region diols and diol-epoxides of benzo(a)anthracene and benzo(a)pyrene. *Biochem. Biophys. Res. Comm.*, 1975, *66*, 693-700.

Malaveille, C., Kuroki, T., Sims, P., Grover, P. L., & Bartsch, H. Mutagenicity of isomeric diol epoxides of benzo[a]pyrene and benz[a]anthracene in *S. typhimurium* TA 98 and TA 100 and in V79 Chinese hamster cells. *Mutation Res.*, 1977(a), *44*, 313-326.

Malaveille, C., Tierney, B., Grover, P. L., Sims, P., & Bartsch, H. High microsome-mediated mutagenicity of the 3,4-dihydrodiol of 7-methylbenz[a]-anthracene in *S. typhimurium* TA 98. *Biochem. Biophys. Res. Comm.*, 1977(b), *75*, 427-433.

Marquardt, H., Baker, S., Tierney, B., Grover, P. L., & Sims, P. The metabolic activation of 7-methylbenz(a)anthracene: The induction of malignant transformation and mutation in mammalian cells by non K-region dihydrodiols. *Int. J. Cancer*, 1977, *19*, 828-833.

Miller, E. C. Studies on the formation of protein-bound derivatives of 3,4-benzpyrene in the epidermal fraction of mouse skin. *Cancer Res.*, 1951, *11*, 100-108.

Miller, E. C., & Miller, J. A. The presence and significance of bound aminoazo dyes in the livers of rats fed p-dimethylaminoazobenzene. Cancer Res., 1947, 7, 468-480.

Miller, E. C., & Miller, J. A. Biochemical mechanisms of chemical carcinogenesis. In H. Busch (Ed.), *Molecular biology of cancer.* New York: Academic Press, 1974. Pp. 377-402.

Miller, J. A. Carcinogenesis by chemicals: An overview (G.H.A. Clowes Memorial Lecture). *Cancer Res.,* 1970, 30, 559-576.

Miller, J. A. Carcinogen activation and inactivation as keys to species and tissue differences in response. Proc. Conf. on Human Epidemiology and Animal Laboratory Correlations in Chemical Carcinogenesis, June, 1977, Mescalero, New Mexico, in press.

Moore, P. D., Koreeda, M., Wislocki, P. G., Levin, W., Conney, A. H., Yagi, H., & Jerina, D. M. In vitro reactions of the diastereomeric 9,10-epoxides of (+)- and (−)-*trans*-7,8-dihydroxy-7,8-dihydrobenzo[a]pyrene with polyguanylic acid and evidence for formation of an enantiomer of each diastereomeric 9,10-epoxide from benzo[a]pyrene in mouse skin. In D. M. Jerina (Ed.), *Drug metabolism and concepts, ACS Symposium Series No. 44.* Washington D.C.: American Chemical Society, 1977. Pp. 127-154.

Moschel, R. C., Baird, W. M., & Dipple, A. Metabolic activation of the carcinogen 7,12-dimethylbenz[a]anthracene for DNA binding. *Biochem. Biophys. Res. Comm.,* 1977, 76, 1092-1098.

Nakanishi, K., Kasai, H., Cho, H., Harvey, R. G., Jeffrey, A. M., Jennette, K. W., & Weinstein, I. B. Absolute configuration of a ribonucleic acid adduct formed in vivo by metabolism of benzo[a]pyrene. *J. Am. Chem. Soc.,* 1977, 99, 258-260.

Newbold, R. F., & Brookes, P. Exceptional mutagenicity of benzo[a]pyrene diol epoxide in cultured mammalian cells. *Nature,* 1976, 261, 52-54.

Remsen, J., Jerina, D. M., Yagi, H., & Cerutti, P. In vitro reactions of radioactive 7β,8α-dihydroxy-9α,10α-epoxy-7,8,9,10-tetrahydrobenzo[a]pyrene with DNA. *Biochem. Biophys. Res. Comm.,* 1977, 74, 934-940.

Sims, P., Grover, P. L., Swaisland, A., Pal, K., & Hewer, A. Metabolic activation of benzo[a]pyrene proceeds by a diol-epoxide. *Nature,* 1974, 252, 326-328.

Slaga, T. J., Bracken, W. M., Dresner, S., Levin, W., Yagi, H., Jerina, D. M., & Conney, A. H. Skin tumor-initiating activities of the isomeric phenols of benzo[a]pyrene. *Cancer Res.,* 1978, 38, 678-681.

Slaga, T. J., Bracken, W. M., Viaje, A., Levin, W., Yagi, H., Jerina, D. M., & Conney, A. H. Comparison of the tumor-initiating activities of benzo(a)pyrene arene oxides and diol epoxides. *Cancer Res.,* 1977, 37, 4130-4133.

Slaga, T. J., Viaje, A., Berry, D. L., & Bracken, W. Skin tumor-initiating the ability of benzo[a]pyrene 4,5-, 7,8-, and 7,8-diol-9,10-epoxides and 7,8-diol. *Cancer Letters,* 1976, 2, 115-122.

Thakker, D. R., Levin, W., Wood, A. W., Conney, A. H., Stoming, T. A., & Jerina, D. M. Metabolic formation of 1,9,10-trihydroxy-9,10-dihydro-3-methylcholanthrene: A potential proximate carcinogen from 3-methylcholanthrene. *J. Am. Chem. Soc.,* 1978(a), 100, 645-647.

Thakker, D. R., Yagi, H., Akagi, H., Koreeda, M., Lu, A. Y. H., Levin, W., Wood, A. W., Conney, A. H., & Jerina, D. M. Metabolism of benzo(a)pyrene. VI. Stereoselective metabolism of benzo(a)pyrene and benzo(a)pyrene 7,8-dihydrodiol to diol epoxides. *Chem.-Biol. Interactions,* 1977(a), 16, 281-300.

Thakker, D. R., Yagi, H., Lehr, R. E., Levin, W., Buening, M., Lu, A. Y. H., Chang, R. L., Wood, A. W., Conney, A. H., & Jerina, D. M. Metabolism of *trans*-9,10-dihydroxy-9,10-dihydrobenzo[a]pyrene occurs primarily by aryl hydroxylation rather than formation of a diol epoxide. *Mol. Pharmacol.,* 1978(b). 14, 502-513.

Thakker, D. R., Yagi, H., Levin, W., Lu, A. Y. H., Conney, A. H., & Jerina, D. M. Stereo-specificity of microsomal and purified epoxide hydrase from rat liver: Hydration of arene oxides of polycyclic hydrocarbons. *J. Biol. Chem.*, 1977(b), *252*, 6328-6334.

Thakker, D. R., Yagi, H., Lu, A. Y. H., Levin, W., Conney, A. H., & Jerina, D. M. Metabolism of benzo(a)pyrene. IV. Conversion of (±)-*trans*-7,8-dihydroxy-7,8-dihydro-benzo(a)-yrene to the highly mutagenic 7,8-diol-9,10-epoxides. *Proc. Natl. Acad. Sci. U.S.A.*, 1976, *73*, 3381-3385.

Toth, B. A critical review of experiments in chemical carcinogenesis using newborn animals. *Cancer Res.*, 1968, *28*, 727-738.

Toth, B., & Shubik, P. Carcinogenesis in AKR mice injected at birth with benzo[a]pyrene and dimethylnitrosamine. Cancer Res., *1967, 27*, 43-51.

Vigny, P., Duquesne, M., Coulomb, H., Tierney, B., Grover, P. L., & Sims, P. Fluorescence spectral studies on the metabolic activation of 3-methylcholanthrene and 7,12-dimethylbenz[a]anthracene in mouse skin. *FEBS Letters*, 1977, *82*, 278-282.

Weinstein, I. B., Jeffrey, A. M., Jennette, K. W., Blobstein, S. H., Harvey, R. G., Harris, C., Autrup, H., Kasai, H., & Nakanishi, K. Benzo[a]pyrene diol epoxides as intermediates in nucleic acid binding in vitro and in vivo. *Science*, 1976, *193*, 592-595.

Whalen, D. L., Montemarano, J. A., Thakker, D. R., Yagi, H., Jerina, D. M. Changes of mechanism and product distribution in the hydrolysis of benzo[a]pyrene 7,8-diol-9,10-epoxide metabolites induced by changes in pH. *J. Am. Chem. Soc.*, 1977, *99*, 5522-5524.

Wislocki, P. G., Chang, R. L., Wood, A. W., Levin, W., Yagi, H., Hernandez, O., Mah, H. D., Dansette, P. M., Jerina, D. M., & Conney, A. H. High carcinogenicity of 2-hydroxybenzo[a]pyrene on mouse skin. *Cancer Res.*, 1977, *37*, 2608-2611.

Wislocki, P. G., Kapitulnik, J., Levin, W., Lehr, R., Schaefer-Ridder, M., Karle, J. M., Jerina, D. M., & Conney, A. H. Exceptional carcinogenic activity of benzo[a]anthracene 3,4-dihydrodiol in the newborn mouse and the bay region theory. *Cancer Res.*, 1978, *38*, 693-696.

Wislocki, P. G., Kapitulnik, J., Levin, W., Yagi, H., Mah, H. D., Jerina, D. M., & Conney, A. H., manuscript submitted for publication.

Wislocki, P. G., Wood, A. W., Chang, R. L., Levin, W., Yagi, H., Hernandez, O., Dansette, P. M., Jerina, D. M., & Conney, A. H. Mutagenicity and cytotoxicity of benzo[a]-pyrene arene oxides, phenols, quinones, and dihydrodiols in bacterial and mammalian cells. *Cancer Res.*, 1976(a), *36*. 3350-3357.

Wislocki, P. G., Wood, A. W., Chang, R. L., Levin, W., Yagi, H., Hernandez, O., Jerina, D. M., & Conney, A. H. High mutagenicity and toxicity of a diol epoxide derived from benzo[a]pyrene. *Biochem. Biophys. Res. Comm.*, 1976(b), *68*, 1006-1012.

Wood, A. W., Chang, R. L., Levin, W., Lehr, R. E., Schaefer-Ridder, M., Karle, J. M., Jerina, D. M., & Conney, A. H. Mutagenicity and cytotoxicity of benzo[a]anthracene diol epoxides and tetrahydroepoxides: Exceptional activity of the bay region 1,2-epoxides. *Proc. Natl. Acad. Sci. U.S.A.*, 1977(a), *74*, 2746-2750.

Wood, A. W., Chang, R. L., Levin, W., Yagi, H., Thakker, D. R., Jerina, D. M., & Conney, A. H. Differences in mutagenicity of the optical enantiomers of the diastereomeric benzo[a]pyrene 7,8-diol-9,10-epoxides. *Biochem. Biophys. Res. Comm.*, 1977(b), *77*, 1389-1396.

Wood, A. W., Goode, R. L., Chang, R. L., Levin, W., Conney, A. H., Yagi, H., Dansette, P. M., & Jerina, D. M. Mutagenic and cytotoxic activity of benzo[a]pyrene 4,5-, 7,8-, and 9,10-oxides and the six corresponding phenols. *Proc. Natl. Acad. Sci. U.S.A.*, 1975, *72*, 3176-3180.

Wood, A. W., Levin, W., Chang, R. L., Lehr, R. E., Schaefer-Ridder, M., Karle, J. M., Jerina, D. M., & Conney, A. H. Tumorigenicity of five dihydrodiols of benzo[a]pyrene on mouse skin. Exceptional activity of benzo[a]anthracene 3,4-dihydrodiol. *Proc. Natl. Acad. Sci. U.S.A.,* 1977(c), *74,* 3176-3179.

Wood, A. W., Levin, W., Lu, A. Y. H., Ryan, D., West, S. B., Lehr, R. E., Schaefer-Ridder, M., Jerina, D. M., & Conney, A. H. Mutagenicity of metabolically activated benzo-[a]anthracene 3,4-dihydrodiol: Evidence for bay region activation of carcinogenic polycyclic hydrocarbons. *Biochem. Biophys. Res. Comm.,* 1976(a), *72,* 680-686.

Wood, A. W., Levin, W., Lu, A. Y. H., Ryan, D., West, S. B., Yagi, H., Mah, H. D., Jerina, D. M., & Conney, A. H. Structural requirements for the metabolic activation of benzo[a]pyrene to mutagenic products. Effects of modification in the 4,5-, 7,8-, and 9,10-positions. *Mol. Pharmacol.,* 1977(e), *13,* 1116-1125.

Wood, A. W., Levin, W., Lu, A. Y. H., Yagi, H., Hernandez, O., Jerina, D. M., & Conney, A. H. Metabolism of benzo[a]pyrene and benzo[a]pyrene derivatives to mutagenic products by highly purified hepatic microsomal enzymes. *J. Biol. Chem.,* 1976(b), *251,* 4882-4890.

Wood, A. W., Levin, W., Ryan, D., Thomas, P. E., Yagi, H., Mah, H. D., Thakker, D. R., Jerina, D. M., & Conney, A. H. High mutagenicity of metabolically activated chrysene 1,2-dihydrodiol: Evidence for bay region activation of chrysen. *Biochem. Biophys. Res. Comm.,* 1977(d), *78,* 847-854.

Wood, A. W., Levin, W., Thomas, P. E., Ryan, D., Karle, J. M., Yagi, H., Jerina, D. M., & Conney, A. H., manuscript submitted for publication.

Wood, A. W., Wislocki, P. G., Chang, R. L., Levin, W., Lu, A. Y. H., Yagi, H., Hernandez, O., Jerina, D. M., & Conney, A. H. Mutagenicity and cytotoxicity of benzo[a]pyrene benzo-ring epoxides. *Cancer Res.,* 1976(c), *36,* 3358-3366.

Yagi, H., Akagi, H., Thakker, D. R., Mah, H. D., Koreeda, M., & Jerina, D. M. Absolute stereochemistry of the highly mutagenic 7,8-diol-9,10-epoxides derived from the potent carcinogen *trans*-7,8-dihydroxy-7,8-dihydrobenzo[a]pyrene. *J. Am. Chem. Soc.,* 1977, *99,* 2358-2359.

Yagi, H., Hernandez, O., & Jerina, D. M. Synthesis of (±)-7β,8α-dihydroxy-9β,10β-epoxy-7,8,9,10-tetrahydrobenzo(a)pyrene, a potential metabolite of the carcinogen benzo(a)pyrene with stereochemistry related to the antileukemic triptolides. *J. Am. Chem. Soc.,* 1975, *97,* 3185-3192.

Yang, S. K., & Gelboin, H. V. Microsomal mixed-function oxidases and epoxide hydratase convert benzo[a]pyrene stereospecifically to optically active dihydrodihydroxy-benzo[a]pyrene. *Biochem. Pharmacol.,* 1976, *25,* 2221-2225.

Yang, S. K., McCourt, D. W., Roller, P. P., & Gelboin, H. V. Enzymatic conversion of benzo-[a]pyrene leading predominantly to the diol-epoxide r-7,t-8-dihydroxy-t-9,10-oxy-7,8,9,10-tetrahydrobenzo[a]pyrene through a single enantiomer of r-7, t-8-dihydroxy-7,8-dihydrobenzo[a]pyrene. *Proc. Natl. Acad. Sci. U.S.A.,* 1976, *73,* 2594-2598.

Yang, S. K., Roller, P. P., & Gelboin, H. V. Enzymatic mechanism of benzo[a]pyrene conversion to phenols and diols and an improved high-pressure liquid chromatographic separation of benzo[a]pyrene derivatives. *Biochem.,* 1977, *16,* 3680-3687.

9. The Carcinogenic Action of Drugs in Man and in Animals

David B. Clayson
Eppley Cancer Institute
University of Nebraska Medical Center
Omaha, Nebraska

We should at this time take great pride in the achievements of the pharmaceutical industry. In Western society, several diseases which were scourges of the young, the adolescent, and the middle-aged have been brought under control by drugs and by the adoption of improved community and individual sanitation. No longer is tuberculosis known, as it was when I was a boy, as the "captain of the kings of death." To have had a bacterial pneumonic infection in the 1930s and to have recovered was, as I think H.G. Wells remarked, a clear indication to make final your last will and testament, for the chances of recovering from a second attack in the succeeding year was remote. Yet, if we read our journals and the outpourings of the popular press, we clearly see that all is not well; the advances are rapidly being forgotten in a sea of recrimination about the safety of a multitude of these products and their over-prescription by the clinician.

I have the feeling that the predestined consequences of our pride, *hubris*, or divine retribution for overweening confidence, have been forgotten, as well as the advantages that have accrued during the past two generations, as man now seeks ever-increasing safety from real, or oftentimes imaginary, environmental chemical hazards. Gratitude for the achievements, which surely must have kept some of us, at least, alive and well long enough to attend this meeting, is forgotten in a sea of recrimination about bad record-keeping, alleged dishonesty with the federal regulatory agencies, or overindulgence of the profit motive, combined with a pathetic public belief that a suitable pill will alleviate the most trivial ailment. I must make it clear, however, that I cannot condone outright dishonesty if it takes place.

Truly, we are now faced with examples of side reactions to drugs, cancer not being the least among them, and in this session, as the use of pharmaceuticals for a wide variety of human conditions has permitted long survivals, a rational overview of human epidemiological observations, combined with the results of safety screening at the single cell or whole organism level, should permit us some feeling for the adequacy of present methods of assessing cancer risk before a drug is introduced onto the market for the treatment of a less than life-threatening ailment. This report attempts to integrate present knowledge from both human and animal studies to judge how well they interrelate to help decide what questions, if any, are answerable by each type of evidence.

CAN HUMAN DRUG EXPOSURES GIVE QUANTITATIVE INFORMATION FOR TRANS-SPECIES EXTRAPOLATION

Hypothetically, the quantity of a drug administered to a particular patient should be available at a higher level of accuracy than with other environmental exposures, such as occupational, food, air and water pollution, or personal habits to carcinogens. Such exposure levels should be more trustworthy with drugs administered solely in the clinic than with those prescribed by the clinician to be used at home or those which may be purchased over the counter. In the latter two categories, the patient may fail to use the prescription, either in whole or in part. Some examples suggest that, even if we can get quantitative information on drug exposure in man, it is unlikely to be helpful in trans-species extrapolation other than at a relatively superficial level.

Chlornaphazin (2-naphthylamine mustard) was introduced by Sir Alexander Haddow and his team shortly after World War II for treatment of leukemia and lymphomas, both of which had a shockingly short prognosis at that time. In Denmark, chlornaphazin was shown in combination with ^{32}P-phosphate to be excellent for the maintenance of patients with polycythaemia vera. The results of the use of this drug are clearly demonstrated by the work of Thiede (Thiede & Christensen, 1969, 1975) who collected a group of 61 patients who had been exposed to this therapy. At the time of his last report in 1975 (see Table 1), he had identified 13 (21%) cases of bladder cancer in this group of whom only 17 (34%) still survived (i.e., patients of the original group of 61). Neither polycythaemia itself nor the additional ^{32}P-phosphate therapy were bladder carcinogens, as shown in groups of other patients surviving for equivalent periods without chlornaphazin. In addition to the patients with bladder tumors, there were 8 (13%) others with abnormal urinary cytology, indicating the probable development of bladder tumors. That is to say, 35% of this small group had developed actual or suspected bladder tumors. The difficulty is that the range of doses of chlornaphazin used was large, from 2-360 g/patient. The latency was very short, from 2.5-11 years with a mean of 6.4 years. Thiede, however, even with this great range of individual exposures, was able to demonstrate some dose relationships in the bladder tumor incidence. Four of 5 patients receiving 200 g or more chlornaphazin developed bladder tumors in 2, 2.6, 4.8, and 6 years (mean latency = 4 yr), compared to three of 31 who received a dose of less than 50 g. The latter developed their tumors 5.8, 9, and 11.3 years (mean latency = 8.7 yr) after the first dose of this drug.

These tumors are most probably a result of the 2-naphthylamine entity in the chlornaphazin. They differ from the occupational tumors mainly in their short latency (6 vs. 18 years) and frequency in the most heavily exposed group. The results of the detailed study of this small group of patients demonstrates: (a) that high doses (total dose, 0.03-5 g/kg body weight) are needed to induce tumors in man in a relatively short time, and (b) that the latency of human tumors is not always as long as those who study occupational human disease would sometimes have us believe (Clayson, 1975). The fact that urinary cytology indicates that slower-growing tumors may be developing in the less severely exposed group indicates clearly that man's long lifespan is disadvantageous as far as exposure to lower doses of carcinogens is concerned.

Similarly, sound data as a result of medical exposure to carcinogens is infrequent. Court Brown and Doll's 1965 survey of the effects of ionizing radiation in the management of ankylosing spondylitis provides a further example. Leukemia was found in this irradiated population. There was evidence of dose dependency, and the authors' main comment about the effects of spinal irradiation concerned the magnitude of the dose required to induce neoplastic disease. This is probably partially a reflection of the tissue irradiated, and the age of the patients. Irradiation for so-called thymic enlargement induces tumors of the thyroid (Hempelmann et al., 1975), while that for tinea capitis (Albert & Omran, 1968) has lead disastrously to head and neck tumors. In utero, diagnostic pelvic irradiation of the mother is stated by Alice Steward and her team (Steward & Kneale, 1970) to be responsible for a variety of childhood tumors, including

TABLE 1
TIME AND DOSE DISTRIBUTION OF 13 BLADDER TUMORS
IN 61 POLYCYTHEMIA PATIENTS RECEIVING CHLORNAPHAZIN

Dose (g)	Number of bladder tumors[a]	(%)	Tumor latency (years)	Number with abnormal cytology	(%)
>200	$\frac{4}{5}$	80	4	$\frac{0}{5}$	0
50-200	$\frac{6}{25}$	24	7.2	$\frac{2}{25}$	8
<50	$\frac{3}{31}$	10	8.7	$\frac{6}{31}$	19

[a]Denominator represents number of patients at risk.

leukemia. This data is controversial, but it is important to note that the incidence of leukemia increased with irradiation in the first, compared to the third trimester of pregnancy, and with the number of films recorded as being taken. Both the differing ages of the tissues affected and the differing characteristics of the radiation employed militate against combining the therapeutic adult and diagnostic fetal irradiation to produce meaningful dose response curves for radiation.

THE LATENCY OF HUMAN CANCER

Clearly, the hope that drug-induced cancer might lead to an understanding of the dose-response curve for human carcinogens is still some distance away. Also, it is apparent the old idea that human environmentally-induced cancer necessarily has a long latency period is open to doubt. This doubt develops more clearly when we examine what happens to renal transplant patients. These patients require immunosuppression to prevent graft rejection. This has been performed by a variety of methods, including the use of antilymphocyte serum, antilymphocyte globulin, azothiaprine, radiation, and suitable alkylating agents. The only tumor known to develop as a consequence of immunosuppression of these patients is reticulum cell sarcoma, mainly of the brain (Hoover & Fraumeni, 1973). The earliest examples of this tumor have been found only 5 months after renal transplantation. Human cancer may sometimes have an exceedingly short latency.

THE NEED TO USE PHYSIOLOGICAL DOSES
OF PHYSIOLOGICALLY ACTIVE AGENTS
IN CANCER INDUCTION

There seems to be an idea that if we are to bioassay, for example, hormonal preparations as carcinogens, these should be used at near physiological doses. The gross endocrine tissue disturbances brought about by, for example, high levels of estrogens, are too well known to need repeating. Yet this concept, particularly with synthetic hormones, runs quite contrary to the present precepts of carcinogen testing, that the maximum tolerated dose (whatever this ill-thought-out term means) should be used to test new chemicals for carcinogenicity. Can human experience with hormone-related tumors help?

Estrogens lead to tumors in three independent situations in man. Diethylstilbestrol (DES) has been used to maintain pregnancy in the face of threatened spontaneous abortion (Smith & Smith, 1949). Oral contraceptives are used extensively by women of child-bearing age. Conjugated estrogens relieve some of the consequencies of menopause. It seems to me unreasonable in any of these cases to equate the levels of estrogen employed with those which can conceivably be called physiological.

According to Herbst (Herbst, Ulfelder, & Poskanzer, 1971), stilbestrol levels given to pregnant patients started at 5 mg daily and in the course of the pregnancy, increased stepwise to 125 mg daily. The consequence of this therapy was first noted by the production of an unusual tumor, clear cell vaginal adenocarcinoma, in the female children after they passed the menarche. The incidence of this tumor at last report was 150-260 in a population estimated to be about 0.5-2.0 million female offspring at risk (Herbst, personal communication to Dr. M. Rustia). Much more common are less dramatic disturbances of the genital tract, including adenosis of the cervical and vaginal epithelium in 50-90% of offspring (Herbst et al., 1975; Stafl & Mattingly, 1974); in males, testicular atrophy (or lack of development) and cystic lesions are reported (Henderson et al., 1976). The doses used, even when reduced to a mg/kg body weight basis (0.08-2.1) scarcely seem physiological, although the recent observation that DES has to be given before the fifth month of pregnancy to induce these deleterious effects may go some way toward redressing the balance (Ulfelder, 1976).

The use of conjugated estrogens, or in some cases, the cheaper DES, to reduce over many years adverse symptoms of the menopause, has been clearly shown in a number of surveys to lead to an increased frequency of endometrial cancer (Kistner et al., 1973; Smith et al., 1975; Ziel & Finkle, 1975). This disease has been stated by one author to be increasing at a rate of 10% yearly in some areas of the United States—a frightening prospect. Again, I question whether a dose of hormone which masks certain of the natural consequences of the menopause can be considered as a physiological dose.

This question has been made more intense by Metzler's 1975 suggestion that DES may be carcinogenic rather than simply hormonal. He bases this suggestion on the idea that the pattern of metabolites obtained from DES is best explained by the formation of an unstable epoxide intermediate (Fig. 1), which by analogy with other unstable epoxides such as those formed from aflatoxin, benzo(a)pyrene, or vinyl chloride, could be carcinogenic. This evidence is extremely unconvincing. My chemical colleagues tell me that the pattern of

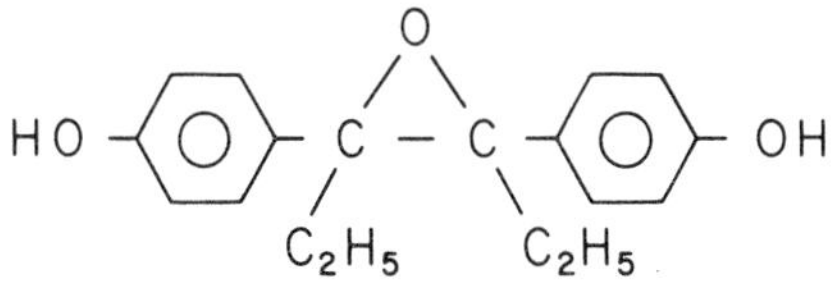

DIETHYLSTILBESTROL   OXIDE

FIGURE 1

metabolites Metzler has so far observed could equally well be explained by other possible metabolic pathways. In contradistinction to the "carcinogenic epoxide metabolites," the DES metabolite is symmetrical about the epoxide group and might therefore be more stable.

Oral contraceptives usually contain a synthetic estrogen and/or a progestogen. Recent evidence from several American sources, the most recent from the American College of Surgeons (Vana et al., 1976), has associated the use of oral contraceptives with the subsequent development of benign liver tumors in young women. In Nebraska, my colleague, Dr. Mahboubi (Mahboubi & Shubik, 1976, unpublished) has now tracked down 21 of these cases in a small population. In all cases, there is evidence of oral contraceptive use. The large survey conducted by questionnaire by the American College of Surgeons has found a much larger number of cases, but a less dramatic association with oral contraceptive use, although still enough to convince them of an association. Whether their search for records of oral contraceptive use was as intensive as that of Dr. Mahboubi is in my mind a very open question, illustrating the benefits of a small, in-depth study against the relatively superficial questionnaire approach.

A disturbing element of these liver lesions, apart from possible arguments whether hormonal doses which suppress any stage of pregnancy can really be considered physiological, is the fact that the consequences appeared predictable from previous animal experiments. The United Kingdom Committee on Safety of Medicines published a report in 1972 stating that oral contraceptives were virtually free from carcinogenic effect. They chose to ignore, with certain oral contraceptives, the clear dose-related association between "benign" liver tumors in rats and the administration of certain of these chemicals. In their defense, a hopefully conscious decision was made to place little emphasis on these tumors at a time when there were even more questions than now about the significance of benign rodent liver tumors. Nevertheless, the apparent association between a low yield of such tumors in humans with oral contraceptive use represents a distressing failure to use the results of animal tests in a proper manner.

ANIMAL EXPERIMENTS

At this stage, it should be becoming clear that we are not making great use of human data in the drug area to help validate our animal experiments at a quantitative level. The reasons for this are that epidemiological techniques, like those using animals, are relatively unrefined and insensitive and the labor required to go into sufficient depth of data collection and analysis to provide possibly hard conclusions at the epidemiologic level, if indeed they are attainable from human populations, would be better spent on multiple investigations of different agents at a much lower level of effort. In investigating the possible effects of drugs in animals, therefore, we are faced with relatively straightforward problems: (a) Is the drug a carcinogen in animals? (b) If so, is there any reason to suspect it will or will not have a similar effect in man? and (c) Does the risk in taking that drug outweigh the benefit derived from its use? The first of these questions is relatively simple to answer, the second, without human exposure data, practically impossible at this time, while the third question should be what drug regulation is all about.

To illustrate some of the problems, I shall mainly discuss some work we have done at the Eppley Institute on two drugs used for the treatment of schistosomal disease, namely niridazole and hycanthone (Fig. 2). Both drugs are potent mutagens in many bacterial strains and should therefore, according to current thought, be suspected of carcinogenicity. Both are teratogenic. Hycanthone was tested because of its expected widespread use in Africa, the Middle East, and South American countries, which had neither the funding nor the facilities to conduct these costly tests on U.S.-produced drugs. Because WHO had requested that niridazole also be tested, we added this to our study.

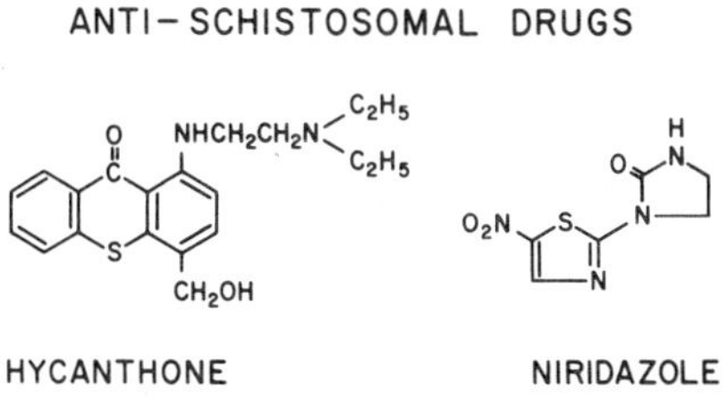

ANTI-SCHISTOSOMAL DRUGS

HYCANTHONE   NIRIDAZOLE

FIGURE 2

Eppley Swiss mice and Syrian golden hamsters were used for both chemicals and MRC rats additionally for niridazole. The effect of *Schistosoma mansoni* infection in mice and hamsters with both chemicals was examined as a possible cofactor. Dr. Yarinsky carried out infestation by his standardized injection techniques. The first conclusion, which is in contradistinction to that earlier found by Bueding with hycanthone, was that schistosomal infection did not significantly modify the response to either drug.

Because these experiments involved several thousands of animals at a considerable variety of dose ranges (Urman et al., 1975; unpublished), it is not possible to discuss all the results. Those with niridazole were very clear-cut. This agent induced significant yields in mice of forestomach papillomas and carcinomas, of lung adenomas and carcinomas, bladder cancer and carcinomas of the mammary gland and ovaries in female mice. Some of these results were dose-dependent, others apparently not, probably because we were too high on the dose-response curve. In addition, we observed the so-called vegetative cells in the bladder submucosa which Friedell and his colleague identified as myoepithelial tumors by ultrastructural examination. In hamsters, niridazole leads to benign tumors of the forestomach and urinary bladder while in rats, a range of kidney carcinomas of various histopathological types has resulted.

These tumors result from feeding niridazole in the diet, and before condemning this drug, it is correct to inquire whether the dose used in our studies is out of proportion to that used in man. It is difficult to assess accurately the total amount used in man because schistosomal reinfection among agricultural workers in heavily irrigated countries is frequent, and therefore these workers will receive repeated courses of treatment to keep their infection suppressed. One further point: niridazole is an unusual immunosuppressive agent insofar as it suppresses the cellular immune response, but has only a transient effect on the antibody response. It is pertinent to inquire what effect, if any, this may have on tumor induction (Mahmoud et al., 1975; Pelley et al., 1975).

The second drug of this series to be tested at the Eppley Institute was hycanthone, a biologically oxidized form of lucanthone (Miracil D). It is extremely effective against *S. mansoni* and *S. hematobium,* a single dose of only 2-3 mg/kg sufficing to cure about 75-80% of the treated population and to reduce the excreted egg count in the remainder also by about 75%. Despite these beneficial effects, hycanthone is a most controversial drug. Its bacterial, though probably not mammalian, mutagenicity, its teratogenicity, and its reputed carcinogenicity have all been strongly expressed by a small group of vocal critics. This drug was tested by i.p. and i.m. injection in mice and hamsters. Hamsters, like rats which have been examined in other laboratories, produced no tumors associated with treatment. In mice, a range of total dose was used varying from 40-800 times the clinical doses on a weight basis. In all groups of animals, there was a rise in the benign liver tumor (hepatoma) incidence from about 0-2% in controls to about 10% in treated animals. Particular care was taken to use standardized criteria for the diagnosis of hepatomas and these will be set out in the published paper. The opinion of more than one pathologist was taken to insure correct diagnosis, and probably these figures are substantially correct. Biostatistically, the prevalence of these tumors on an age-adjusted prevalence basis, which seems the correct approach since they are not killing lesions, was examined. It was concluded that none of the results in males and no results in infected female mice were statistically significant at the 5% level. In noninfected female mice treated by either the i.m. or i.p. route, significance was achieved at the 95% and 92% level, respectively. Dose-relatedness was also looked for within the groups, but not found.

I do not believe that at this stage in carcinogen testing, we can afford to ignore completely the possible 5-fold increase in hepatoma incidence when making public health decisions. Nevertheless, if I had schistosomal disease, I would prefer hycanthone to niridazole treatment. My major concern with these results is that in all 16 separate analyses of liver tumor prevalence, that is, male versus female, infected versus noninfected mice, the i.m. versus the i.p. route, and the possibility of dose-relatedness within each group, the probability that the two positive results arose by chance is still an open question.

As with all other forms of carcinogenicity testing, one must be concerned that results in man and animals may differ. Presently, we recognize the ability of the effective antituberculosis drug, isoniazid, to induce lung adenomas in a wide variety of mice which are susceptible to this tumor (Juhàsz, Balò, & Kendrey, 1957). In man, despite the fact that this drug has been effectively and extensively used since 1953, a period of 24 years, I know of no convincing evidence of its carcinogenic effect in man. The work by Ferebee (1970), for example, has concentrated on prophylactically-treated patients to exclude the possible confounding effects of other treatments in tubercular patients, but at the last report in 1970, was quite negative.

Unfortunately, we know of no sure way to differentiate accurately between those drugs and other chemicals which induce cancer in both animals and man and those which although effective in animals, are ineffective in man. Prudence, therefore, dictates that we should take great care in using animal carcinogens to attempt to treat human disease. This standard of care should increase the more trivial the ailment being treated, but even with such serious diseases as cancer, caution cannot be dispensed with because as therapy improves, and survival times increase, the opportunities for developing a second, but unrelated, tumor also markedly increase. For example, Arseneau and colleagues (Arseneau et al., 1972; Canellos et al., 1975) showed that treatment of Hodgkin's disease with irradiation *or* chemotherapy led in each case to a *4-fold* increase in the probability of developing a second tumor, whereas both treatments together led to a 14.5-fold increase, compared to a similar segment of the general population.

How, then, should we regard the increase in mouse lung adenomas and lymphomas induced by Flagyl (metronidazole) (Rustia & Shubik, 1972), which is widely used in this country to treat infective vaginitis, which although not life-threatening, affects the patient adversely through the induction of extreme itching? Should the induction of hepatomas in mice combined with the thyroid tumors which Dr. Rustia (unpublished) has recently observed in old (2 year +) griseofulvin-treated rats be sufficient to stop the use of this valuable fungicide in the treatment of human fungal infection?

Even more to the point, we may ask whether there are circumstances in which the use of drugs leads to a permanent or semipermanent change in the way animals or humans handle other drugs? Again my colleague, Dr. Rustia (unpublished), has provided an example. Transplacental diethylstilbestrol followed after birth by the administration of DMBA leads in hamsters to the rarely seen mammary carcinoma in this species in about 70% yield. Do other drugs have a similar effect? How do we allow for such vagaries in risk-benefit evaluation?

In this paper, questions have been asked which may be relevant to the use of both animal and epidemiologic data in the risk assessment of drugs. A drug-by-drug review of the present evidence has been avoided because this is adequately covered in the literature (Clayson, 1972; Fraumeni & Miller, 1972;

Clayson & Shubik, 1976). There are still many problems to be solved before meaningful trans-species extrapolation from animals to man is possible and consequently, real risk-benefit analyses based on hard animal data can be carried out with real precision for man.

REFERENCES

Albert, R.E., & Omran, A.R. Follow-up study of patients treated by x-ray epilation for tinea capitis. I. Population characteristics, post-treatment illnesses and mortality experience. *Arch. Environ. Hlth.*, 1968, *17*, 899-918.

Arseneau, J.C., Sponzo, R.W., Levin, D.L., Schniper, L.E., Bonner, H., Younge, R.C., Cannellos, G.P., Johnson, R.E., & DeVita, V.T. Non-lymphomatous malignant tumors complicating Hodgkin's disease: Possible association with intensive therapy. *New Engl. J. Med.*, 1972, *287*, 119-122.

Canellos, G. P., DeVita, V.T., Arseneau, J.C., Whang-Peng, J., & Johnson, R.E. Second malignancies complicating Hodgkin's disease in remission. *Lancet*, 1975, *1*, 947-949.

Clayson, D.B. Carcinogenic hazards due to drugs. In L. Meyler & H.M. Peck (Eds.), *Drug-induced diseases* (Vol. 4). Amsterdam: Excerpta 1972. Pp. 91-109.

Clayson, D.B. Epidemiology of bladder cancer. In E.H. Cooper & R.E. Williams, (Eds.), *The biology and clinical management of bladder cancer.* 1975. Pp. 65-86.

Clayson, D.B., & Shubik, P. The carcinogenic action of drugs. *Cancer Det. Prev.*, 1976, *1*, 43-77.

Court Brown, W.M., & Doll, R. Mortality from cancer and other causes after radiotherapy for ankylosing spondylitis. *Brit. Med. J.*, 1965, *2*, 1327-1332.

Ferebee, S.H. Controlled chemoprophylaxis trials in tuberculosis: A general review. *Bibl. Tubercul. Res.*, 1970, *26*, 28-106.

Fraumeni, J.F., & Miller, R.W. Drug-induced cancer. *J. Natl. Cancer Inst.*, 1972, *48*, 1267-1270.

Hempelmann, L.H., Hall, W.G., Phillips, M., Cooper, R.A., & Ames, W.R. Neoplasms in persons treated with X-rays in infancy. Fourth survey in 20 years. *J. Natl. Cancer Inst.*, 1975, *55*, 519-530.

Henderson, B.E., Benton, B., Cosgrove, M., Baptista, J., Aldrich, J., Townsend, D., & Mack, T.M. Urogenital tract abnormalities in sons of women treated with diethylstilbestrol. *Pediatrics*, 1976, *58*, 505-507.

Herbst, A.L., Poskanzer, D.C., Robboy, S.G., Friedlander, L., & Scully, R.E. Prenatal exposure to stilbestrol: A prospective comparison of exposed female offspring with unexposed controls. *New Engl. J. Med.*, 1975, *292*, 334-339.

Herbst, A.L., Ulfelder, H., & Poskanzer, D.B. Adenocarcinoma of the vagina. Association of maternal stilbestrol therapy with tumor appearance in young women. *New Engl. J. Med.*, 1971, *284*, 878-881.

Hoover, R., & Fraumeni, J.F. Risk of cancer in renal-transplant recipients. *Lancet*, 1973, *2*, 55-57.

Juhàsz, J., Balò, J., & Kendrey, G. Über die geschwulsterzeugende Wirkung des Isonicotinsäurehydrazide (INH). *Z. Krebsforsch.*, 1975, *62*, 188-196.

Kistner, R.W., Krantz, K.E., Lebherz, T.B., Lewis, G.L., Reagan, J.W., Smith, J., Tobin, J.G., & Weid, G.L. Endometrial cancer: Rising incidence, detection and treatment. *J. Reprod. Med.*, 1973, *10*, 53-74.

Mahboubi, E., & Shubik, P. Benign liver cell adenomas in women using oral contraceptives. *Cancer Letters,* 1976, *1,* 331-338.

Mahmoud, A.A.F., Mandel, M.A., Warren, K.E., & Webster, L.T., Jr. Niridazole. II. A potent long-lasting suppressant of cellular hypersensitivity. *J. Immunol.,* 1975, *114,* 297-283.

Metzler, M. Metabolic activation of diethylstilbestrol: Indirect evidence for the formation of a stilbene oxide intermediate in hamster and rat. *Biochem. Pharmacol.,* 1975, *24,* 1449-1453.

Pelley, R.P., Pelley, R.J., Stavitsky, A.B., Mahmoud, A.A.F., & Warren, K.S. A potent long-lasting suppressant of cellular hypersensitivity. III. Minimal suppression of antibody responses. *J. Immunol.,* 1975, *115,* 1477-1482.

Report of the Committee on the Safety of Medicines. Carcinogenicity tests of oral contraceptives. London: HMSO, 1972.

Rustia, M., & Shubik, P. Induction of lung tumors and malignant lymphomas in mice by metronidazole. *J. Natl. Cancer Inst.,* 1972, *48,* 721-729.

Smith, D.C., Prentice, R., Thompson, D.J., & Herrmann, W.L. Association of exogenous estrogen and endometrial carcinoma. *New Engl. J. Med.,* 1975, *293,* 1164-1167.

Smith, O.W., & Smith, G.V.S. Use of diethylstilbestrol to prevent fetal loss from complications of late pregnancy. *New Engl. J. Med.,* 1949, *241,* 562-568.

Stafl, A., & Mattingly, R. F. Vaginal adenosis: A precancerous lesion? *Am. J. Obstet. Gynecol.,* 1974, *120,* 666-673.

Stewart, A., & Kneale, G.W. Radiation dose effects in relation to obstetric x-rays and childhood cancers. *Lancet,* 1970, *1,* 1185-1188.

Thiede, T., & Christensen, B.C. Bladder tumours induced by chlornaphazine. A five-year follow-up of chlornaphazine-treated patients with polycythaemia. *Acta Med. Scand.,* 1969, *185,* 133-137.

Thiede, T., & Christensen, B.C. Blaeretumorer Inducede af Klornafazinbehandling. *Ugeskrift fur Laeger,* 1975, *137,* 661-666.

Ulfelder, H. The stilbestrol-adenosis-carcinoma syndrome. *Cancer,* 1976, *38*(suppl), 426-431.

Urman, H.K., Bulay, O., Clayson, D.B., & Shubik, P. Carcinogenic effects of niridazole. *Cancer Letters,* 1975, *1,* 69-76.

Vana, J., Murphy, G., Arnoff, B.L., & Bakder, H.W. Study of association between liver tumors and oral contraceptive use. Commission on Cancer, American College of Surgeons, Interim Report, November 15, 1976.

Ziel, H.R., & Finkle, W.D. Increased risk of endometrial carcinoma among users of conjugated estrogens. *New Engl. J. Med.,* 1975, *293,* 1167-1170.

10. Sex Steroids and Hepatic Growth

E. T. Mays
University of Kentucky
Lexington, Kentucky

INTRODUCTION

DR. WYNDER: David, we appreciate this challenging overview on an obviously important societal issue. Our next speaker belongs to what our colleague Bob Miller at the NCI calls the alert clinicians who make on the basis of a few cases important epidemiological observations.

In this regard, I would like to second what David said; namely, that if we had better records in our clinical cancer centers, the comprehensive cancer centers, we could make some sense of these observations much earlier. And I urge all of us who have an influence on these comprehensive clinical cancer centers to see to it that better records are kept.

I hope, Dr. Mays, that in your discussion you will touch on a few issues that are of general interest to us; namely, are there differences in types of oral contraceptives that relate to hepatomas, benign hepatomas? You know it has been suggested that this may be related only to sequential estrogens. We would like to know from you what the total number of cases now is in the world and what may we expect to see in years to come.

I would be interested to hear whether we can identify the high risk patient. Are there women that are particularly prone to these oral contraceptives in terms of benign hepatomas? Finally, perhaps, you might want to comment on a point also stressed by David Clayson; namely, their risk-benefit analysis.

Clearly, it relates to increased hepatomas, clearly we know it increases a woman's risk for stroke, clearly we know that together with cigarette smoking, it increases risk for myocardial infarction. But, what about the benefits, what

197

about population control, what about death from abortions, and how are we going to make decisions of these kinds?

DR. MAYS: Dr. Wynder, Dr. Shubik, ladies and gentlemen. I'm honored to address you today. For a surgeon to come before an audience such as this is a downright distinction.

After 20 years of practicing medicine I'm totally convinced that the health of our citizens is clearly related to what we do to and for, or don't do to and for, ourselves. I think a conference such as this is keenly appropriate. Not only the external environment that each of us comes in contact with daily, but also the internal milieu that is a part of each of us is modified, altered, and changed frequently by what we do, or don't do to, and for ourselves—this is our greatest health problem.

After looking at those aromatic, polycyclic curves this morning, let's see the first slide and see some real curves. In 1968 I operated on this young lady. She was brought to the hospital after collapsing while preparing a meal for her family. She was in a state of shock when brought in by the police ambulance. Of historical interest to this group: she was taken to the same hospital where a few years later we began to see the cases of angiosarcoma from vinylchloride exposure at the B. B. Goodrich plant in Louisville, Kentucky.

Next slide. When I cut open her abdomen I encountered this large tumor which had been palpable preoperatively in the upper part of her abdomen. In fact, she looked almost 9 months pregnant. This gives you an idea of the size of this tumor. You're looking now at the abdomen cut open through a vertical midline incision and this represents the left lobe of the liver; the incision has been extended into her chest cavity through the eighth intercostal space. Here, you see in the left lobe of the liver—this large hepatic tumor. Next slide. This is a resected surgical specimen, the entire left lobe of the liver, including the large tumor. This is a rather large tumor and was quite impressive. It required major (and extremely risky) surgery to remove this tumor from the young lady. Next slide.

Now this is the one I want you to remember. My wife says I repeat myself a lot, and I'll be doing that this morning because I want to get this point across and I want you to remember this very well. The right lobe of her liver can be seen here. It is entirely normal to inspection, to blood chemical measurements, and to direct palpation with the hands. The right lobe of her liver is entirely normal. Now keep this in your mind, because later I'll show you how this young lady fits into the total picture. She'll be coming back to see us in just a few minutes, but in the meantime remember that when we removed the entire left lobe of the liver, the right lobe was normal as best our medical technology could determine in this day and age.

When she came back to the office, after she was well, she looked at me very suspiciously and said, "Doctor, do you think that these birth control pills I've been taking had anything to do with my liver tumor?" I said, "No! No way!" (This was 1968, remember.) "There's no evidence we know of in medicine today that would even suggest your liver tumor was due to the birth control pills. You were probably born with it, and it's just been growing all these years." All of us know that primary hepatocyte tumors are often congenital, and they're often found in the very young.

I gave her this information, and then instructed her to go home and continue taking her birth control pills.

I thought perhaps I should look into the question a little more carefully to be sure I had not given her the wrong information. Going to the medical library, I pulled out a number of articles. At the Mayo Clinic, which should see a fairly representative picture of what's going on in the United States, in nearly a half century of experience they had only 6 primary, benign hepatic tumors composed of hepatocytes. Terminology has been quite confusing over the years, but the thing I want to point out to you this morning is that these were tumors composed primarily of hepatocytes and in almost a half century of experience at the Mayo Clinic only 6 were seen.

Well this encouraged me and made me realize that I was in step with most physicians. These were just simply rare tumors and this young girl just happened to be one of those people who had a rare tumor. Next slide.

But then it began to happen. A few miles away, one of my former surgical residents encountered a young lady in the hospital in the middle of the night. She had pain in her abdomen. He examined her and sent her home with an analgesic.

She went home. During the night the pain increased, she became dizzy and had to go back to the emergency room the next morning at 8 o'clock. He was called again to see her, and this time she was in obvious hypovolemic shock with a distended abdomen, lowered blood pressure, and pale, cold, clammy skin. When he opened her abdomen, he found a massive hemoperitoneum of 2-3 liters.

He obviously thought it was a ruptured tubal pregnancy as it would be in most young ladies this age. He made a lower abdominal incision, and saw that the tubes and ovaries were normal. After finding nothing there, he made an upper abdominal incision and looked at the spleen because this would be the next most common source of interperitoneal bleeding. The spleen was normal. Finally, looking at the liver, he found the source of bleeding and controlled it with sutures.

He called me on the phone and told me he found this large tumor in the right lobe of the liver, and asked if the patient could come over and have it resected. She came to our hospital, and we removed the right lobe of the liver. Here, you can see this large, pale, yellowish-tan tumor with obvious rupture and hemorrhage into the liver as well as into the free peritoneal cavity.

From this point a number of interesting and frightening events began to happen. We do not have time to go into them now, but within a short time my colleagues and I had operated on 13 young women, most of them having experienced a catastrophic event: interarperitoneal hemorrhage. We reported our findings in the AMA Journal. Because our interest by then was aroused, we developed a repository of tissue and data to expedite morphologic delineation of these tumors and to study the potential biologic characteristics of the tumor.

As of today we have about 180 of these tumors in our tumor registry. We're only going to talk about one hundred of them this morning, because this data is reported in the February 1977 issue of the *Journal of the National Cancer Institute*. We'll limit our comment to those carefully studied patients. Any participant in the conference who wants to look up that information, as we'll move through these slides rather quickly, can do so.

Next slide. Four different cell types of tumors have been uncovered. The peculiarities of naming hepatocyte tumors over the years came into play. It's very difficult in certain stages to tell these tumors one from another. But my pathologist colleague, Dr. William Christopherson, who's been working with me on this problem, feels that he can differentiate between focal nodular hyperplasia and adenoma.

Adenomas, as some of you know, are characterized by having only hepatocytes, no bile duct epithelium, and a well-formed capsule, whereas focal nodular hyperplasia is composed of bile duct epithelium, hepatocytes, and a considerable number of fibrous septae. And in the third type of tumor, hepatoma, the malignant hepatocytes have bizarre nuclear patterns, as you see here.

About 20 percent of the patients did present with hemoperitoneum. This was a catastrophic event easily recognized. And those of our patients who were operated on are alive and well today and have been followed for from 3 months to 14 years.

But in other reported cases there have been a number of deaths from bleeding. This catastrophe caught everyone's eye. It's interesting—as the years have gone by—to see what happens to young women who faint and fall over.

We have had nurses in the hospital die with a belly full of blood and be written off as having used drugs or overdosing on drugs. One of these patients was a nurse who worked in the operating room in a small, rural hospital who fainted while on duty and was put in bed. The following day, she finally had to be operated on and was found to have a ruptured primary hepatic tumor.

And so the story goes on with rather frightening details. Some of the women would make their way to the emergency room only to be sent home with aspirin and die during the night of their hemoperitoneum.

In later years, however, as this information has been disseminated, we are seeing more and more patients presenting with primarily abdominal mass: the liver has grown to a size that is easily palpable by examination.

The American College of Surgeons survey showed 12% of patients had presented with hemoperitoneum. In our patients we've had a larger percent (almost 20% of our patients) presented primarily with a catastrophe. Next slide.

The duration of pill use in months is listed here. I will not go into detail on this, because it gets a little confusing. Most of the patients used the pill for 5-7 years. There are always those who fall outside the normal bell-shaped curve of distribution. Some of those with the very worst malignant tumors used the pill for six months to one year. Perhaps this information may be helpful in deciding whether or not the risk-benefit analysis mentioned a few minutes ago is worth it. Next slide.

The type of drug that these women had been using is listed here. The first thing that catches your eye is that mestranol is the most common estrogen component. After the publication of Brian Henderson and Hugh Edmonson (NEJM), the question arose in everybody's mind as to whether mestranol is more responsible than other estrogens. I think this requires us to go look at several areas. First of all the marketing method and influence it has on what pill women use must be considered. Mestronol was the very earliest drug markedted. It had been in use much longer than other estrogens. Anyone using oral contraceptives would most likely have used this particular drug rather than ethinyl estradiol. The other thing we need to know is about the metabolism of estrogen in the human body.

The two major estrogens that we—that humans—produce are estradiol and estrone. The final common pathway of their action on the cell is completely dependent upon the estrogen receptor protein in the cytosol of the cell. This has primarily been worked out in the breast. It's well known now that for estrogen to manifest its classic effect physiologically, it must be bound to this cytosol protein. This estrogen-protein complex is transferred to the nucleus where it translocates and initiates DNA formation and other protein synthesis.

The interesting thing about these two estrogens which are the most common in oral contraceptives is that mestranol is simply the methyl ester of ethinyl estradiol. It has no activity in vivo and vitro in the classic sense, because it cannot be bound and has no capacity to unite with the cytosol estrogen-binding protein. Mestranol is first demethylated to ethinyl estradiol and then bound to protein where it initiates a physiologic effect.

Some of these women had been using the conjugated equine estrogen, premarin. When you think of the relative potency of estrogens, their estrogenic hormonal effect comes down to the final common pathway, and depends on how readily they are bound to the estrogen-binding protein. Nearly all estrogens have equal potency in regard to their physiological hormonal effect, because it depends upon estrogen-binding protein in the cytosol.

We'll leave that for some discussion and argument later on. The other drugs you see listed here. One patient had a thecoma. As most of you know this is an estrogen-producing tumor of the ovary. Such a tumor produces about the same effect as a person ingesting oral contraceptives.

Primary tumors composed of hepatocytes have not been a common occurrence but have been a perennially problem in patients who are pregnant. Blood estrogen levels peak in pregnancy. The liver is exposed to about the same concentration as a patient on oral contraceptives. Even before the advent of oral contraceptives as commonly used in this country, there was a suggestion that when the internal hormonal milieu was changed, either by pregnancy or by estrogen-producing tumors, a small percentage of such women exposed to increased blood values of sex steroids would develop tumors composed of hepatocytes.

We should not focus on any one drug but on the sex steroids in general. We have had one male, and others have reported about a dozen males using testosterone for various reasons who developed primary hepatic tumors. There was a report in 1965 about a young man developing a primary hepatic tumor who had taken testosterones for Fanconi's anemia. We need to look at the sex steroid ring itself and measure its effect upon the human liver. Next slide.

This is a patient I just operated on last month who went to see her family doctor because she could feel a large mass in her abdomen. You can see why: it's a rather impressive sized tumor. This is not the liver you're looking at, this is the tumor. Please note: all her liver function tests were normal. Here's the surgical specimen. Next slide. And the cut surface shows a large, whitish-gray scar in the center.

This central scar is supposed to denote focal nodular hyperplasia, but under the microscope this was not fibrous tissue but soft, gelatinous areolar tissue. This tumor was an adenoma. I show it to you to help you realize we're not talking about small nodules; we're talking about mammoth tumors that occur in the human liver. Next slide.

The histology has varied. You see there's a lot of mitotic activity, but the hepatocytes are not grossly abnormal. In fact they look almost like normal hepatocytes and it's hard to tell them from the normal liver. Next slide.

But the startling thing that caught our attention were the changes in the blood vessels. You see this small hepatic artery has intimal proliferation. We feel that they may play a role in the pathogenesis of this entire disease. They occur both in the arteries and in the veins. About 12 cases have been reported in which these changes occurring in the outflow veins, the hepatic veins, have caused Budd-Chiari syndrome. In 12 patients that have been reported, women were ingesting oral contraceptives. At first we could not determine whether these changes were due to hemorrhagic infarction and destruction of the liver, or whether the blood vessel changes were induced by the sex steroids themselves. After looking up investigations done in other laboratories, I find that, indeed, sex steroids had an effect upon blood vessels. They cause intimal proliferation in arteries, and they cause endothelial proliferation in veins. We can draw together the entire picture of complications of oral contraceptives. If these changes occur in the blood vessels of the liver, the patient develops hepatic tumor; if they develop it in the brain, the patient presents with a stroke; or if they develop in the heart, the patient presents with a myocardial infarction. Moreover, if they develop in the intestinal tract, the patient presents with gangrene of the intestine; and if they develop in veins of the leg, the patient presents with thrombophlebitis. You recognize each of these as being reported complications of oral contraceptives in this country today. This patient would never have been entered in our registry had it not been for someone having an interest in her death. This young lady died at a University hospital in the United States of infectious hepatitis. Had it not been for an autopsy and had it not been for some of us investigating autopsy material, this would have gone on record for ever and ever in the archives of medicine as a patient with infectious hepatitis. She was a young female. She started her vacation trip from Portland, Oregon. She went to her family doctor before leaving, because she was feeling poorly. Her symptoms were vague. Her vacation was coming due and asked her doctor, "Should I go on my vacation?" He said, "Yes, go ahead. I can find nothing wrong." She came to Indiana to visit relatives. While in Indiana her disease progressed rapidly and she became jaundiced. She went to see her physician in Indiana, and he found bilirubinemia and markedly enlarged liver with evidence of severe liver failure.

In the hospital in Indiana she deteriorated rapidly and was transferred to a university hospital. In about 10 days to 2 weeks, her liver failure worsened, and she died. Her case report and her physical examination were signed out as infectious viral hepatitis. But I had the interest to investigate. Here, you can see that this young lady did not have viral hepatitis, but she had a malignant hepatocellular carcinoma that grew rapidly and killed her. I went back and contacted her husband, called her family physician, in Portland, obtained her records, and found out she'd been on oral contraceptives for the 19 months prior to her death.

What is unfortunate is that so many of these cases are being put aside as due to some other cause. Some of the tumors have been well encapsulated, others have not. This young lady presented primarily with chest pain and was evaluated with about six hospital admissions in a period of 18 months.

Next slide. Here's the gross tumor in the right dome of the liver which caused this young lady chest pain. That was her only complaint. Most of the doctors who saw her felt that she was a chronic complainer because for 18 months she'd been telling them that whenever she took a deep breath it hurt. A selective hepatic arteriogram finally uncovered this large tumor and it was resected. Next slide. This is a close-up showing the fibrous components and scarring of these large tumors. Next slide. How do you diagnose these tumors? This is a liver scan done with Technetium. This is another young lady who would never have been entered in our tumor registry had it not been that she wanted a tubal ligation. She'd been on the pill about 7 years and she requested a tubal ligation. Her gynecologist did the band-aid operation, a laparoscopic banding of both tubes. He turned the laparotoscope around and looked at the liver. It was enlarged but he could tell nothing more about it.

After the operation he called in an internist who did a liver scan; here you see in this totally asymptomatic lady with normal hepatic function and two large tumors. And this is what makes the problem of finding out how many tumors of the liver there actually are. The true incidence of this disease is going to be immensely difficult to measure. How many other women are running around with these hepatic tumors totally asymptomatic, we do not know. The liver scan is one of our main clinical tools for detecting these tumors, since women do not show derangements on our chemical studies of the blood.

Next slide. This is the arteriogram of the tumor I showed you three slides ago, the large tumor taken from the young girl who had chest pain. The catheters are in the common hepatic artery, the contrast medium is injected, and it shows the hepatic arterial tree. The right hepatic artery divides into posterior and anterior branches. At this point notice that instead of being like the limbs on a tree and fading out gradually, there is suddenly a break off, demonstrating the lesions I showed you microscopically a few minutes ago.

Next slide. Here is an arteriogram of the large malignant tumor, two of them, in fact, one here and one here. This young lady was a farmer's wife, collecting hen eggs one night when she fell over in a state of shock with a belly full of blood. She died on the operating table while surgeons tried to resect these two large cancers of the right lobe of the liver.

Liver scan and hepatic arteriography are our main tools in diagnosis. That's why it's so difficult to uncover these tumors. Arteriograms are not innocuous procedures. You cannot go around doing hepatic arteriograms and liver scans on all women taking the pill.

Next slide. Earlier I asked you to remember the young lady in the bikini. I showed you the right lobe of her liver. I told you how she'd inquired, "Doctor, did these birth controls pills cause my tumor." She did just as the doctor told her: she went home and for the next seven years she took the oral contraceptives, bought herself a new bikini, and finally came back to the office and said, "Doctor, my right side is hurting." I show you this to show you the scar she had acquired in trying to rid herself of a disease caused by the oral contraceptives.

Next slide. She said, "My pain is just like it was before." We did a liver scan, and sure enough (this is the right lobe of her liver, the left side has been removed entirely as I showed you at the first of the discussion) seven years later after ingesting oral contraceptives, another tumor. We operated upon her, biopsied the tumor, and histologically it was similar to the one removed seven years earlier.

I realized the ideal model in medicine is the animal model in the laboratory. You try to produce a certain finding. And, of course, the ideal experiment and the scientific method is to use laboratory animals and discover what happens in them when exposed to oral contraceptives.

This young lady convinced me more than any statistical studies (and more than any animal studies) that oral contraceptives most likely cause primary benign hepatic tumors.

And if I had 100 patients that we had—as in this case unintentionally—

given them oral contraceptives, removed their liver tumors and then prescribed oral contraceptives for them for the next seven years, and found new tumors—if we had 100, or 1,000, or one million, it still would not convince some people. I remind you many of our major discoveries in medicine have been made with only a small series or a small sampling of animals or humans with disease. When it's significant, it's usually there. While I have only one such patient she does teach us keenly about the particular relationship between sex steroids and tumors. Next slide. I presented our first small group of patients at the American College of Surgeons Meeting in Miami in 1971. It caused our cancer commission to survey the hospitals associated with the American College of Surgeons Cancer Program. The National Cancer Advisory Board provided impetus in that they recommended to the American College of Surgeons that this be done. The final conclusion of the survey, which was just published in this last month's Bulletin of the American College of Surgeons, was the same as mine in 1971. Next slide. They surveyed hospitals participating in the cancer program of the American College of Surgeons. From this survey, they found 528 benign and malignant liver tumors. One hundred sixty-six of these were in males. That left 362 in females. You can see there was an obvious increase in benign tumors in the users of oral contraceptives, when compared to the nonusers. It's very difficult to do any kind of epidemiologic studies on these women. A lot of them don't know the name of the pill they were taking. An equal number don't remember how long they took it. Many never inquired from their doctor as to the number or the name of the pill they were taking. It's most likely a lot of these unknowns would probably fall into this group. But this is just a problem of human nature. This study, and a number of other studies, have all concluded with the statement that before women are given oral contraceptives they should have an evaluation of liver function. What I've tried to impress on you is that the first lady had a normal *right* lobe of the liver and normal liver function. All the women studied in our survey and in the material I presented to you this morning had normal livers. None had cirrhosis. It doesn't make sense to say on our drug-marketing processes that physicians should screen the patient for liver disease and if patients have liver disease, don't use oral contraceptives.

Next slide. We've heard a lot this morning about carcinogens, and it may be that estrogens act as direct carcinogens. I doubt this very much. It would be ironic for Mother Nature to do this to us, to give us carcinogens that also provide us with so much pleasure. More than likely, it's a cocarcinogen and this correlates more closely with what we know about the effects of estrogen physiologically. In oophorectomized mice which are given a carcinogen for mammary cancer, they do not develop mammary cancer. In the animal studies where estrogen is withdrawn, they do not develop endometrial cancer. Hormones probably excite epithelial cells of the breast and uterus to growth processes. Vitamin A is stored in the liver. There's been a lot of work lately on the role of vitamin A in the development of cancer in epithelial cells.

Anyone who's been operating on either the animal liver or the human liver will be impressed—as I am—that the human liver is perennially primed for marked, and astonishingly rapid, mitotic activity. Within 24 hours after a partial hepatectomy, DNA begins to replicate. There's a rapid series of events that take place to restore liver mass.

While most of my colleagues have been looking at what we call the porto-trophic factors or substances that cause regenerative hyperplasia, I have been more interested in what have been called chalones. These are mitotic inhibitors. They've been demonstrated in a number of animal livers. If sex hormones block the mitotic inhibitors, then hepatic hyperplasia can go on unchecked for some time.

Next slide. We had a lot of evidence showing we should have expected this phenomenon. Dr. Bonser showed that isolated nodules do occur in the liver of rats treated with mestranol and other synthetic estrogens. She presented her report to the British Committee on the safety of medicines.

Second, in clinical medicine we've known for years that the male with cirrhosis develops feminization, that his estradiol and estrone levels in the blood are increased, that he develops breast tissue much like a female, and that he loses his hair. We've also known for years that cirrhotics are persons who develop hepatic growths. In the United States when you have a malignant hepatocellular carcinoma, it will nearly always occur in a cirrhotic liver. That's why I pointed out this morning that all of these women have had normal livers.

While hepatic tumors in women on oral contraceptives are an interesting phenomenon that has developed and caught everyone by surprise, it really might have been expected from the very beginning. Thank you.

Discussion

DR. WYNDER: Thank you, Dr. Mays. It so happens that some of the interested people in epidemiology have been surgeons rather internists, and I wonder what this means in terms of our background and training. There's one comment that I'm sure will come up in the discussion, Dr. Mays, and that Dr. Greenwald will make: obviously, we must present control data. The utilization of oral contraception is very high in the population: 80% of our patients in New York between 20 and 29 use the pill. Obviously, one needs to develop a ratio of risk that requires an identification of the control population, and while it seems to me that there is good evidence that oral contraception hormones do relate to benign hepatomas, I would like to believe on the basis of your own data that there are other environmental factors which relate just as well and I think we need to study them.

How do estrogens relate to different animal tumors? I'm sure Dr. Shellenberger will tell us the dilemma that we have with estrogens and related carcinogenesis. The ideal model my own staff would like us to believe is where clearly we know that estrogens and production ratios are important but not in the absence of a specific carcinogen.

And I would concur with Dr. Mays that probably the hormones act as tumor promoters. Or is the monkey the ideal animal or must we rely on man or in this case woman? We hope that Dr. Shellenberger will give us this final answer before lunch, before the discussion.

11. Estrogens and Animal Cancer

T. E. Shellenberger
Department of Health, Education, and Welfare
National Center for Toxicological Research
Jefferson, Arkansas

INTRODUCTION

Steroidal and nonsteroidal estrogens have been used extensively as oral contraceptives, as drugs in human therapy (usually in disorders of the female endocrine system and/or treatment of appropriate hormone dependent tumors in males or females), and as anabolic agents of food (meat) production. In addition, low levels of many, naturally occurring chemicals of estrogenic activity exist in foods consumed by humans. Thus, humans may be exposed to estrogens for a variety of reasons over a wide range of dose levels and time periods.

Estrogens, therefore, present unique toxicological problems necessitating a review of the endpoints elicited in laboratory animals in relation to endpoints found epidemiologically in humans. The present review is directed to a brief summation of the voluminous literature on the carcinogenic effects of estrogens in animals. The role of estrogens in human disease is to be covered separately in this conference and is mentioned herein only as background. For the most part, animal studies are evaluated or reviewed with respect to tumorigenic processes in the liver, pituitary, kidney, mammary gland, and reproductive tract with little but passing comment on species differences and/or differential effects due to route of exposure.

ESTROGENS AND HUMAN CANCER

There is epidemiological evidence for the role of estrogens and human cancers which I will briefly summarize. The synthetic estrogen, diethylstilbestrol (DES), for example, has been implicated in the causation of adenocarcinomas of the vagina, cervix and endometrium of young adult females who were exposed in utero (Herbst et al., 1971). Reported results during the 1970-71 period show approximately 250 cases of adenocarcinoma out of the 500,000 to 2 million women who were administered this drug during pregnancy as an abortion preventative; however, an incidence of 70-80% adenosis was found in the resulting female offspring as they approached adulthood; obviously, not all adenosis led to adenocarcinomas—at least not to date. Dose levels were as low as 1.5 mg and dose intervals were as short as 7 days; generally the most dramatic positive effects were noted when DES was given during the first 18 weeks of pregnancy. Allegedly, endometrial adenocarcinomas have resulted from the use of conjugated estrogens and sequential preparations of oral contraceptives; this latter association resulted in the withdrawal of approval of these products. Oral contraceptives have also been linked to the possible appearance of benign liver adenomas in humans. The role, however, of estrogens in human mammary tumors remains unknown and unproven at this point in time. As a direct carcinogen, estrogen exposure has not been proven to result in mammary tumors, as a promoter or cocarcinogen; however, estrogen must be further evaluated to establish if any causal relationship exists between mammary tumors, estrogens, and other mammary carcinogens.

ESTROGENS AND CANCER IN EXPERIMENTAL ANIMALS

The literature on estrogen-induced tumors in animals has been reviewed elsewhere (IAPC Monograph, 1974). Pertinent key literature citations were selected to illustrate the relevancy of lesions induced in the target organs of animals and to those in humans.

Liver

The role of estrogens in inducing hepatic tumors in experimental animals is not resolved as yet. The status of in vivo bioassays regarding potential hepatic lesions or tumors produced by oral contraceptives in mice and rats was summarized in a 1972 report "Carcinogenicity Tests of Oral Contraceptives" by the Committee on Safety of Medicine. The report covers results obtained in tests with a series of estrogens and progestins in several strains each of rats and mice. It concluded that all treated animals showed the typical pathologic changes known to occur following prolonged administration of estrogens or progestins. The extensive tests reported therein did not support the previous work showing liver damage progressing to nodule hyperplasia and increased hepatomas from prolonged administration of oral contraceptive preparations to mice. This report further stated:

In rats, there is an increase in benign hepatoma formation in a few groups but even in these groups it is observed only with doses which are from 200 to 400 times greater than the equivalent dosage in women. A variability is observed between male and female involvement even with the same compound in the high dosage groups. Though some strains of rats do show slight increase in incidence of hepatoma, other strains do not.

In a separate 2-year study with Sprague-Dawley rats, administration of chlorotrianisene (CTA), DES, and conjugated equine estrogens did not result in hepatotoxic effects, carcinogenesis, or bile retention (Gibson et al., 1967).

The problem, therefore, of possible hepatoma induction by estrogens in rodents remains unresolved at this time, and the significance of the observations in humans must, consequently, be investigated further in experimental animals.

Pituitary

The pituitary, in conjunction with the hypothalamus, is considered to be a target tissue susceptible to, and responsive to, estrogen stimulation. This response can be stimulated in the case of prolactin or reduced in the case of LH; responses are variable depending on species-specific feedback mechanisms (Neumann & Elger, 1972). That the pituitary can respond to estrogens by hyperplasia and neoplasia, therefore, is not totally unexpected.

Subcutaneous injection of DES in intact or castrate rats, produced increased pituitary weight within 6 days (Table 1), with more dramatic increases in intact animals than in castrates (Benas, 1956). In a separate study (Jacobi et al., 1975), a single subcutaneous dose of 20 mg/animal of DES diproprionate was reported to have produced enlarged pituitaries, but there were no marked abnormalities observed in the tissues or changes in tissue prolactin and growth hormone; whereas, in grossly enlarged tissues (concluded to be tumors) pituitary concentrations of prolactin and growth hormone were low. Likewise, estrone-acetate, as subcutaneous injections, and DES, as implants, produced marked enlargement of the pituitary (Orosz et al., 1970).

TABLE 1
EFFECT OF DIETHYLSTILBESTROL (DES)[a]
ON PITUITARY WEIGHT OF RATS[b]

Group	Number animals/gr	Length of dosing (days)	Pituitary wt./BW (mg/g) intact	castrate
Control	16	0	0.027 ± 0.004	0.045 ± 0.001
DES	8	6	0.062 ± 0.001	0.070 ± 0.003
DES	8	16	0.170 ± 0.001	0.140 ± 0.001
DES	6	26	0.182 ± 0.001	0.152 ± 0.007

[a]Subcutaneous injection of 250 μg in 0.05-ml olive oil/rat every other day for 6, 16, or 26 days.
[b]Taken from Benas (1959).

In Kirkman's (1959) long-term feeding study, DES, at dietary levels of 0.2 mg/kg/day for 18 months or 0.02 mg/kg/day for 24 months, significantly increased pituitary weights in female rats (Table 2); males did not respond to these dose levels, and CTA and conjugated equine estrogens (CEE) did not induce pituitary weight increases under the conditions of the study.

Tumorigenic responses were also reported in the above studies. Pituitary tumors were classified as "mammotropic" in five cases and "somatropic" in one case (IARC Monograph, 1971). Pituitary tumors appear to be related, in part, to estrogen activity, dose level and duration, as well as species and strain. Estrone-acetate produced tumors in both outbred and inbred albino rats, whereas a 25-mg implant of DES produced only hyperplastic enlargement (Orosz et al., 1970). However, DES and conjugated equine estrogens, in feeding studies, produced pituitary tumors in Sprague-Dawley rats, whereas, CTA was ineffective (Gibson et al., 1967). Pituitary adenomas, mainly chromophobic, were reported in long-term feeding studies in mice at high levels with estrogens (Committee on Safety of Medicines, 1967); in these studies, mestranol and ethynylestradiol produced tumors in the three strains of mice tested. In rats, the spontaneous incidence of pituitary adenoma varied widely by strain, but, in general, the rats did not show a rise in incidence of estrogen-induced pituitary adenoma.

TABLE 2
RELATIVE PITUITARY WEIGHTS OF RATES GIVEN ORAL
ESTROGENS FOR 2 YEARS (MG/KG)[a]

Dosage (mg/kg/day)	Compound[b]	18-month duration		24-month duration	
		Number animals	Pituitary weight (mg)	Number animals	Pituitary weight (mg)
Males					
0	—	5	0.023	9	0.151
2.00	CTA	6	0.025	12	0.028
0.20	DES	9	0.460	—	—
0.02	DES	—	—	14	0.092
0.70	CEE	6	0.039	5	0.078
Females					
0	—	5	0.037	12	0.049
2.00	CTA	6	0.027	11	0.041
0.20	DES	6	1.321[3]	—	—
0.02	DES	—	—	14	0.212[c]
0.70	CEE	6	0.059	6	0.103

[a]From Gibson et al. (1967).
[b]CTA, Chlorotrianisene; DES, diethylstilbestrol; CEE, conjugated equine estrogens.
[c]$p = <0.05$.

Kidney

Estrogen-induced renal tumors in the hamster are well known and have been reviewed elsewhere (Kirkman, 1959, 1972); for the most part, these tumors can be routinely produced in males by injection or pellet implantation of DES, estradiol, or estrone (Kirkman, 1972) (Table 3). Renal tumors will not be induced by estrogens in intact females; however, tumors can be induced in female hamsters if estrogen treatment is started: (a) after ovariectomy, (b) at times of lowest progestrone secretion, (c) before reproductive maturity, (d) in female with "masculinized" pituitary (testosterone-treatment neonatally), or (e) in females maintained in male environments (Kirkman, 1972).

Dimethyl ether of DES (DES DME), when injected subcutaneously for 12 months, produced a high incidence of renal tumors in male hamsters (Lacomba & Gabaldon, 1971) but, the glucuronide (DESGA) was not effective. A tumor incidence of 80% (eight in 10 animals) was observed in the animals injected 3 times/wk with DES DME in an 11.2 mM suspension (0.2 ml) in vehicle. The DESGA in the same concentration and identical treatment regime (11) produced no tumors (0 in 12 animals). Interestingly, subcutaneous injection of a bromoergocryptine (CB-154) markedly inhibited renal-tumor incidence in estrogenized male hamsters (Hamilton et al., 1974). The adenohypophysis of DES-treated animals showed considerable enlargement of the intermediate lobes and increased numbers of prolactin cells in the anterior lobes; these changes were significantly inhibited by CB-154.

The growth of renal tumors in male hamsters is obviously a complex process, and one that at least partially can be reduced by removing the estrogen stimulation (McGregor et al., 1960). In this study, regression was complete within 1 month in 60% of the animals following treatment with DES with 10 months.

TABLE 3
ESTROGEN-INDUCED RENAL TUMORS IN INTACT MALE HAMSTERS[a]

Treatment	Number animals	Method of administration	Renal tumors No.	%	Metastases No.	%
None	61	—	0	0	0	0
DES	245	Injected and/or pellets[b]	177	73	50	28
Estradiol	15	Pellets	15	100	6	40
Estrone	8	Pellets	7	88	1	15
Total (Estrogen treated)	268		199	74	57	99

[a]Kirkman (1959).

[b]Subpannicular injection of 0.6 mg every 2nd day followed in some cases by 20-mg pellets implanted subpannicularly; in other cases, pellets only.

For some of the animals, some factor other than removal of excess estrogen appeared to be involved in the regression process.

Hamster kidney tumor cells have been grown in culture in order to determine effects of estrogens on these cultures (DeKernion & Fraley, 1971); in these studies, DES failed to stimulate tumor cells in culture. Based on the results of this study, the authors concluded that the mode of action of DES in initiating and maintaining hamster kidney tumors is not simply the result of a direct effect of hormones on cells, and noted instead that there may be unidentified stromal or humoral factors—probably important constituents in the complex series of events leading to cell transformation.

Mammary Gland

The role of estrogens toward the development of mammary carcinomas in the C_3H mouse deserved special attention. Figure 1 shows the results reported by Gass et al. (1964). In Gass's study, 6.25-1000 ppb dietary levels of diethylstilbestrol were fed to C_3H female and male mice with mammary tumor virus (MTV^+) as well as to a castrate strain-A males for 18 months. The problem encountered by this experiment is shown at the low end of the dose-response curve; at 6.25 ppb, there was an incidence of 48% tumors in the female C_3H mice. This was significantly different from the 33% incidence in the control mice. However, at 12.5 and 25 ppb, the incidence of tumors was roughly 43% in both groups which was not significantly different from the controls. If tumor response at the three dietary levels (6.25, 12.5, and 25 ppb) is combined, the combined results are significantly different from the controls. There are several possibilities to explain the lack of a consistent dose-response at this low end of the study. Simply, the tumor incidence in the control group may be low, or that of the 6.25 ppb group may have been higher than would be encountered in a replicate experiment. However, it is also conceivable that the dose levels at this range represent or proximate physiological levels; normal variations would be, or could be, expected at this area of the dose-response curve. In a separate experiment, now in progress at NCTR, preliminary data indicate a dose-dependent incidence of mammary tumors in C_3H female MTV^+ mice due to dietary levels of diethylstilbestrol (Fig. 2) and estradiol (Fig. 3) (Norvell & Shellenberger, 1977; Highman et al., 1977a). Although the dose level producing tumors in the estradiol-fed animals is markedly higher than those fed diets containing DES, it is interesting to note that the natural estrogen is indeed producing mammary tumors in these mice. These results suggest that—in mammary tissue, at least—carcinogenicity of chemicals possessing estrogen activity may be due solely to the estrogenic activity.

In a subsequent experiment (Gass et al., 1974) (Table 4), male C_3H mice, having a low titer to mouse MTV^+ factor, were fed diets containing diethylstilbestrol at 250 ppb which, when fed for 18 months produced a 10% incidence of

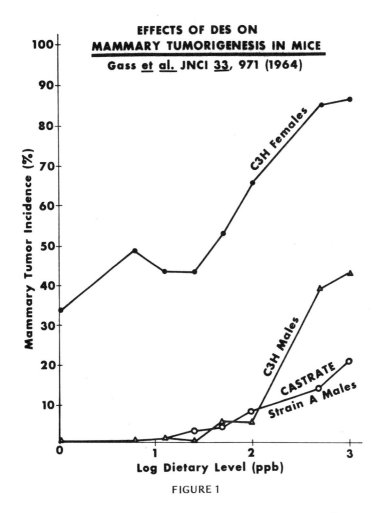

EFFECTS OF DES ON
MAMMARY TUMORIGENESIS IN MICE

Gass et al. JNCI 33, 971 (1964)

FIGURE 1

tumors in the MTV⁻ animals and a 72% incidence in the MTV⁺ animals. Although this data is obtained with males, it demonstrates that the virus is a necessary prerequisite for the induction of mammary tumors in the C_3H mouse following estrogen stimulation. In the NCTR experiment noted above (Norvell & Shellenberger, 1977; Highman et al., 1977a), DES, when fed at dietary levels as high as 500 pbb to low-titer MTV female C_3H mice, failed to produce a significant increase in tumor incidence when compared to the controls after approximately 20 months of exposure (unpublished data from an ongoing experiment).

Experimental results, therefore, demonstrate that although estrogen stimulation does produce mammary tumors in the C_3H mouse, the incidence and time-to-tumor is markedly enhanced by the presence of MTV. Mammary tumorigenesis, however, in C_3H mice is also influenced by the circulating levels of prolactin

TABLE 4

INCIDENCE OF MAMMARY ADENOCARCINOMAS IN
CASTRATED C_3H/ANF AND C_3H/AN MALE MICE[a]

DES dietary level (ppb)	Mouse substrain	Observation period (months)	Tumor incidence No.	%
0	$C3H/AnF(MTV^-)$	12	0/30	0
0	"	18	1/50	2
250	"	12	0/30	0
250	"	18	5/50	10
0	$C3H/An(MTV^+)$	12	0/30	0
0	"	18	0/50	0
250	"	12	9/30	30
250	"	18	36/50	72

[a]From Gass et al. (1974).

which are elevated in mice following estrogen stimulation. Results obtained in C_3H mice exposed to the chemical CB-154 to suppress prolactin release by the pituitary are summarized in Table 5 (Welsch & Gribler, 1973). In this study, the compound, CB-154, bromoergocryptine was injected subcutaneously at a daily dose level of 0.1 mg for 12 months; the CB-154 was dissolved in ethanol and brought to volume with saline. The resultant was a 0.9% sodium chloride solution with not more than 2.5% ethanol. A portion of the animals was sacrificed

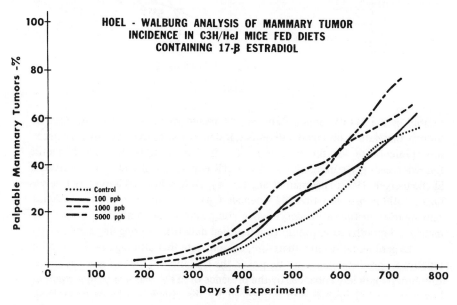

FIGURE 2

216

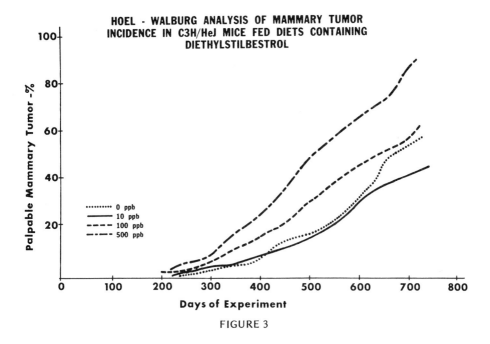

FIGURE 3

at the end of the 12-month treatment period (14 months of age), and the remainder 10 months later. After the 12-month treatment, there was marked suppresion of hyperplastic alveolar nodules in the animals treated with the ergot drug; several of the 10 animals sacrificed at this period were free of tumors, compared to only one of 10 controls. The effects observed at the second sacrifice period were less pronounced. However, the results of this study definitely suggest that the role of prolactin is very important in the etiology of the C_3H mouse mammary tumorigenesis.

In a subsequent report (Brooks & Welsch, 1974) from the same laboratory, the bromoergocryptine, CB-154, significantly reduced the incidence of hyperplastic alveolar nodules and the inguinal gland ratings in nulliparous ovariectomized and hysterectomized mice that were subsequently exposed to estradiol in drinking water (Table 6). Estradiol was added to the drinking water at a level of 0.5 mg/ml (i.e., approximately equivalent to 2.5 mg/day).

In related experiments (Quadri & Meites, 1971), bromoergocryptine injection markedly induced regression of spontaneous mammary tumors in older rats; a subsequent report (Meites, 1972) reviewed the roles of estradiol and prolactin in mammary tumors superimposed on treatment with the mammary carcinogen, DMBA. The results with rodents definitely suggest that prolactin is extremely important in the etiology of mammary tumors following estrogen stimulation. The role, however, of prolactin in mammary tumorigenesis in humans has not been resolved; an excellent review was published on the state-of-the art knowledge of prolactin in humans (Perez-Lopez & Robyn, 1974). Although much re-

TABLE 5

EFFECT OF TREATMENT (1 YEAR) OF 90 YOUNG
C$_3$H/HeJ NULLIPAROUS MICE ON DEGREE OF MAMMARY
GLAND DEVELOPMENT AND NUMBER OF
MAMMARY HYPERPLASTIC NODULES[a]

Treatment	No. mice examined	Mean inguinal mammary gland development	No. of nodules	% mice free of nodules
		After 14 months		
Control	10	3.6[b]	3.0 ± 0.5[b,c]	10[b]
CB-154	10	1.0[b]	0.4 ± 0.2[b,c]	70[b]
		After 24 months		
Control	16	3.8	14.6 ± 1.7	0
CB-154	15	3.3	6.9 ± 0.6	7

[a] Modified from Welsch and Gribler (1973).

[b] $2p < 0.001$, control/CB-154 treated.

[c] Mean ± S.E.

TABLE 6

THE EFFECTS OF CB-154 TREATMENT IN ESTROGEN-STIMULATED
C$_3$H/HeJ MICE ON NORMAL, HYPERPLASTIC, AND NEOPLASTIC
MAMMARY GLAND DEVELOPMENT[a]

	Treatment[b]		
	17β-Estradiol	17β-Estradiol plus CB-154	P
No. mice beginning of study	55	59	
No. mice end of study	20	27	
Mean body weight	28.6 ± 0.9	27.8 ± 0.5	
No. of tumors	25	19	<0.05
No. of mice with tumors	24	19	
Mean latency period (months)	7.7 ± 0.7	8.8 ± 0.8	
Mean number HAN	19.3 ± 2.0	3.5 ± 0.6	<0.001
Mean-range inguinal gland ratings	4.3 (1.5-6.0)	1.6 (1.0-3.0)	<0.001

[a] Taken from Brooks and Welsch (1974).

[b] 17β-Estradiol in drinking water and CB-154 as daily s.c. injection for 12 months.

mains to be learned about prolactin in humans, current data suggest that estrogen stimulation produced much less elevation of serum or blood prolactin in man than in experimental animals.

Mammary tumorigenesis in mice is a complex process involving multiple factors including prolactin levels and viral interaction. Although the applicability of this data to the human situation of mammary tumorigenesis is unknown, it would appear that the use of the C_3H mouse mammary-tumor endpoint is a crude animal model system for direct translation to potential effects in humans, i.e., the direct estrogen effect. Additional refinement of this animal model system, however, may render it an appropriate tool for investigating the effect of estrogens as cocarcinogens, promoters of carcinogenesis, or possible direct carcinogens. At this stage of development, the primary role of the mammary-tumor endpoint in C_3H mice following estrogen stimulation appears to be that of direct comparison of structure-activity relationships and relative potencies.

Reproductive Tract

Lesions of the reproductive tract of both male and female mice have been produced by subcutaneous in utero injections or by neonatal exposure to various estrogens. A 1963 study of DES in neonatal mice following subcutaneous injections was conducted by Dunn and Green. In this study, eight litters of neonatal C_3H and 10 litters of neonatal BALB/c mice were injected subcutaneously with 0.1 cc of 2% DES suspended in physiologic saline (0.9% sodium chloride), i.e., 2 mg/animal. Surviving animals were held for 13-27 months, but survival was very low. In 14 of the 21 surviving male mice, epididymal lesions consisting of vacuolization of tubular cells were observed as well as single or multiple cysts, often bilateral. The results obtained in this study were of marginal usefulness because of high dose levels and the limited number of animals in each group or age. Somewhat similar results were obtained with CD-1 mice. Pregnant CD-1 females received subcutaneous injections of DES at dose levels of 0.01, 0.1, or 1.0 μg/mg/mouse/day during days 9-16 of gestation (McLachlan et al., 1975a, 1975b). Surviving animals were maintained after parturition and examined periodically. In male offspring, lesions of the genital tract were observed at the highest dose level. Such lesions consisted primarily of epididymal cyst, inflammation and cryptorchism, as well as nodular masses in the seminal vesicles and/or prostate; 60% of these males proved to be sterile in mating trials with untreated females. These effects were not observed at the four lowest dose levels.

These workers (Dunn & Green, 1963) also noted reproductive tract lesions in female mice; concretions or stones were observed in the vagina of surviving females, as well as carcinoma of the uterine and cervical and vaginal tissues. Granular cell myoblastoma was observed in the uterine-cervix of two animals. The impact of these results was weakened, principally by the use of very high dose levels, the small number of animals on study, as well as the route of exposure (subcutaneous injection). The reproductive capacity of the females exposed in utero to the selected range of dose levels showed dose-dependent decreases in in reproduction, measured as decreased ova production after subsequent stimulation; in addition, these workers reported a low incidence (< 10%) of cancer of the vagina, cervix, and/or uterus.

Forsberg (1975) described in detail lesions in three female mice exposed to DES during the first 5 days postpartum in which DES was injected subcutaneously into the newborn pups at a dose of 5 μg/day/animal. Lesions described for the three NMRI female mice consisted of extensive adenosis in most of the cervical wall, epidermization of glandular epithelium, evidence of cancerous development, and hyperplasia of vaginal squamous epithelium. The description of lesions in these mice is very similar to those reported in the young adult female humans exposed in utero to DES. Forsberg also quotes some of his earlier results obtained with estradiol exposure:

> Earlier, it has been shown that estradiol injected for 5 days after birth inhibits proliferation of the columnar, cervical, and vaginal epithelium, before its transformation into squamous epithelium. At the same time, there is an increased mytotic rate in the uterine epithelium. Mytotic-rate inhibition in the cervical and upper vaginal region is paralleled with the appearance of areas with remaining columnar epithelium, interspersed in normal squamous epithelium. After puberty, this columnar epithelium forms downgrowths into the stroma, giving a picture of adenosis. Castration at puberty prevents the glandular downgrowths. Later, it was demonstrated that diethylstilbestrol injected neonatally resulted in the same epithelial changes as those caused by estradiol. (p. 101)

It is interesting to note the speculation that the uterine-cervical changes seen in neonatal mice receiving injections of an estrogen are identical whether the chemical was estradiol, the natural estrogen, or diethylstilbestrol, the synthetic nonsteroidal chemical. Speculatively, is the similarity of action of response based simply on the estrogen activity of the chemical rather than some other unique property of the compound or compounds? If, indeed, the lesions of the reproductive tract of female mice are due entirely to estrogenic potency or activity, then the protocols used in toxicological evaluations of estrogens should be developed, considering that these compounds have physiological activity in addition to potential carcinogenic activity. Also, results suggest that chemicals possessing estrogenic activity may, under the proper circumstances, produce lesions up to, and including, carcinoma of the reproductive tract of female mice.

In our study (Highman et al., 1977a), pathological lesions at several sites including the reproductive tract of C_3H mice have been observed in a long-term feeding study with DES and 17β-estradiol at dietary levels of 10, 100, or 500 ppb, or 100, 1000, or 5000 ppb, respectively (Table 7). In addition, preliminary histopathological results have been obtained on over 400 mice (C_3H/HeJ and C_3HeB/FeJ), sacrificed or that died during the first 15 months. At the high

TABLE 7
INCIDENCE (%) OF PATHOLOGIC CHANGES IN MICE GIVEN DIETHYLSTILBESTROL (DES) OR 17β-ESTRADIOL (E₂) FOR 52 WEEKS[a]

Agent (ppb)	No. of mice	Cervix			Uterine horns				Mammary		Osseous hyperplasia
		Mucoid stroma	Adenosis[b] +	>+	Glandular hyperplasia	Adenomyosis	Hyaline changes	Marked ovarian atrophy	HAN's	Tumors	
					C₃H/FeJ (MTV⁺) Mice						
0	47	15	11	0	23	2	4	20	0	4	0
10 DES	32	26	14	0	19	3	3	35	3	0	3
100 DES	38	31	33	6	79	46	39	53	5	8	3
500 DES	48	93	9	89	100	93	85	100	14	7	82
100 E₂	35	17	17	0	24	6	12	15	0	0	0
1000 E₂	36	34	15	0	62	6	19	29	3	6	16
5000 E₂	48	100	38	36[c]	96	81	96	91	9	8	82
					C₃HeB/FeJ (MTV⁻) Mice						
0	18	6	11	0	11	17	11	6	0	0	0
10 DES	39	5	18	0	5	6	3	0	0	0	3
100 DES	18	33	59	0	89	33	50	80	0	0	6
500 DES	37	92	48	21[c]	95	84	95	90	0	0	97

[a]From Highman, et al. (1977)b.

[b]Refers to mice with adenosis limited to upper third of cervix and >+ to those with adenosis extending into lower two-thirds.

[c]Significantly different from group on line 4 by chi square test. p <0.01. The other groups were not subjected to a statistical analysis.

221

dietary levels of both estrogens, the cervix often showed stromal mucoid changes and adenosis associated with foci of low stratified or columnar epithelium lining the cervical canal. Uterine horns showed marked hyperplasia which often penetrated the muscularis. Twelve adenocarcinomas variably involving the uterine horns, corpus, and cervix have been observed in both DES and estradiol-fed animals; some lesions appeared from endometrial glands and some from areas of adenosis. Similar lesions, although less frequent or severe, were observed in animals at the lower dietary levels. No lesions were seen in either strain or at any dose level prior to 52 weeks or in the controls.

Lesions of the reproductive tract have also been reported in rats following subcutaneous injections of diethylstilbestrol into pregnant and/or lactating Sprague-Dawley females (Vorherr et al., 1976). Nine pregnant rats received subcutaneous doses ranging from 0.15 to 1.5 mg/kg of DES in oil from Days 6-20 of gestation; three females received the same dose levels during lactation. Six of the 9 pregnant rats aborted following DES administrations. Three of the 19 surviving pups were exposed in utero and during lactation. These animals were regularly examined 9-26 months following parturition. In males, inhibition of testicular growth and descent, as well as abnormalities of both Wolffian derivatives, was commonly observed. In the females, abnormal development of urogenital sinuses was common, and included lesions described as vaginal adenosis, endometrial squamous metaplasia, vaginal squamous carcinoma in 2 females, as well as endometrial and ovarian adenocarcinoma in 2 other female offspring.

Reproductive tract lesions have also been produced in hamster progeny following oral doses of DES during the latter stages of gestation (Rustia & Shubik, 1976). DES, at levels of 20 or 40 mg/kg on Days 14 or 15 of gestation, produced hyperplastic and neoplastic lesions in most female progeny. These lesions were described variously as cervical polyp, cervical squamous-cell papilloma, mixed mesodermal tumor, vaginal squamous-cell papilloma, Cowper-gland adenoma, and uterine adenocarcinoma. Of male progeny, 20% developed spermatic granulomas of the epididymis and testes. The incidence and severity of these lesions was less pronounced at the 20-mg/kg dose level.

Uterine vaginal lesions have also been reported in monkeys, specifically the squirrel monkey (McClure & Graham, 1973). Ten adult female squirrel monkeys received four 60-mg pellets of DES; animals were sacrificed 5, 9, 11, or 14 months after pellet implantation. Malignant uterine mesotheliomas were observed in 7 of the 10 female squirrel monkeys. In the other 3 animals, early proliferative lesions of the uterine serosa were observed, and 2 of the animals had extra genital serosal lesions in the adrenals, spleen or mesentery.

Lesions, therefore, reported in the reproduction tract of humans (vaginal clear-cell carcinoma in female off-spring following in utero exposure to DES) as well as probable endometrial carcinomas from use of oral contraceptives, have generally been confirmed in animal models. Similar lesions have been seen in mice, rats, hamsters, and squirrel monkeys following a variety of exposures including implants, subcutaneous injection, and oral dietary exposures to several estrogenic chemicals including DES and estradiol. With some exceptions, most animal studies have generally been undertaken with high dose levels injected into a relatively small number of animals. Additional studies are needed using oral exposures and dietary feedings, a wider range of dose levels including low levels and species/strains. In addition, basic studies are needed to follow the kinetics of cell differentiation in the reproductive tract in fetal and neonatal animals following exposure to several estrogens. In this manner, it may be possible to differentiate mechanism, i.e., a "true carcinogenic process," versus a possible "teratogenic process" involving functionally altered cell differentiation.

OVERVIEW

Reproductive tract lesions observed in humans are also evident in several species of laboratory animals that have been treated with both natural and synthetic estrogens. Hepatic lesions in humans have not been observed unequivocally in animal models. Oral contraceptives produced benign liver lesions at high doses in the males only of some strains of rats; results in mice were inconclusive. Obviously, more research is needed in this area. Estrogen-induced pituitary tumors are not uncommon in rodents, and renal tumors can be induced in hamsters; these endpoints as seen in laboratory animals apparently do not correlate with responses observed in humans. Estrogenic induction of mammary tumors in mice and rats is known, but interpretation of the induction mechanism is complicated by the interaction of viruses and prolactin. The relationship of estrogens to human mammary tumors has not been resolved. Estrogen-induced endpoints in humans, with only one or two exceptions, have been reproduced in experimental animals. On the other hand, some lesions in animals have not, to date, been reported in humans. Estrogens, however, must be considered carcinogenic on the premise that exposure of an animal, and even humans, to an estrogen produced: (a) increase in incidence of a tumor occurring spontaneously, (b) a decrease in the latent period for tumor induction, or (c) an increased incidence of a rare spontaneous tumor event.

But, is this a suitable basis for carcinogenic evaluations of hormonally active (specifically estrogenic) chemicals? Protocols for evaluating carcinogenicity of estrogens in experimental animals must be reevaluated. Can estrogenic chemicals, even in conjunction with other materials such as progestins, be evaluated in animal models using, by rote, simple multiples of anticipated human exposures? How can results with estrogens be interpreted if the carcinogenic endpoint is complicated by other hormonal factors such as prolactin, or by viruses? Should toxicologic testing protocols be modified to reflect relative potencies of hormonally active agents in the various experimental animals? Answers to these questions will have a significant impact on endocrine toxicology.

However, there are even more important questions to be resolved. Are estrogens carcinogenic because of estrogenic activity or because of some other unique property akin to more classical concepts of chemical carcinogenicity? Are estrogens direct-acting carcinogens or are they functioning in a more complex manner as moderators, i.e., initiators, promoters, or cocarcinogens? If the latter is the case, how can these actions be evaluated? If these events can be titrated, what impact, if any, will they have on regulatory concepts and procedures?

These complex questions have not been resolved. The preponderance of data suggests that carcinogenic activity is related to estrogenic potency, but a direct permanent action on genetic material cannot be ruled out. This dichotomy can best be illustrated by the lack of resolution of the etiology of mammary tumors in experimental animals. The basic problem was simply and eloquently stated by Dr. Roy Hertz in response to questions posed during hearings in the U.S. Senate before the Subcommittee on Monopoly of the Select Committee on Small Business, January, 1970:

> Question: It is your testimony then that estrogens in and out of themselves are not the sole cause (of breast cancer).
>
> Dr. Hertz: Not the sole cause.
>
> Question: It is your testimony that there are other causes.
>
> Dr. Hertz: I think that they (estrogens) are to breast cancer what fertilizer is to the wheat crop. They are not the seed.

REFERENCES

Benas, A. Increased pituitary weight produced by stilbestrol in intact and castrated rats. *Endocrinol.*, 1956, *65*, 529-31.

Brooks, C.L., & Welsch, C.W. Inhibition of mammary dysplasia in estrogen-treated C3H/HeJ female mice by treatment with 2-bromo-α-ergocryptine. *Proc. Soc. Exp. Biol. Med.*, 1974, *145*, 484-7.

Committee on Safety of Medicines. *Carcinogenicity tests of oral contraceptives.* London: Her Majesty's Stationery Office, 1972.

DeKernion, J.B., & Fraley, E.E. Growth characteristics of the stilbestrol-induced hamster kidney tumor. *J. Surg. Oncol.*, 1971, *3*, 507-15.

Dunn, T.B., & Green, A.W. Cysts of the epididymis, cancer of the cervix, granular cell myoblastoma and other lesions after estrogen injection in newborn mice. *J. Natl. Cancer Inst.*, 1963, *31*, 425-55.

Forsberg, J.G. Late effects in the vagina and cervical epithelia after injections of diethylstilbestrol into neonatal mice. *Amer. J. Obstet. Tynecol.*, 1975, *121*, 101-4.

Gass, G.H., et al. Carcinogenic dose-response curve to oral diethylstilbestrol. *J. Natl. Cancer Inst.*, 1964, *33*, 971-7.

Gass, G.H., et al. Carcinogenic effects of oral diethylstilbestrol on C3H mice with and without the mammary tumor virus. *J. Natl. Cancer Inst.*, 1974, *53*, 1369-70.

Gibson, J.P., et al. Comparative chronic toxicity of three oral estrogens in rats. *Toxicol. Appl. Pharmacol.*, 1967, *11*, 489-510.

Hamilton, J.M., et al. Inhibitory effect of 2-Br-α-Ergocryptine-Methanesulfonate on renal carcinogenesis in the male hamster. *J. Natl. Cancer Inst.*, 1974, *52*, 1929-30.

Herbst, A.L., et al. Adenocarcinoma of the vagina: Association of maternal stilbestrol therapy with tumor appearance in young women. *N. Engl. J. Med.*, 1971, *284*, 878-81.

Highman, B., et al. Pathologic changes in mice induced by diethylstilbestrol and 17-β-estradiol. *Toxicol. Appl. Pharmacol.*, 1977(a), *41*, 1178-1179. Abstract.

IARC. *IARC Monograph Vol. 6, Sex Hormones.* Lyon, France, 1974.

Jacobi, J., et al. Induction of pituitary tumors in male rats by a single dose of estrogen. *Horm. Metab. Res.*, 1975, *7*, 228-30.

Kirkman, H. Estrogen-induced tumors of the kidney. IV. Incidence in female Syrian hamsters. *NCI Monograph*, 1959, *1*, 59-91.

Kirkman, H., Hormone-related tumors in Syrian hamsters. *Progr. Exp. Tumors Res.*, 1972, *16*, 201-240.

Lacomba, T., & Gabaldon, M. Biochemical studies of diethylstilbestrol induced kidney tumors in the golden Syrian hamster. *Cancer Res.*, 1971, *31*, 1251-56.

McClure, H.M., & Graham, C.E. Malignant uterine mesotheliomas in squirrel monkeys following diethylstilbestrol administration. *Lab Animal Sci.*, 1973, *23*, 493-8.

McGregor, R.F., et al. Estrogen-induced kidney tumors in the golden hamster. I. Biochemical composition during tumorigenesis. *J. Natl. Cancer Inst.*, 1960, *24*, 1057-66.

McLachlan, J.A., et al. Effect of prenatal exposure of mice to diethylstilbestrol on reproductive tract function in the offspring. *Toxicol. Appl. Pharmacol.*, 1975(a), *33*, 190. Abstract.

McLachlan, J.A., et al. Reproductive tract lesions in male mice exposed prenatally to diethylstilbestrol. *Science*, 1975(b), *190*, 991-2.

Meites, J. Relation of prolactin and estrogen to mammary tumorigenesis in the rat. *J. Natl. Cancer Inst.*, 1972, *48*, 1217-24.

Neumann, F., & Elger, W. Critical considerations of the biological basis of toxicity studies with steroid (sex) hormones. In E.J. Plotz & J. Haller (Eds.), *Methods in Steroid Toxicology.* Geron-X, 1972.

Norvell, M.J., & Shellenberger, T.E. Mammary tumorigenesis in female C3H mice fed diets containing diethylstilbestrol or 17-β estradiol. *Toxicol. Appl. Pharmacol.*, 1977, *41*, 179. Abstract.

Orosz, A., et al. Effect on thyroid function of long-term oestrogen treatment at high dose level in the rat. *Acta physiologica Academia Scientarum Hungaricae*, 1970, *37*, 273-280.

Perez-Lopez, F.R., & Robyn, D. Minireview: Studies on human prolactin physiology. *Life Sciences*, 1974, *15*, 599-616.

Quadri, S.K., & Meites, J. Regression of spontaneous mammary tumors in rats by ergot drugs. *Proc. Soc. Exp. Biol. Med.*, 1971, *138*, 999-1001.

Rustia, M., & Shubik, P. Transplacental effects of diethylstilbestrol on the genital tract of hamster offspring. *Cancer Letters*, 1976, *1*, 139-46.

Vorherr, H., et al. Teratogenesis and carcinogenesis in rat offspring after transplacental and transmammary exposure to diethylstilbestrol (DES). Abstract, presented at the 60th Annual Meeting, Fed. Amer. Soc. Exp. Biol., April 12-16, 1976, Anaheim, Calif.

Welsch, C.W., & Gribler, C. Prophylaxis of spontaneously developing mammary carcinoma in C3H/HeJ female mice by suppression of prolactin. *Cancer Res.*, 1973, *33*, 2939-46.

Day Two—Morning Discussion

DR. WYNDER: Thank you, Dr. Shellenberger. We have about 25 minutes for discussion, and perhaps we could start with the mechanistic considerations first, and then go to the drugs and hormones. I'd like us to bear in mind the title of the conference, "Human Epidemiology and Animal Laboratory Correlation in Chemical Carcinogenesis." When we look at the title, let's look at the end point for which we'll be judged by future generations. In other words, what will happen to the incidence of cancer 10, 20 or 30 years from now? If the incidence does not decline, in fact, if for certain cancers it will increase, we will certainly have not done our job effectively.

Now with this reminder, I would like the first discussant to call on an old friend of ours—Professor Truhaut—to comment on the first two papers. I would like to say, Dr. Truhaut, as I have watched the intensity with which you have watched the various lecturers, I wish some of our young people could watch you to see how you listen to every lecture, how you take notes, how you look at the slides. I think, if all of our young people would work with this kind of energy toward solving our problems, we would be much better off.

DR. TRUHAUT: Thank you, Mr. Chairman, for your very kind words. I must confess that I was hesitant to take the floor for two reasons. The first one is that it is very difficult for me to express my ideas, because I have to hunt for the right words, but fortunately you are friends and you are patient with me.

The second reason is more important. As is the case with specialists we could be defined as having some, but not many, gaps in our knowledge. I have only a few gaps in my ignorance, and for this reason I hesitate to comment about the two very excellent papers we listened to this morning. I congratulate my two colleagues on these presentations.

But, Professor Jim Miller, you said about chemical carcinogenicity that we ought to realize at once that there is a similarity in chemical structure among chemical carcinogens. Already we have read all your excellent published papers and we became enthusiastic, because if there is any rationale, it is that there is some homogeneity about the mechanisms of reaction.

But my question is the following: I think this stresses the fact that there are two main categories of carcinogens. The first is those directly acting on molecular sites such as nucleic acids, proteins, or even simpler compounds such as methionine. The second category includes those chemicals which need first a metabolic activation, giving a so-called proximal or ultimate carcinogen, which finally reacts at the sites you mentioned.

But in my view there is another category of carcinogens. I call them secondary carcinogens. There are those compounds which really act in two stages. There is a need for a first stage, a stage in which there are physiological modifications, and even the induction of some pathological conditions which are necessary, absolutely necessary, for the second stage of the development of carcinogenicity. And among those I have to mention, as you did, some examples.

The first one I will mention is the class of hormonal compounds. These chemicals are good examples of the application of the concept, benefit versus risk, because I think that if we would not have had a normal back ground of these chemicals, we would not have entered life and even would not be here, because there would have been no possible reproductive function manifested. But what is important is that in my view there is a necessary physiological background for the compounds, and it is only when there is a change leading to an unbalanced amount of those compounds that there is a possibility for manifestation of carcinogenic potential. Of course, this is true so far regarding the whole group of hormonal compounds because they act indirectly. Among the examples I will mention are those compounds which act as bladder carcinogens by producing stones in the bladder, and also the compounds which might act (in my view) by inducing at the level of the liver some hepatotoxic effect, beginning with hypertrophy, and this is also a first stage. And finally, as a first example, as you did Professor Miller, I will mention some trace elements like selenium. It is really impressive to note that at very minute doses selenium is an essential element, but at higher, but still very minute, doses selenium is able to induce tumors. In this case you have really two curves. The first one is really a curve which represents beneficial effects, and for this secondary carcinogen I think that there are two or three consequences.

The first consequence in my view is that if there is a third category of carcinogenic compounds—and there might be others, we still don't know—an important concept is to keep in mind that every chemical compound should be evaluated for carcinogenic potential as well as for toxic potential on its own merit. It is very dangerous to have an absolute theory which puts all these things in the same basket. This is my first comment.

My second comment is that for this secondary carcinogen you have to realize that there is a need for a first stage. In this stage, there is not only a dose-effect relationship, but clearly there is a threshold. This is very important, because to apply a concept like zero threshold, zero risk is, in my view, not scientific at all.

At the beginning of my professional life I was very rigid about chemical carcinogenity, but becoming older I don't know if I am becoming more reasonable or if I am becoming less cautious. To my two colleagues, Professor Miller and Dr. Conney, I ask the following question: What do you think about the third category of carcinogens? I might have made a mistake, and maybe you can answer that. The so-called secondary carcinogens are those acting on genetic material, those which are truly genetic compounds. Thank you very much, Mr. Chairman; I was very long, I hope you will excuse me.

DR. MILLER: Thank you, Professor Truhaut; you've raised a number of important considerations. First of all, we've never intended this electrophilicity theory (as you called it) to be an absolute one. Certainly not. A very good example of (a secondary carcinogen) is a proposed food additive which emerged 45 years ago; they fed it at an extremely high level in the diet, actually, believe it or not, up to 25% of the diet. This additive was oxidized to oxalic acid, and as you might guess, it formed calcium oxalate stones in the bladder and people got tumors. We can do the same thing by dropping a glass bead in the bladder, and so on. I don't look upon this as a chemical carcinogen.

This may actually relate to endogenous carcinogens, for all we know, metabolites, perhaps, of tryptophan, and the continual removal of the transitional cell epithelium by mechanical means by the stones perhaps could be considered a promoter. That's the kind of theory I like to think of in this case.

Now in this case I would point out that if this theory is correct, then the tryptophan metabolites like 3-hydroxykynurenine and 3-hydroxyanthranilic acid have a potential, as aromatic amines of developing electrophiles.

So now, with hormones, I think, it's been amply demonstrated from what we've heard this morning; I certainly look upon these as permissive agents in a sense, and it may well be that they're acting essentially as promoters. I don't know if I covered all the points but I think that's enough.

DR. KENSLER: I've been quite interested in nitrilotriacetic acid, which was proposed as a detergent substitute for phosphates. In both man and animal it's been shown with reasonably good mass balance not to be metabolized, although in the environment it is degraded into the diacetic nitrilocompound which can be turned into a nitrosocompound which Lijiniski tested and found to be inactive as a carcinogen.

Recently, when treating at levels of 20,000 ppm in the rat, this material induced what would appear to be a significant level of cancers in the urinary tract. Now this compound is inactive in the Ames test. It is a sequestering agent and we do have metal carcinogenesis; it would appear that this might be another category where, if you grossly overloaded the system you could produce metal imbalance, which by some mechanism or other—that's the one you're talking about—might produce cancer.

And as Al Kolbye is worried about losing all solvents, it seems to me if you push sequestering agents high enough you might lose all sequestering agents, but in any case what do you think about this situation?

DR. MILLER: Sorry, I forgot to mention that part of Professor Truhaut's comments, and I'm glad you brought that up. I mentioned the handful of carcinogenic metal ions which, if given at high enough levels like cobalt ion, cadmium ion, beryllium ion, chromium ion, often produce tumors at subcutaneous sites. Some of these ions are nutrients at micro, while at very high levels they appear to be carcinogenic. These metal ions, of course, are electrophiles per se, but they don't enter generally, to my knowledge, into forming covalent bonds. They form fairly strong electrostatic bonds, and I think the work that Larry Loeb at the Institute of Cancer Research in Philadelphia has been doing in recent years on the effect of these metal ions on decreasing the fidelity by which DNA template is replicated is perhaps a very possible mechanism of metal carcinogenesis.

DR. KRAYBILL: Concerning valence state, this is an elementary question, but I'd like to ask you about chromium. This has bothered me for some time. The hexavalent chromium, as we all know, is identified as a carcinogen, yet trivalent chromium in the body, I believe, can be converted to hexavalent. Trivalent chromium of course is, according to Mertz, a component in the glucose tolerance factor, and is essential. Why the difference here between the hexavalent and trivalent?

DR. MILLER: I don't really know. It's perfectly true that the body is barely able to reduce hexavalent to trivalent chromium, and my feeling about this is, if you start out with trivalent chromium it never gets in the cell, it gets trapped on the way, because it's the one that binds protein and, quite likely, phosphate groups and nucleic acids. But if you give the hexavalent, which can get through the cell, and then inside the cell it gets reduced to trivalent, that's what I regard as the carcinogen there.

DR. KENSLER: I'll be very brief. Dr. Truhaut a moment ago said something which I thought was extremely interesting. I wish I could remember exactly the way he expressed it. Interesting and provocative, and I think we should keep it in mind in this meeting. He asked, in effect, "Did God deliberately give women estrogen, knowing it was a carcinogenic agent?" Well, I think you might ask this about all those agents which have been discussed here which are naturally occurring, synthesized within the mammalian bodies and in their food supply and are mutagenic, whether or not they're carcinogenic.

I heard an extremely interesting lecture by Medawar, and if he is right then the answer is even necessary. It is necessary to increase the very low, ordinary rate of mutation for the survival of the species. He pointed out that without a reasonably high rate of mutation there'd be no adaptation to a changing environment, and we wouldn't be here today.

And I think that we're dealing with factors which do increase the risk of cancer long after the reproductive age is over, when it doesn't matter in the least for the survival of the species, and in so doing, increases the chance of survival of a species with environmental changes.

The idea of trying to eliminate mutagenic agents, I think, is a little short of stupidity.

Which is better, to have animals die of cancer at the end of the reproductive age, or in the case of estrogen, not reproduce and have the species die out, or in the case of other mutagenic agents, not be able to adapt to a changing environment?

I don't think we should condemn mutation in those things which increase it.

DR. BUTLER: Dr. Conney, you presented two extremely interesting papers on entirely separate entities. I was wondering if the effects of these are, in fact, to induce neoplasms in an animal? Which of the facts you're talking about, the nutritional and environmental or the metabolic, could be considered to be rate-limiting standards, if there is such an effect? The other smaller thing was in your first paper concerning idiosyncratic reactions with drugs. These reactions are extremely common and quite a problem. Do you think the things you've been describing could form any basis for this?

DR. CONNEY: I think that there are many aspects to this. First, an overriding aspect is the individual differences among people. There are large differences among people which could be and definitely are genetically and environmentally caused, and we don't know yet the relative role that environment and genetics play.

This is an area that needs further attention. It's going to be important, knowing this individuality, to focus on individual environmental carcinogens, knowing the steps that cause metabolic activation and those that cause formation of the reactive intermediate—DNA and RNA protein—to determine among individuals what is the relative formation of each of these, and I think this is going to be a challenge of the future.

It's not known what the rate-limiting step is in terms of genetics or environmental effects and also the same can be said for nutrition. The relative role that this plays in explaining individuality is really not known.

DR. WYNDER: Let us adjourn for lunch where are guest luncheon speaker will be Dr. Delbert Barth of the EPA.

12. EPA's Environmental Carcinogen R & D Program

Delbert S. Barth

Deputy Assistant Administrator for
Health and Ecological Effects
Office of Research and Development
U.S. Environmental Protection Agency

EPA is particularly concerned about environmental carcinogens and their adequate control to protect public health. Many of the laws which EPA implements contain explicit or implicit authorities related to environmental carcinogens. The latest law with the broadest authorities is the Toxic Substances Control Act.

Examples of specific problems of immediate concern include (1) kepone in the James River and Chesapeake Bay, (2) trace amounts of chlorinated hydrocarbons in drinking water supplies, and (3) asbestos in air and in surface waters. In each case, the question is, "What additional regulatory action, if any, should be taken to afford adequate protection to public health?" In each case, the answer to this question requires knowledge of the risk to humans associated with the existing environmental levels of the pollutants of concern. One of the functions of the Office of Research and Development of EPA is to compile a data base on the basis of which the required risk assessment may be performed. For environmental carcinogens, this is always a difficult task due to a variety of reasons the most important ones of which are probably related to the variable latent period between exposure to environmental carcinogens and appearance of frank disease, as well as the fact that pertinent toxicologic data in experimental animals have usually been obtained at massive dose levels compared to existing environmental exposure levels. In addition, pertinent human epidemiologic data are usually nonexistent, sparse, or of doubtful significance due to possible confounding cofactors such as cigarette smoking, possible combination effects from exposure to complex mixtures of many other environmental pollutants, residence changes, job changes, uncontrolled demographic factors in general, etc.

In spite of all the difficulties cited above, we must develop the best research and development program we can devise with the general objective of

231

providing data bases to enable meaningful risk assessments for environmental carcinogens. The remainder of this presentation will outline in general terms the approach we are taking, give a brief status report on results of efforts to date, and point out the direction we hope to take in the future.

The first step in our approach is to take advantage of all the work already done or underway by other governmental agencies. The principal other agencies with which we already have or will seek interagency agreements in this area include: the National Cancer Institute, National Institute of Environmental Health Sciences, National Institute of Occupational Safety and Health, National Center for Health Statistics, National Center for Toxicological Research, and Center for Disease Control. The purpose of these agreements is to establish a more formal mechanism to enable improved information exchange as well as to allow for transfer of funds so that the best qualified agency may manage or carry out portions of the total program.

The experimental approach for acquiring new data contemplates balanced efforts in epidemiology, with special attention to exposure assessment, toxicology, and measurement methods development. Initially, the epidemiologic studies will be retrospective, with emphasis on comparing geographical regions with high mortality rates for a selected cancer type to matched geographical regions with low rates. Exposure assessment will retrospectively estimate exposure by all significant routes of entry for selected known or suspected environmental carcinogens. Retrospective emission inventories for the selected pollutants will be compiled to serve as input data for estimating total integrated exposures for periods up to 20-25 years.

Our program began as a contract program in fiscal year 1976 with the understanding that the first year of the program would be devoted to a systematic compilation of selected nationwide existing data and then more specific existing data for selected pilot study areas. On the basis of these data, then, hypotheses will be formulated and final study areas, cancer types, and pollutants of concern will be selected for the next phase of the epidemiologic program.

In the future, we hope to design and carry out some new epidemiologic studies to test hypotheses developed in the current effort. We ultimately hope to shift our measured end point from cancer mortality to cancer incidence. We also hope to develop some prospective epid miologic studies in the future. Concomitantly with the beginning of new epid miologic studies, supportive toxicologic and measurement method development will be initiated. The end product sought is a systematic approach to development of the required data bases for performing reliable risk assessment for environmental carcinogens.

It is fully understood that the program briefly described above must be long term. It will take many years to develop the required data bases for the known high priority, or high estimated risk, environmental carcinogens. In the meantime, we fully expect that new, or newly recognized, high estimated-risk environmental carcinogens will be identified. We sincerely hope that the systematic approach now being devised will enable more cost effective risk assessments to be done in the future.

13. Estrogens and Human Cancer

Peter Greenwald
Cancer Control Bureau
New York State Department of Health

We will cover the evidence on estrogens at the three stages of life; that is, in utero estrogen exposure, exposure during the fertile years, and in older women. In part, this updates some of our previously published work (Greenwald et al., 1971, 1973, 1977; Greenwald, Caputo, & Wolfgang, 1977). In addition, I would like to briefly describe some of our current work on prostate cancer. Most of the people attending this conference are men. We talked about studies on mice and women, and should also include men. Prostate cancer is the third leading cause of cancer deaths among men. Most likely, several people in this room already have the so-called latent form of prostate cancer and others of us will have it.

IN-UTERO ESTROGEN EXPOSURE

Table 1 lists the young women who developed vaginal cancer in New York State since 1950. We have gone to great depth to obtain information about their exposure to diethylstilbestrol (DES), starting with a controlled study in 1971[1]. You might note from Table 1 that there are 26 patients; for 22 we could establish definite or possible exposure to estrogens.

There was aggregation by birth years, 1950 to 1957 with a peak in 1952 to 1953—the time of peak use of estrogens. The age range for those with definite or possible exposure is 14 to 23 years.

One of our problems in retrospective epidemiologic studies is definitely establishing the exposure. I'd like to mention several examples to you (see p. 236) to illustrate these problems:

[1] This study was supported in part by Grant 12707 from the National Cancer Institute.

TABLE 1
VAGINAL AND CERVICAL CANCER AFTER MATERNAL USE OF SYNTHETIC ESTROGENS IN PATIENTS REPORTED IN THE NEW YORK STATE CANCER REGISTRY, 1950-1975

Case No.	Year of birth	Age (year) at diagnosis	Maternal synthetic estrogen therapy during pregnancy		
			Time started	Time ended	Drug & dose
			Definite exposure		
1	1950	23 (1973)	3 mo.	Unk.	Stilbestrol, 10 mg/day increased to 25 mg/day in 4th mo. and 35 mg/day in 5th mo.
2	1951	15 (1965)	5 wk.	Delivery	Stilbestrol, 5 mg/day initially, increased 5 mg/wk to 125 mg/day
3	1952	15 (1968)	Conception	Delivery	Stilbestrol 0.1 mg/day until 3rd week, then 5 mg/day to 100 mg/day.
4	1952	17 (1970)	3 mo.	6 mo.	Dienestrol, 5 mg/day; t estrone (intramusc) for 2 doses at 3rd mo; progest. & thyroid 3rd mo to delivery
5	1952	18 (1970)	2½ mo.	5½ mo.	Stilbestrol 25 mg/day 2½ mo to 5½ mo.
6	1952	19 (1971)	2½ wk.	3½-4 mo.	Stilbestrol, 5 mg tablets initially & 25 mg later
7	1952	19 (1971)	3 mo.	9 mo.	Stilbestrol, 75 mg/day from 3rd mo to 7 mo, decreased beginning 7 mo to 50 mg/day and at middle of 8 mo to 25 mg/day
8	1952	19 (1971)	3 mo.	Delivery	Stilbestrol, 100 mg/day
9	1953	17 (1970)	2½ mo.	5 mo.	Stilbestrol, possibly 65 mg/day; also 28 "estrogen" shots from 2½ mo. to 4½ mo.
10	1953	17 (1970)	Unk.	Unk.	Stilbestrol, dosage unknown
11	1953	20 (1973)	2 mo.	Unk.	Stilbestrol, oral, given under Smith schedule
12	1954	17 (1972)	3 mo.	9 mo.	Stilbestrol, dosage unknown
13	1954	18 (1972)	OB record confirms use of Stilbestrol. Mother recalls one shot in first or 2nd month of pregnancy, then pills for one month.		Stilbestrol, dosage unknown

TABLE 1 (continued)

| Case No. | Year of birth | Age (year) at diagnosis | Maternal synthetic estrogen therapy during pregnancy | | |
			Time started	Time ended	Drug & dose
14	1954	18 (1973)	12 wk.	24 wk.	Stilbestrol, 1.5 mg/day
15	1955	14 (1969)	13 wk.	35 wk.	Stilbestrol, increasing dosages from approx. 20 mg/day to no more than 150 mg/day
16	1955	18 (1973)	During 1st trimester	Unk.	Stilbestrol, 5 mg/day
17	1955	19 (1974)	12 wk.	13 wk.	DES, dosage unknown
18	1956	17 (1973)	Unk.	Unk.	Premarin 1.25 mg, Proluton (intramuscularly)
19	1957	15 (1973)	8 wk. 18 wk.	17 wk. Delivery	Stilbestrol, 25 mg/day Stilbestrol, 50 mg/day

Possible exposure

20	1953	16 (1970)	3 mo.	4 mo.	Mother states she took a drug during pregnancy. Unconfirmed by records
21	1953	17 (1971)	3 mo.	Delivery	Possibly Stilbestrol, dosage unknown
22	1953	20 (1973)	Unk.	Unk.	Mother states she took a drug during pregnancy. Unconfirmed by records

No known exposure

23	1950	21 (1971)	None		Mother states that no drugs were taken during pregnancy. Obstetric records negative
24	1951	21 (1973)	3 mo.	3 mo.	Mother states that she was given one injection. OB states that his records were destroyed but he never gave anything but progestrone in cases of threatened abortions
25	1952	14 (1966)	1st trimester	Continued 90 days	Probably Provera, dosage unknown
26	1959	8 (1967)	None		Mother states no drug taken. Obstetric records negative

a. Patient 6 (Table 1). The mother felt that she had taken some drugs during pregnancy. The physician was very cooperative; we read his records and the hospital records. There was no evidence whatever of estrogen use and he denied that he had given it, based on his records. Finally, we were able to identify the pharmacist, who had maintained his records for many years. He found two prescriptions for DES written during the mother's pregnancy in 1952.

b. Patient 9. The obstetrician had died and his records were destroyed. There was a note on the delivery record that DES had been given. We could tell nothing regarding the dose. One of the few benefits of our tax system may be record keeping; the mother had retained her bill indicating DES and the number of pills. Since she remembered the color of the pills, we were able to estimate her total dosage.

c. There was another patient, not shown in Table 1, actually one of the first reported with adenocarcinoma of the vagina. This 30-year-old woman was born in 1940. I was very interested in her because she was a twin, a dizygous twin, both female. The affected twin had died. I actually did the reverse of what we usually do. I went to find the unaffected twin sister first and interviewed her, rather than first seeing the hospital records. She lived in St. Lawrence County far north of Syracuse and north of the Adirondacks, and it turned out that she was raised on a very rural, primitive farm having no running water. While interviewing her mother with the twin sister present, the mother said, for the first time, and with some feelings of guilt, that she had attempted an abortion during that pregnancy.

This was in 1940 before DES use. In spite of a good effort, we couldn't trace the physician, who had left the area many years before. We did finally find a nurse who worked for him, an alert, elderly lady residing in a nursing home. The best she could recall was that the physician generally used some sort of solution squirted against the cervix. She didn't know what it was, but probably not permanganate.

Well, after getting all of this information, I obtained the hospital records. It turned out that there was a new, inexperienced record-room clerk. The actual diagnosis was adenocarcinoma of the cervix, not classified as such because the clerk felt that since the cancerous cervix was removed, it couldn't be listed as the affected organ. Cervical adenocarcinomas are relatively more common and are not included in this study.

The evidence about DES may be summarized by indicating the evidence which I think supports a cause-and-effect relationship:

1. The vast majority of mothers took DES. This was unlike controls and unlike what we know about the majority of mothers at that time. There was a strong statistical association.

2. All of the mothers whose daughters had vaginal cancer took it during the earlier months of pregnancy. If this was a spurious cancer association, we would not expect a relationship to trimester of pregnancy.

3. There was a regular induction period. The years of diagnosis were at ages 14-23 years. This, again, was consistent with an etiologic factor.

4. There was aggregation by date of birth in the early 1950s, the time of peak use of synthetic estrogens. Furthermore, when we looked at some of the mothers' records to find out whether DES could have contributed to the cancer in the absence of a threatened abortion, we found that a number of the women did not actually have a threatened abortion. They might have had spotting at a previous pregnancy, or another reason for DES use, so we felt that it was not necessary to have the combination of factors.

5. There was a common histology which tends to be consistent with a single etiology.

6. The hypothesis is biologically plausible and is supported by multiple investigators finding the same thing. There are no strong alternative hypotheses. In sum, what we have is a convergence and coherence of varying lines of evidence.

I think if you recall Dr. Kraybill's first slide, you will see that the logic that we used in epidemiology is similar to that in carcinogenesis. It is not a mere association which makes us believe in probable causality, but this convergence and coherence of many lines of inference. One thing we did not have is a dose-response. We tried to find this by comparing mothers whose children got vaginal cancer with other mothers who took DES and whose children did not develop cancer. It turned out that dosage levels were so uniformly high in both groups, that we couldn't set up gradients for analysis.

Figure 1 is a histogram that shows the number of cases diagnosed per year in upstate New York. Based on this figure, we are reassessing our estimate of what is likely to happen in the future. It looks like the number of new cases per year has peaked, and hopefully is on the decline.

We have also analyzed data relating to the question of whether cancers might have developed in boys or girls other than the vaginal and cervical adenocarcinomas (Greenwald et al., 1973). This study showed no association with other cancer types. However, the testicular cancer group is so heterogeneous that it may merit further study.

Well, then, for the magnitude of the problem. Thus far only vaginal and cervical cancers have been established as related to DES. There is strong evidence of causality. There have been approximately 15,000 exposed in the United States per year in the 1960s—a greater, but undetermined, number in the 1950s. There are over 300 cases now in the United States, and it appears that the number of new cases per year may have leveled off, or perhaps be on the decline.

ORAL CONTRACEPTIVES AND BREAST CANCER

Next, we're going to take up the question of whether there's a risk of breast cancer from oral contraceptives. You see in Fig. 2 the time trends in breast cancer incidence rates and oral contraceptives use rates.

You can see that the breast cancer incidence rate has been climbing gradually over the years. The dashed line is contraceptive sales figure rates de-

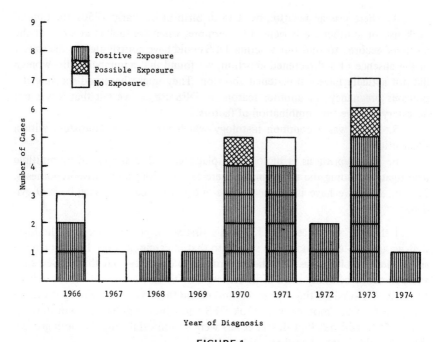

FIGURE 1

Number of Vaginal and Cervical Cancer Cases by Year of Diagnosis and Exposure to Synthetic Estrogens for Patients Reported to the New York State Cancer Registry, 1950-1975.

rived from a Department of the Census survey of industry giving the wholesale dollars of sales for different drugs in the United States. Figure 2 shows no parallelism in trends.

There have been six case-control studies of breast cancer and oral contraceptives (Arthes, Sartwell, & Lewison, 1971; Vessey, Doll, & Jones, 1975; Boston Collaborative Drug Surv. Program, 1973; Henderson et al., 1974; Stavraky & Emmons, 1974; Fasal & Paffenbarger, 1975). These are summarized in Table 2. By and large, they were done by good investigators with careful attention to case ascertainment and control selection. If you look down the right hand column of Table 2 showing the estimated relative risks, you see that there is no association observed in these case-control studies between oral contraceptives and breast cancer.

Now, there is one major caution. Oral contraceptives came into use about 1960. They weren't widely used until the mid 1960s. The maximum follow-up in these studies is generally less than 10 years. Dr. Louis Hemplemann (1976) in Rochester, who has been studying radiation-induced breast cancer, does not find an increase until after 15 years. Dr. Robert Hoover (1976), working with Dr. Gray in Louisville, published an unconfirmed study showing a slight increased risk of breast cancer after long-term estrogen use. Again no difference was observed until after 15 years.

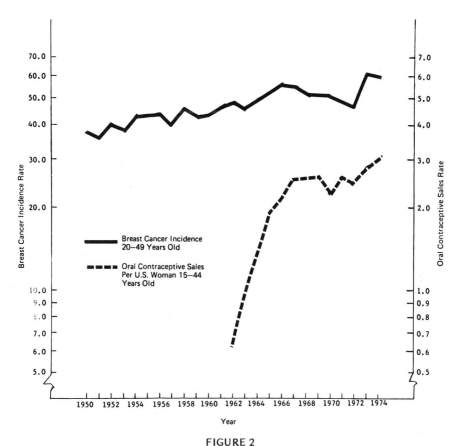

FIGURE 2

Trend in use of Oral Contraceptives as Compared to Breast Cancer Incidence Rate Per 100,000 Women of Ages 20-49 Years, New York State, Exclusive of New York City, 1950-1974.

So it does not appear to me that there is any way that we can draw a conclusion about safety, because of this short duration of follow-up. There is, however, some reason to be concerned about selected subgroups or oral contraceptive users. Table 3, taken from the work of Fasal and Paffenbarger (1975) shows the risk in their study according to the months that estrogens were used. If you look at the second line, at the 25-48 month (2-4 year) duration of use, the relative risk is 1.9. Drs. Fasal and Paffenbarger felt that this might suggest that oral contraceptives could accelerate existing breast cancer. They said "accelerate" because with a causal relationship you would normally expect a longer duration to yield a higher risk. This acceleration possibility is unconfirmed, but it does raise a concern that should be analyzed further.

More striking is Table 4 from the same study showing the risk to women who had prior benign disease. Women with prior benign disease who took oral contraceptives for more than 6 years have an 11-fold increase in risk. Small

TABLE 2

ABSENCE OF ASSOCIATION OF ORAL CONTRACEPTIVES WITH BREAST CANCER
CASE-CONTROL EPIDEMIOLOGIC STUDIES

Investigators & place	Cases	Controls	Oral cont. use rate		Estimated relative risk[a]
			Cases[a]	Controls[a]	
Arthes, Sartwell, & Lewison (1971), Baltimore	Johns Hopkins Hosp. patients, 15-75 yrs; N = 119	Other surgical patients; matched on age, race, marital status, time of admission; N = 119	0.05	0.06	0.85
Vessey, Doll & Jones (1975), London	5 London hospitals; married patients 16-45 yrs; N = 322	Same hospitals; medical or surgical wards; married, matched on age & parity; N = 412	0.36	0.38	0.89
Boston Collaborative Drug Surveillance Program (1973)	24 hospitals; patients, 20-44 yrs; N = 23	Selected other patients; 20-44 yrs.; N = 842	0.13	0.20	0.60
Henderson et al (1974), Los Angeles	Los Angeles cancer registry, patients up to 65 yrs; N = 307	Outpatient without malignancy; Matched on age, race, socio-economic status; N = 307	0.19	0.22	0.74
Stavraky & Emmons (1974), Ontario	Ontario Cancer Foundation Clinic; Premenopausal; N = 95	Clinic patients with other types of cancer or benign disease; N = 106	0.32	0.30	1.05
Fasal & Paffenbarger (1975), Berkeley	19 Hospitals; Patients up to 50 yrs; N = 452	2 other patients/case, 1 medical, 1 surgical; matched on age, race, religion, hospital, residence; excluding gynec., obstet., thromboemboli, mental disorders, N = 872	0.50	0.46	1.1

[a]When not given, estimates were calculated from the papers.

TABLE 3
RELATIVE RISK OF BREAST CANCER
ACCORDING TO DURATION OF ORAL
CONTRACEPTIVE USE[a]

Duration of use (months)	Summary of Chi-square analysis		
	Number of subjects	Relative risk	P
1-24	999	1.0	1.0
25-48	802	1.9	<0.01 ←
49-96	862	1.1	0.83
97 and over	743	1.4	0.48

[a]From Fasal and Paffenbarger (1975).

TABLE 4
RELATIVE RISK OF BREAST CANCER FROM USE OF
CONTRACEPTIVES, BY DURATION OF USE AMONG
WOMEN WITH PRIOR BIOPSY FOR BENIGN
BREAST DISEASE[a]

Duration of use (months	Biopsy		
	Number of subjects	Relative risk	P
Ever-use, All	136	1.5	0.40
1-24	105	1.2	0.99
25-48	91	1.3	0.99
47-92	91	1.2	0.85
73 and over	90	11.2	0.04 ←

[a]From Fasal and Paffenbarger (1975).

numbers of study subjects in these categories limit the statistical power and thus our confidence in these results, but an 11-fold increase is very striking.

One last thing about breast cancer: in addition to six reports on breast cancer and oral contraceptives, there are six studies by competent investigators on benign breast disease and oral contraceptives (Boston Collaborative Drug Surv. Program, 1973; Fasal & Paffenbarger, 1975; Vessey, Doll, & Sutton, 1972; Sartwell et al., 1973; Kelsey et al., 1974; Nomura & Comstock, 1976). Two of these show no difference and four show what is interpreted by the investigators as a protective effect.

I only mention this to tell you that I don't believe it. The reason I don't believe it is that one of my colleagues in Albany, Dr. Dwight Janerich (1977), has been studying prescribing habits of physicians in relation to benign breast disease and oral contraceptives. In New York State, if there is a history of benign disease, one third of physicians will not prescribe oral contraceptives. There are some who do just the opposite. They give contraceptives. Further, if benign breast disease develops, 47% of the physicians will stop the oral contraceptives. So the question is whether the investigators were too far out of touch with the clinical doctors and whether what they called a protective effect was merely a manifestation of prescribing habits.

This has an important clinical implication. If doctors give oral contraceptives because they think it will protect against benign disease, they may be doing more harm than good.

MENOPAUSAL ESTROGEN USE
AND ENDOMETRIAL CANCER

We'll go on now to the question of menopausal estrogen use and endometrial cancer. A striking problem in assessing this question, especially in trying to compare cancer trends from registries to drug use trends is that we have very inadequate information on the extent of drug use in the United States, and specifically on how different segments of our population use the various drugs. There's just very, very little information on drug use patterns.

TABLE 5
ENDOMETRIAL CANCER CASES AND INCIDENCE RATE
FOR NEW YORK STATE, EXCLUSIVE OF NEW YORK CITY
1960-1974, AS COMPARED TO ESTROGEN SALES
IN THE UNITED STATES

	Endometrial cancer		Estrogen sales	
Year	Upstate NY number	Incidence rate per 100,000 women	U.S. wholesale dollars	Rate per woman age 45-64 yrs
1960	749	15.49	—	—
1961	777	15.81	—	—
1962	848	16.98	15,422,000	0.81
1963	791	15.56	18,427,000	0.95
1964	807	15.65	21,009,000	1.06
1965	893	16.90	25,583,000	1.28
1966	962	17.90	34,700,000	1.70
1967	1030	18.82	40,226,000	1.93
1968	900	16.21	44,699,000	2.11
1969	979	17.30	46,519,000	2.16
1970	957	16.64	50,489,000	2.31
1971	1057	17.99	57,619,000	2.60
1972	1130	18.76	64,423,000	2.88
1973	1423	23.38	69,832,000	3.11
1974	1594	25.95	77,083,000	3.41
1975	—	—	82,777,000	3.64

Table 5 shows the incidence of endometrial cancer and the estrogen sales rates. Endometrial cancer rose by about 68% since 1960, with over 80% of the rise in the past 5 years. Table 5 excludes so-called "Stage 0" *in situ* cancer, and the rise is present for all stages. In New York State, the endometrial cancer rise is present for all age groups, most marked in the 45-64-year age group.

Sales of estrogens (wholesale dollars) from 1962, where we first could obtain data to 1975, rose by 437%. Now the consumer cost only rose by 25%, so that's not an inflation effect; it's a real major increase in consumption. There are some supporting data for this. Dr. DeNuzzo of the Albany College of Pharmacy each year has his pharmacy students visit about 100 different pharmacies and abstract 100 consecutive prescriptions. He then evaluates the rank order of prescription drug sales.

In 1968 the estrogenic drug "Premarin" was the 36th most commonly prescribed drug. In 1975 it was 19th (DeNuzzo, 1973, 1976). Assuming a 1.5-mg tablet with women taking the drug 3 out of 4 weeks in a cyclical fashion, we would estimate that presently 14% of United States women over 45 now take estrogens. Of course, this could be a much higher percent with women taking it for shorter periods in the year. A good survey in the Seattle area by Stadel and Weiss (1975) shows that 51% of menopausal women used estrogens at some time.

If estrogens are inducing endometrial cancer as suspected, we have the question of whether the disease may be less malignant than the usual endometrial cancer. While incidence has risen, mortality has been falling gradually. This is a paradox. We don't have a good explanation, but it could be due to less severe disease or problems with pathologic diagnosis.

One piece of evidence incriminating estrogen, then, is the parallelism in time trends between drug use and cancer. There's a second piece of evidence suggesting a true association. Some time ago, endometrial cancer was studied among women with functional ovarian tumors that presumably secrete estrogen (Mansell & Hertig, 1955). Twelve of 32 Boston patients with these tumors developed endometrial cancer. At the Mayo Clinic, women with polycystic ovaries known to be associated with high estrogen levels as well as androgen levels were studied for the occurrence of endometrial cancer (Jackson & Dockerty, 1957). Seventeen of 45, or 38%, had endometrial cancer.

Dr. Hoover (Hoover et al., 1976) at the National Cancer Institute studied breast cancer patients in Connecticut and analyzed whether second primary cancers of the endometrium were more common in those women who had an initial course of hormone therapy as compared to breast cancer patients who did not have an initial course of therapy. The risk of a second primary endometrial cancer was 2-3 times greater in those having initial hormone therapy.

There are four case-control studies that have been published thus far on endometrial cancer (Smith et al., 1975; Ziel & Finkle, 1975; Mack et al., 1976; Gray et al., 1977), summarized in Table 6. The findings were all the same. If you look down the right-hand column at relative risk and take the more sensitive

TABLE 6
ENDOMETRIAL CANCER ASSOCIATED WITH ESTROGEN USE
CASE-CONTROL EPIDEMIOLOGIC STUDIES

Investigators & place	Cases	Controls	Estrogen use rate		Estimated relative risk
			Cases	Controls	
Smith et al. (1975); Seattle	Selected hospitals; N = 317	Other gynecologic cancer; matched for age, year of diagnosis; N = 317	0.48	0.17	4.5 (7.5 with matched pair analysis)
Ziel & Finkle (1975), Los Angeles	Kaiser Foundation Health Plan members; N = 94	Other Kaiser Health Plan members; matched for age, duration in plan, residence; N = 188	0.57	0.15	7.6
Mack, et al. (1976), Los Angeles	Affluent retirement Community; N = 63	Same community; matched for age, marital status; post-hysterectomy excluded; N = 252	0.89	0.50	8.0
Gray et al. (1977)	One physician's practice; N = 205	Hysterectomy, matched on age, parity, year of surgery; N = 205	0.16	0.06	3.1

statistical test for the first reference, you'll see that the relative risks for the first three are around 7, and the last, 3.

There have been some criticisms of these studies. The first by Smith et al. (1975) used cervical cancer patients and other gynecologic cancer patients as controls. Endometrial and cervical patients come from different socioeconomic groups, and there was a question of whether socioeconomic status confounded the results. This concern was not present for the other studies. Another question was the absence of pathologic confirmation by a research pathologist. Some of this is being corrected by work in progress.

The case-control study by Gray, Christopherson, and Hoover (1977) compensates for some of the deficiencies of the earlier three and comes up with the same findings.It's a study based on Dr. Gray's practice. Dr. Gray is a gynecologist who had a large practice over many years. Two hundred and five of his patients had developed endometrial cancer. These were matched with 205 of his other patients who had hysterectomies. They were also matched on age, marital status, parity, and weight. Matching on hysterectomy status is important, because the earlier studies were challenged in that the controls excluded hysterectomy; also, it was thought by some that hysterectomy patients might more frequently have estrogen, resulting in selective exclusion of estrogen users from the controls. This could not happen in the Gray study.

In addition, all the patients with hysterectomy have pathology examinations, thus providing the first study in which pathologic examination was present for the controls. Some controls in this last study also had uterine bleeding, another interesting addition, since the control group still used less estrogen.

Thus far, we have reviewed three pieces of evidence, the parallelism in drug use and endometrial cancer trends, disease associations with diseases that have high estrogen levels being associated with endometrial cancer, and four case-control studies with high relative risks and consistent results. Further, there are now data on dose response. For example, Dr. Gray and his associates (1977) found that after 10 years of estrogen use, the relative risk for endometrial cancer was 11.5%, a major increase with longer use.

In summary, we have a convincing suspicion of causality for estrogens and endometrial cancer. The biggest remaining doubt rests with the certainty of the pathologic diagnosis in studies to date, and whether estrogen-associated endometrial cancer is the same type of disease. The real magnitude of the problem is uncertain and further work is in progress on this. The impact of many more hysterectomies on the patients obviously affects endometrial cancer trends, and works in a way that would tend to minimize the extent of risk from estrogens.

PROSTATE CANCER

Prostate cancer is a difficult subject area. Our knowledge of prostate cancer is very rudimentary. Unfortunately, there still are many major cancer sites, (for example, prostate, pancreas and ovary), where very few epidemiologic studies have been done. Few investigators have made an effort to study these major causes of death.

A number of years ago, as part of my doctoral thesis, I was studying the question of whether there were factors preceding prostate cancer that implicated hormones indirectly and decided to look at anthropological measurements (Greenwald et al., 1974). Well, we were very fortunate that two anthropologists as their life project did very careful anthropologic measurements of undergraduates at Harvard during the early part of this century. They extensively noted body measurements, took nude photographs, and rated all of these using anthropometric scales. The scales chosen discriminate most effectively between men and women. These included body hair distribution and scales known as gynandromorphy, androgyny, and somatotype. All data were, of course, rated without knowledge of who would later get prostate cancer.

Harvard follows nearly all of their alumni. I analyzed anthropologic information about the 270 dying with prostate cancer as compared to controls, including additional information such as age at first child, age at last child, and other things about life-style.

Well, this study was totally negative. We could find nothing in this group but considered that the exposures were related to younger times of life—mostly prior to college age, but including up to age 40 or so.

If we look at the age distribution of prostate cancer, we see a disease of older men. The youngest person we can find in New York State with the adenocarcinoma of the prostate is age 34. The vast majority are over 60 or even over 70. Thus we wondered whether the etiologic factors for prostate cancer might not really be operative until the late middle-aged period and whether we ought not to focus down in our further efforts on, say, the 40-64 age group.

Well, one of the observations about prostate cancer that has been consistently reported from fairly crude vital records studies is that the mortality is higher among widowers and divorced men (King, Diamond, & Lilienfeld, 1963). This is also true of some other cancers. And we thought even though the increase is only about 20%, it might be worth doing an inexpensive study to see whether we could decide where to focus further research. We were interested that widowers—with reportedly high prostate cancer mortality—frequently go through major changes in life-styles when their wives die. These changes are great enough that epidemiologic study is quite feasible.

Therefore, we began looking at duration of widowerhood. If a carcinogenic effect occurs after widowerhood, we thought the duration might be longer among cases than controls, because of the usual lengthy period of cancer induction.

This also came out to be negative, except that we could find certain artifacts in the classification that would explain this higher rate among widowers. There may be an interesting finding with respect to an associated hypothesis, however, which we are exploring further. It appears that predeceased wives of prostate cancer widowers may have had high rates of breast and endometrial cancer. The sample size was too small to make a definitive decision about this in our preliminary study, and work is continuing. If this holds up, it will indicate possibilities of common carcinogenic exposures during marriage, or of people with similar risks marrying each other. Consistent with these ideas is the observation by Dr. Wynder (Wynder, Mabuchi, & Whitmore, 1971) of parallelism in international correlations between the cancers of the endocrine dependent sites.

Thank you.

REFERENCES

Arthes, F.G., Sartwell, P.E., & Lewison E.F. The pill, estrogens and the breast. Epidemiologic. aspects. *Cancer,* 1971, *28,* 1391-1394.

Boston collaborative drug surveillance program. Oral contraceptive and venous thromboembolic disease, surgically confirmed gallbladder disease, and breast tumours. *Lancet,* 1973, *1,* 1399-1404.

U.S. Dept. of Commerce, Bureau of the Census. Current industrial reports: Pharmaceutical preparations except biologicals, 1962 through 1975, Series MA-28G(62)-1 through MA-28g(75)-1. Washington, D.C., 19 .

DeNuzzo, R.V. 20th Annual prescription survey by the Albany College of Pharmacy. *Medical Marketing Media,* 1976, *11,* 17-34.

DeNuzzo, R.V. 1972 Prescription survey by the Albany College of Pharmacy. *Medical Marketing Media,* 1973, *8,* 13-26.

Fasal, E., & Paffenbarger, R.S. Oral contraceptives as related to cancer and benign lesions of the breast. *J. Natl. Cancer Inst.,* 1975, *55,* 767-773.

Gray, L.A., Christopherson, W.M., & Hoover, R. N. Estrogens and endometrial carcinoma. *Obstet. Gynec.,* 1977, *49,* 385-389.

Greenwald, P., Barlow, J.J., Nasca, P.C., & Burnett, W.S. Vaginal cancer after maternal treatment with synthetic estrogens. *N. Eng. J. Med.,* 1971, *285,* 390-392.

Greenwald, P., Caputo, T.A., & Wolfgang, P.E. Endometrial cancer after menopausal use of estrogens. *Obstet. Gynecol.,* 1977, *50,* 239-243,

Greenwald, P., Damon A., Kirmiss, V., Polan, A.K. Physical and demographic features of men before developing cancer of the prostate. *J. Natl. Cancer. Inst.,* 1974, *53,* 341-346.

Greenwald, P., Nasca, P.C., Burnett, W.S., Polan, A.K. Prenatal stilbestrol experience of mothers of young cancer patients. *Cancer,* 1973, *31,* 568-572.

Greenwald, P., Nasca, P., & Caputo, T.A., & Janerich, D.T. Cancer risks from estrogen intake. *N.Y.S. J. Med.,* 1977, *77,* 1069-1074.

Hemplemann, L.H.. et al. Personal communication, December, 1976.

Henderson, B.E., Powell, D., Rosario, J. An epidemiologic study of breast cancer. *J. Natl. Cancer Inst.,* 1974, *53,* 609-614.

Hoover, R., Fraumeni, J.F., Jr., Everson, R. & Myers, M.H. Cancer of the uterine corpus after hormonal treatment for breast cancer. *Lancet,* 1976, *1,* 885-887.

Hoover, R. et al. Menopausal estrogens and breast cancer. *New Engl. J. Med.,* 1976, *295,* 401-405.

Jackson, R.L., & Dockerty, M.B. The Stein-Leventhal syndrome: Analysis of 43 cases with special reference to association with endometrial carcinoma. *Am. J. Obstet. Gynecol.,* 1957, *73,* 161-173.

Janerich, D.T., Glebatis, D.M., & Dugan, J.M. Benign breast disease and oral contraceptive use. *JAMA*, 1977, *237*, 2199-2201.

Kelsey, J. L., Lindfors, K.K., & White, D. A case-control study of the epidemiology of benign breast diseases with reference to oral contraceptive use. *Internat J. Epidemiol*, 1974, *3*, 33-340.

King, H., Diamond, E., & Lillienfeld, A.M. Some epidemiologic aspects of cancer of the prostate. *J. Chronic. Dis.*, 1963, *16*, 117-153.

Mack, T.M., Pike, M.C., Henderson, B.E. et al. Estrogens and endometrial cancer in a retirement community. *N. Engl. J. Med.*, 1976, *294*, 1262-1267.

Mansell, H. & Hertig, A.T. Granulosa-theca cell tumors and endometrial carcinoma: A study of their relationship and a survey of 80 cases. *Obstet. Gynecol.*, 1955, *6*, 385-395.

Nomura, A., & Comstock, G.W. Benign breast tumor and estrogenic hormones: a population-based retrospective study. *Am. J. Epidemiol.*, 1976, *103*, 439-444.

Sartwell, P.E., Arthes, F.G., & Tonascia, J.A. Epidemiology of benign breast lesions. lack of association with oral contraceptive use. *New Engl. J. Med.*, 1973, *288*, 551-554.

Smith, D.C., Prentice, R., Thompson, D.J. et al. Association of exogenous estrogen and endometrial carcinoma. *N. Engl. J. Med.*, 1975, *293*, 1164-1167.

Stadel, B.V., & Weiss, N.S. Characteristics of menopausal women: A survey of King and Pierce counties in Washington, 1973-1974. *Am. J. Epidemiol.*, 1975, *102*, 209-216.

Stavraky, K., & Emmons, S. Breast cancer in premenopausal and postmenopausal women. *J. Natl. Cancer Inst.*, 1974, *53*, 647-654.

Vessey, M.P., Doll, R., & Jones, K. Oral contraceptives and breast cancer. *Lancet*, 1975, *1*, 941-943.

Vessey, M.P., Doll, R., & Sutton, P.M. Oral contraceptives and breast neoplasia: A retrospective study. *Brit. M. J.*, 1972, *3*, 719-724.

Wynder, E.L., Mabuchi, K., & Whitmore, W. F. Epidemiology of cancer of the prostate. *Cancer*, 1971, *28*, 344-360.

Ziel, H.K., & Finkle, W.D. Increased risk of endometrial carcinoma among users of conjugated estrogens. *N. Engl. J. Med.*, 1975, *293*, 1167-1170.

Discussion

DR. WYNDER: Peter, we are grateful for this overview. It's clear that even in epidemiology we have to learn more, and one of the things that we recognize where we need to know more is that we have our own limitations. Therefore, as I will say to you tomorrow, we must go into an area that we call metabolic epidemiology, where we're studying man himself in the laboratory. So clearly, there are only so many questions that we can ask; and one out of 15 women are destined to develop cancer of the breast. There must be some environmental factors to which all women are exposed rather than some to which only a few are exposed. The same really applies to prostate cancer. Prostate cancer, as Peter (Greenwald) properly said, is again one of those areas that has been neglected by the scientific community.

In part this is true because we do not have a satisfactory animal model. Well, people in my lab say: "What are we going to do? We don't have any mice or rats with which to study." Well, if you don't have them, go right to man, and this is precisely what is being done. As Peter said, one of the best leads in this country is the high rate of prostate cancer among the blacks, a fact well confirmed by the U.S. Census Survey.

I can report to you that we have just completed 200 interviews on prostatic cancer patients and find no difference between positives and controls. So again we recognize that either we don't ask the right question or the answer is just not available. What we need to do now is go to metabolic studies, studying hormones in blacks and whites, and studying hormones in Japanese and Americans, at all different ages. I was glad to hear earlier about trace metals, and I'm amazed how little work has been done on prostatic tissue in the laboratory. So these are all the kind of areas that have to be examined in the future. Perhaps some of you may want to discuss these trace elements as we go into the discussion period.

14. On the Absence of Carcinogenicity to Man of Phenobarbital

Johannes Clemmesen
S. Hjalgrim-Jensen
The Danish Cancer Registry, The Finsen Institute

Phenobarbital, introduced in the treatment of epilepsy around 1920, represented a forward step, unforgettable to those who have seen the side effects of the previous therapeutic methods. Nevertheless, had this drug been proposed today in the United States it would have been forbidden, because experiments on a total of 800-900 rodents suggest that it may produce cancer in mice and perhaps in rats.

Evidence on experience from man, particularly when negative, does not enjoy corresponding publicity nor favor when quoted (e.g. I.A.R.C. Monogr., apl., 1977), for which reason the following pages will be rather extensive, having been disregarded by two major clinical journals when presented in a somewhat more condensed form.

In a previous study by Clemmesen, Fuglasang-Frederiksen & Plum, (1974a), it was demonstrated that 9,136 patients admitted for epilepsy at the Danish Epilepsy Center Filadelfia, Dianalund, during the years 1933-62 did not experience any statistically significant increase in risk of malignant neoplasms, apart from the excess of tumors of the central nervous system, clinically expected among this category of patients.

While it was generally admitted that this result did justify the use of phenobarbital, some minor deviation of observed values from those expected called for critical remarks by Schneiderman (1974). While accepting the idea that less active sexual lives might explain a deficit in cases of cervical uterine cancer, Schneiderman would expect a reverse trend for mammary carcinoma. However, since values for the latter also fell short of the expected, he attributed this deficit to oversight of breast cancers by the physicians at Filadelfia. Medically impossible as this would be in any hospital in Denmark, not to speak of the high standard at Filadelfia, it may be added that, as originally suggested by Rigoni Stern in 1842, this counterbalance of the two neoplasms does not apply in Denmark, (Clemmsen, 1951) if indeed anywhere, with the exception of Israel and Japan, when taken together (Clemmesen, 1976).

Superficially, it might seem more essential when Schneiderman pointed to the slight, nearly statistically significant, excess of 5 cases of liver cancer against 2.5 expected. However, as originally communicated, one male patient (identical with the one case developed within ten years from admission) had received an injection of radioactive thorium dioxide (Thorotrast) in preparation for angiography with a view to a possible brain tumor. As this compound is known to cause liver carcinoma and leukemia (Faber, 1973) and Clemmesen (1975) scrutinized records and found a total of 3 Thorotrast receivers among the 5 liver cancer cases. From a statistical viewpoint, it might, perhaps, have been more relevant to suspect (Clemmesen, 1976b) that the general trend for observed values to fall short of the expected, might be due to an inflation of the latter by missing information on some cases dropping out of the study by death, emigration etc.

Consequently, when it had become possible to extend the study period five more years, and since it proved within reach to establish a follow-up on a personal basis, the present investigation was undertaken.

EARLIER STUDIES

Saltzstein and Ackerman (1959) made a review of scattered reports on lymphadenopathies occurring in conjunction with therapeutic use of various hydantoin derivatives. Furthermore, they contributed a number of histologically well-documented cases, and concluded that cessation of therapy could be followed by remission of the lymphadenopathy, which they considered an allergic response. Hyman and Sommers (1966) and Gams, Neal, and Conrad (1968) found some cases developing into malignant lymphomas or Hodgkin's disease (Dorfman and Warnecke (1974), while others have regarded this association as accidental.

In recent years, major congenital malformations have been found in children born of epileptic mothers treated with anticonvulsants (Speider and Meadow, 1972; Nelson and Forfar, 1971), and the possibility of an association between teratogenic and oncogenic effects has drawn the attention of clinicians to these observations (Editorial, 1971, 1972, 1974). Because anticonvulsant therapy mostly covers a considerable part of a lifetime and often involves heavy doses, the question is of considerable consequence.

However, results from animal experiments appear controversial.

RATS

Phenobarbital was first studied by Peraino, Fry, and Staffeldt, (1971). They found no ill effects in Sprague-Dawley rats fed phenobarbital, and simultaneous feeding of this drug with the hepatocarcinogen 2-acetylaminofluorene (AAF) even reduced the effect of the latter. Contrarily, sequential feeding of this carcinogen and phenobarbital resulted in a significant increase in hepatomas, a paradox with parallels in other cocarcinogens.

In a later study Peraino et al. (1975) confirmed that phenobarbital (and DDT) could increase tumor incidence in rats previously fed AAF for a short period, while this was not the case for phenylhydantoin. Out of 45 rats fed phenobarbital only, one showed an area of hyperplasia in the liver.

Rossi et al. (1977) used Wistar rats and reported noninfiltrating nodular growths in 13 out of 36 male and 9 out of 29 female rats.

Schmähl and Habs, 1976, who administered phenobarbital as intraperitoneal injections to Sprague-Dawley rats, saw two malignant tumors in their 62 test animals and four among their 69 controls.

MICE

Before the publication of the rather negative experience on rats, Thorpe and Walker (1973) had fed phenobarbital, 500 ppm, and various related compounds to CF-1 mice with spontaneous liability to liver tumors. In the livers they found some cases of simple nodular growths of parenchymal cells and some areas of papilliform and adenoid growth of tumor cells, sometimes associated with lung metastases. The authors doubted, however, if this increase in the frequency of spontaneous tumors reflected a genuine carcinogenic potential to man. Peraino et al. (1973) also found an increase and earlier appearance of liver tumors in C3H mice fed on phenobarbital, while Ponomarkov et al. (1976) found similar results in studies on CF-1 mice (cf Table 1).

To judge from experimental evidence it therefore seems questionable whether the mouse is an adequate testing object for carcinogenicity in man, and equally problematic if phenobarbital can be assumed to possess a carcinogenic potency of its own.

BACKGROUND AND ORGANIZATION

The neuropsychiatric hospital Filadelfia, in Dianalund, Denmark, was founded in 1897 by Dr. A. Sell as a religious home for epileptics. At the beginning of the present study period in 1933, it had developed into a modern center for epilepsy

253

TABLE 1
HEPATIC TUMORS IN ANIMALS FED
PHENOBARBITAL, 500 PPM

Mice				Hepatic adenomas & carcinomas (number and percent)	
Thorpe & Walker (1973)	Male	Controls	45	24	—
CF-1 Mice		Phenob.	30	80	—
	Female	Controls	45	23	—
		Phenob.	30	75	—
Peraino et al. (1973)	Male	Controls	54	59.3	—
C3H Mice		Phenob.	53	96.2	—
	Female	Controls	55	10.9	—
		Phenob.	44	88.6	—
Ponomarkov et al. (1975)	Male	Controls	44	27.3	—
CF-1 Mice		Phenob.	98	78.5	—
	Female	Controls	47	0	
		Phenob.	73	61.6	—
Rats					
Peraino et al. (1975)		Controls	108	28.7	—
Sprague-Dawley Rats		+ Phenob.	108	78.7	—
		+ Diphenylhyd.	102	27.4	—
Rossi et al. (1976)	Male	Controls	36	0	
Wistar Rats		Phenob.	36	36.1	(Ben.)
	Female	Controls	35	0	
		Phenob.	34	26.4	(Ben.)
Schmaehl & Habs (1976)		Controls	69	5.8	—
Sprague-Dawley Rats (intraperitoneal injections)		Phenob.	62	3.2	—

treatment in Denmark. With the same chief physician, H. P. Stubbe Teglbjærg, in charge from 1928 to 1959, the epilepsy department kept this position until the late 1950s when treatment became less centralized. A gradual change of therapy after 1960 has tended to shorten the stay in hospital, and with the decentralization of treatment, the center's share of patients became one of more serious cases.

Besides a series of monographs for the doctorate (Faurbye, 1974; Hendriksen, 1923; Munch-Petersen, 1929; Teglbjaerg, 1936; Yde, 1938) the standard of Filadelfia is evidenced by the early dates for introduction of new antiepileptic drugs. Naturally, a study period covering decades must comprise some changes in therapy, but in the present case they have been few. The general principles of therapy were reviewed by Stubbe Teglbjærg (1957).

The basic drug, phenobarbital, was introduced at Filadelfia about 1920, in highly individualized doses between 100 and 300 mg, given mainly in the evening. Phenylhydantoin, as reported by Faurbye (1939), was given during the daytime in doses of 100 to 400 mg, while primidone (Jørgensen, 1954) was administered in doses of 0.5 to 1.5 g. It may be recalled that primidone is converted into phenobarbital, according to some calculations, at an average of 24.5%.

A detailed analysis of 233 case records from 1933 to 1952 confirmed these treatment regimens. Out of 27 patients who died in the hospital during the early 1970s, 23 had received a total dose of between 1 and 4½ kg of anticonvulsants.

Patients at Filadelfia were, as far as possible, occupied in special workshops, and whatever the degree of success in single cases it was attempted to offer protection of patients against promiscuity, alcohol, and tobacco. Due to the considerable variation in the duration of the stay at Filadelfia, it would be futile to adjust for variations in cancer morbidity risk with degree of urbanization by residence before admission, and calculations of risk have been based on morbidity rates for all of Denmark, as given in the reports of the Danish Cancer Registry.

Also, the Registry worked under unchanged conditions during the study period, being in charge of the same person, acquainted with everyday work at Filadelfia from short-term appointments during 1930-1932. The Registry works on the basis of notifications of all cases of cancer diagnosed at Danish hospitals or at postmortems, supplemented with information from death certificates which are all passed on to the Registry by the National Health Service.

METHODS

Taking a more individual approach than the statistical calculation of cancer risk involved in admission for epilepsy, we checked for the follow-up the files for patients discharged less than four weeks after admission, deleting those for which a diagnosis of epilepsy was not sustained.

By the courtesy of the efficient people's registries, various local officials, the cancer register, and the death files, it proved possible to follow a total of 8,078 patients out of the original 9,136 admissions covered by the statistical study of Clemmesen et al. (1974). With the exception of 199 persons followed to the month of last "contact," all patients were followed to their death or to December, 1972, thus covering five more years than the earlier study. It may prove difficult to attain a closer coverage through a longer and more stable period of therapy.

Because the manifestation of carcinogenic effect often takes an average of one to two decades from the beginning of exposure of patients admitted at Filadelfia during 1933, 42 were included in our studies with a view to long-term observation, although the taped death files and those of the Cancer Registry only begin with 1943. For the necessary deletion of names of patients deceased before that year, in the statistical study we had to rely on hospital information only. In the present follow-up, however, it was possible to make use of the population registers, which resulted in some, although not significant, reduction of expected rates.

CALCULATIONS

As in the statistical survey, the principle of analysis has been a comparison of the number of cancer cases observed among the epileptic patients with the cases expected among corresponding numbers of average persons of corresponding sex and quinquennial age group within the pertinent secular 5-year period.

The expected number of cancer cases was calculated as average annual incidence for each secular quinquennium for the anatomical site in question, multiplied by the man-years under observation within the secular 5-year period. Man-years were counted as the sum of individual observation periods beginning with admission and ending with the month of death, or December 31, 1972, or in 199 cases, the month of last information.

Because treatment for less than 10 years could hardly be expected to cause any significant increase in cancer cases, tables were worked out separately for patients when observed for less and for more than 10 years.

RESULTS

Cases of epilepsy diagnosed as due to brain tumors within the month of admission or developed following removal of a brain tumor were primarily excluded from the studies. However, since these tumors often present with epilepsy years

TABLE 2
FOLLOW-UP OF EPILEPTIC PATIENTS
ADMITTED 1933-62, THROUGH 1943-72

	Males	Females
Total Admissions: 9,136	4,794	4,342
Exclusions		
Aliens	80	80
Deaths before 1943	80	51
Not traceable at all	115	225
Twice registered (errors in data)	34	72
Diagnosis of epilepsy not sustained	217	104
Total exclusions	606	651
Followed until trace was lost	80	119

TABLE 3
FOLLOW-UP OF PATIENTS ADMITTED TO FILADELFIA FOR EPILEPSY AND RECORDED WITH THE REGISTRY FOR CANCER WITHIN 10 YEARS FROM ADMISSION, GIVEN ACCORDING TO QUINQUENNIUM OF NOTIFICATION

	1943/47		1948/52		1953/57		1958/62		1963/67		1968/72		Total	
	Obs.	Exp.	Obs.	Exp.	Obs.	Exp.	Obs.	Exp.	Obs.	Exp.	Obs.	Exp.	Obs.	Exp.
Males														
Oral cavity & pharynx	1	0.3	–	0.3	–	0.4	–	0.4	–	0.3	1	0.1	2	1.7
Digest. syst. exc. liver	2	1.6	–	1.8	4	2.3	2	2.8	2	2.1	1	0.6	11	11.1
Liver (exc. biliar. pass.)	–	0.1	–	0.1	–	0.1	–	0.1	1	0.1	–	0.0	1	0.4
Respiratory system	–	0.5	–	0.7	1	1.2	2	1.8	7[a]	1.7	–	9.6	10	6.4
Breast	–	0.0	–	0.0	–	0.0	–	0.0	–	0.0	–	0.0	–	0.1
Male genital organs	–	0.4	1	0.5	1	0.8	3	1.0	1	0.9	1	0.3	7	3.8
Urinary system	–	0.2	1	0.3	1	0.6	3	0.8	1	0.8	–	0.3	6	3.1
Skin	1	0.4	–	0.6	1	0.8	–	1.0	2	0.9	–	0.3	4	4.0
Brain & nervous system	7[b]	0.3	5[b]	0.3	2	0.4	6[b]	0.6	6[b]	0.4	1	0.1	27[b]	2.1
Other organs	–	0.1	–	0.1	–	0.2	–	0.2	1	0.2	1	0.1	1	0.8
Unspecified organs	–	0.1	–	0.1	–	0.1	–	0.1	–	0.0	–	0.0	–	0.3
Connective tissue	–	0.1	–	0.1	–	0.1	–	0.1	–	0.1	–	0.0	–	0.4
Lymphatic & haemat. tissue	–	0.43	1	0.54	–	0.8	1	1.1	1	0.8	–	0.2	3	3.8
Metastases	–	0.1	1	0.1	–	0.1	–	0.2	–	0.1	–	0.0	1	0.6
All malignant neoplasms	11[c]	4.4	9	5.5	10	7.7	17	10.1	22	8.4	4	2.6	73[b]	38.7

TABLE 3 (cont.)

Females	1943/47		1948/52		1953/57		1958/62		1963/67		1968/72		Total	
	Obs.	Exp.	Obs.	Exp.	Obs.	Exp.	Obs.	Exp.	Obs.	Exp.	Obs.	Exp.	Obs.	Exp.
Oral cavity & pharynx	—	0.1	—	0.1	—	0.1	1	0.2	—	0.1	—	0.0	1	0.6
Digest. syst. exc. liver	—	1.0	—	1.0	1	1.3	1	1.7	2	1.5	3c	0.6	7	7.2
Liver (exc. biliar. pass.)	—	0.1	—	0.04	—	0.06	—	0.03	—	0.05	—	0.02	—	0.25
Respiratory system	—	0.1	1	0.2	—	0.2	—	0.3	1	0.3	—	0.2	1	1.2
Breast	—	1.3	1	1.5	3	1.9	—	2.2	2	2.0	—	0.7	5	9.6
Uterus	1	1.5	3	1.8	1	2.5	1	2.8	2	2.1	2	0.6	9	11.4
Other female genital organs	—	0.4	2	0.5	1	0.7	—	0.8	2	0.7	2c	0.2	8c	3.4
Urinary system	—	0.1	—	0.1	—	0.2	1	0.3	—	0.3	—	0.1	—	1.2
Skin	—	0.3	—	0.4	1	0.6	—	0.7	—	0.7	2	0.3	4	2.9
Brain & nervous system	2c	0.2	2	0.3	4a	0.4	9b	0.4	1	0.3	—	0.1	18b	1.7
Other organs	1	0.1	1	0.1	—	0.2	—	0.2	2c	0.2	—	0.1	3	0.8
Unspecified organs	—	0.1	1	0.1	1	0.1	—	0.1	—	0.1	—	0.0	2	0.4
Connective tissue	—	0.0	1	0.1	—	0.1	—	0.1	—	0.1	—	0.0	1	0.4
Lymphatic & haemat. tissue	1	0.3	—	0.4	2	0.5	—	0.6	—	0.5	—	0.2	3	2.3
Metastases	—	0.1	—	0.1	—	0.1	—	0.1	—	0.1	—	0.0	—	0.5
All malingant neoplasms	5	5.7	11	6.6	14	8.9	13	10.5	10	8.9	9a	3.0	62c	43.7

a $P < 0.01$.
b $P < 0.001$.
c $P < 0.05$.

TABLE 4
FOLLOW-UP OF PATIENTS ADMITTED TO FILADELFIA FOR EPILEPSY AND RECORDED WITH THE REGISTRY FOR CANCER OVER 10 YEARS FROM ADMISSION, GIVEN ACCORDING TO QUINQUENNIUM OF NOTIFICATION

	1943/47 Obs.	1943/47 Exp.	1948/52 Obs.	1948/52 Exp.	1953/57 Obs.	1953/57 Exp.	1958/62 Obs.	1958/62 Exp.	1963/67 Obs.	1963/67 Exp.	1968/72 Obs.	1968/72 Exp.	Total Obs.	Total Exp.
Males														
Oral cavity & pharynx	—	0.1	—	0.3	—	0.5	2	0.8	2	1.2	1	1.6	5	4.4
Digest. syst. exc. liver	1	0.6	2	1.9	3	3.3	5	5.5	10	8.7	8	12.5	29	32.5
Liver (exc. biliar. pass.)	—	0.02	—	0.06	—	0.1	—	0.2	4[b]	0.4	3[c]	0.6	7[c]	1.3
Respiratory system	—	0.2	2	0.7	—	1.7	4	3.5	7	6.8	17	11.2	30	24.0
Breast	—	0.0	—	0.0	—	0.0	—	0.0	—	0.1	—	0.1	—	0.2
Male genital organs	—	0.1	1	0.5	1	0.9	1	1.7	5	3.1	4	4.8	12	11.1
Urinary organs	—	0.1	—	0.4	—	0.8	1	1.6	2	3.3	2	5.6	5[a]	11.7
Skin	—	0.1	—	0.6	1	1.2	1	1.9	5	3.7	5	5.5	12	13.0
Brain & nervous system	—	0.1	3[b]	0.26	2	0.5	2	0.8	2	1.1	3	1.6	12[a]	4.3
Other organs	—	0.0	—	0.1	—	0.2	2	0.3	—	0.4	—	0.6	1	1.6
Unspecified organs	—	0.0	—	0.1	—	0.1	—	0.1	—	0.1	—	0.2	—	0.6
Connective tissue	—	0.0	1	0.1	—	0.1	—	0.1	—	0.2	—	0.1	—	0.6
Lymphatic & haemat. tissue	—	0.1	—	0.4	2	0.8	1	1.4	2	2.3	3	3.2	8	8.1
Metastases	—	0.0	—	0.1	—	0.1	—	0.3	2	0.4	—	0.7	2	1.7
All malignant neoplasms	1	1.6	9	5.3	9	10.2	18	18.3	41	31.7	46	48.1	124	115.1

TABLE 4 (cont.)

	1943/47		1948/52		1953/57		1958/62		1963/67		1968/72		Total	
	Obs.	Exp.	Obs.	Exp.	Obs.	Exp.	Obs.	Exp.	Obs.	Exp.	Obs.	Exp.	Obs.	Exp.
Females														
Oral cavity & pharynx	—	0.0	—	0.1	—	0.2	—	0.3	1	0.4	—	0.5	1	1.4
Digest. syst. exc. liver	—	0.4	2	1.4	—	2.5	5	4.4	9	6.5	5	9.7	21	25.0
Liver exc. biliar. pass.	—	0.0	—	0.1	—	0.1	—	0.1	1	0.2	2	0.3	3	0.8
Respiratory system	—	0.0	2	0.2	1	0.3	—	0.6	4	1.3	3	2.5	7	5.0
Breast	1	0.4	3	1.7	2	2.9	3	5.0	8	8.0	9	11.9	23	30.0
Uterus	—	0.5	3	1.8	2	3.3	6	5.7	5	8.0	3a	9.4	20	28.6
Other female genitals	—	0.1	1	0.5	—	1.1	1	1.7	1	2.7	1	3.9	6	10.1
Urinary organs	—	0.0	—	0.2	—	0.4	1	0.7	1	1.3	1	2.2	4	4.8
Skin	—	0.1	1	0.4	1	0.8	—	1.4	4	2.8	5	4.3	10	9.9
Brain & nervous system	1	0.1	1	0.2	1	0.4	2	0.7	1	1.0	2	1.3	8	3.6
Other organs	—	0.0	—	0.1	—	0.2	—	0.3	1	0.5	1	0.7	2	1.8
Unspecified organs	1	0.0	—	0.1	1	0.1	1	0.2	—	0.2	—	0.3	2	1.0
Connective tissue	—	0.0	—	0.1	1	0.1	—	0.1	—	0.1	—	0.2	1	0.5
Lymphatic & haemat. tissue	—	0.1	—	0.3	—	0.5	2	0.9	1	1.4	3	2.1	6	5.2
Metastases	—	0.0	—	0.1	—	0.1	—	0.3	—	0.4	1	0.6	1	1.6
All malignant neoplasms	3	1.9	10	7.0	7	13.0	22	22.6	37	34.8	36a	49.9	115	129.2

a P < 0.05.
b P < 0.01.
c P < 0.001.

before they are diagnosed—in Teglbjærg's estimate (1957) in 60%—we must expect a considerable excess of observed versus statistically expected numbers for this site, and, as confirmed by the tables, decreasing with time after admission. Still it is noticeable for how many years the epileptic syndrome may anticipate the causative tumor.

As it will appear from the tables the logical subtraction from totals of the numbers for tumors of the central nervous system reduces considerably any excess of observed over expected numbers.

The second site showing an excess of cancer cases is the liver ($P < 0.001$) 10 years or more after admission, contrasted to the group treated for less than ten years, which may suggest a carcinogenic effect. This is explained by the fact that, out of the total of 11 cases, 8—all histologically verified—had received injections of thorium dioxide (Thorotrast). It may be added that the only patient who developed liver carcinoma, and additionally myelogenous leukemia, within ten years from admission had received Thorotrast elsewhere nine years before coming to Filadelfia. Another patient among the liver cancer cases had developed myelosclerosis.

Thus it appears that if we subtract the liver cancer cases associated with Thorotrast injections we are left with three cases, which is close to the number expected.

One remaining significant deviation of observed from expected numbers in the group treated for more than ten years is a deficit in cases observed ($P < 0.05$) for the male urinary system. Another deviation is found in the excess of 8 cases against 3.4 expected ($P < 0.05$) for other female genital organs, thus balancing against the deficit of only 6 cases against 10.1 expected among patients treated less than ten years. For the uterus and female breast, there are consistent, though not significant, trends of fewer cases than expected. The significant deficit ($P < 0.05$) for these sites found in the earlier statistical study appears to have been reduced in the individual follow-up.

DISCUSSION

In the estimate of the scattered occurrence in Tables 3 and 4 of differences marked as statistically significant, it should be recalled that according to chance alone such markings will occur with exactly the frequency they indicate. Non-significant deviations may or may not reflect medical or biological realities. However, the considerable overall correspondence between observed and expected numbers should not encourage one to overestimate the medical significance of deviations for single groups. In considering, e.g., secular variations for the male urinary system or for other female genital organs, it is advisable to turn attention, for conclusive evidence, to totals, particularly those for more than ten years of treatment.

TABLE 5
LIVER CANCER CASES

Males

1. No. 28-364   Born Oct. 12, 1903; epilepsy diagnosed 1936; admitted 1957; thorium dioxide 440 rad. Mar. 28, 1948; died Nov. 23, 1964; myelogenous leukemia of chronic type; cholangiocarcinoma; cirrhosis hepatis.

2. No. 11-002   Born Oct. 10, 1915; epilepsy diagnosed ca. 1926; admitted 1936; thorium dioxide, 1938; death certified Apr. 7, 1965; Neopl. malign. hepatis.

3. No. 17-123   Born Sep. 14, 1930; epilepsy diagnosed and admitted 1942; Thorium dioxide, Nov. 30, 1942; Died July 17, 1967; Cholangiocarcinoma.

4. No. 97-83   Born Oct. 15, 1905; epilepsy diagnosed and admitted 1933; died Apr. 18, 1967; adenocarcinoma hepatis, probably cholangiocarcinoma.

5. No. 20-475   Born Jan. 14, 1912; epilepsy from 1937, diagnosed in England, 1944; admitted 1945; Thorium dioxide, 20 ml., Jan. 28, 1946; removal of angioma racemosum, ca. 1952; biopsy: adenocarcinoma of peritoneum and liver; died Sept. 28, 1971.

6. No. 16-132   Born June 28, 1900; epilepsy from ca. 1907; admitted 1941; thorium dioxide, 30 ml., Feb. 13, 1943; died Sept. 26, 1968; necropsy: Angiosarcoma hepatis; meningeoma, thorium dioxide deposits.

7. No. 10-740   Born Feb. 14, 1913; hydrocephalic; epilepsy (post-traumatic) from 1927; admitted 1936; died Nov. 28, 1969; necropsy: adenocarcinoma colloides hepatis primaria; adenoma gland. thyroid.

8. No. 11-982   Born Jan. 21, 1915; admitted 1937; thorium dioxide, 50 ml., 1938; died Apr. 16, 1967; necropsy: angiosarcoma hepatis, cirrhosis.

Females

9. No. 23-198   Born Mar. 3, 1899; epilepsy diagnosed 1946; admitted 1948; died July 7, 1964; necropsy: primary liver cancer (no histology).

10. No. 11-633   Born Aug. 28, 1907; epilepsy from ca. 1921; admitted 1937; removal of racemose venous angioma in left temporal region after angiograph; died Sept. 17, 1971; multiple liver tumors; liver deposits of thorium dioxide.

The extension of the study period by 5 years, together with the reassessment of data, has added strength and clarity to conclusions drawn from the previous statistical survey. As foreseen (Clemmesen, 1976b), some trends for most sites of cancer to fall short of expected numbers have been reduced, with the disappearance of statistical significance ($P < 0.05$), particularly for the uterus and female breast.

Contrarily, as would also be expected, the slight, though not significant excess for the liver (5 obs./2.5 exp.) ascribed to the effect of thorium dioxide has, with the extension of the study period, become significant (11 obs./2.1, exp., $P < 0.001$), for more than 10 years after injection of the compound. With 3 non-Thorotrast cases against an expectation of about 2.8 it seems difficult to argue for any measurable effect of phenobarbital on the occurrence of liver cancer, when the neoplasms developed in the Thorotrast-exposed livers belong to the histological types usually found in such cases.

In a preliminary report on 1,005 Danish patients having received Thorotrast injections, Faber (1973) found 756 survivors from the neurosurgical disease for which angiography had been done, with 312 later deaths, of which 28 had hepatic neoplasms, hemangioendotheliomas, and hepatocarcinomas. A further 11 died from leukemia, but the ratio of the two diseases does not appear to be the same everywhere, judged from the *Proceedings of III International Meeting*, Copenhagen, 1973, and we have no means of estimating to what extent our 8,078 patients may have been exposed to Thorotrast in some hospital or other.

With a view to the possible risk of leukemia and lymphomas ascribed to anticonvulsants by some authors, it should be specified that the patients treated for less/more than 10 years show the following totals: for males, 3/3 leukemias, 0/4 lymphomas, and 0/1 mycosis fungoides; for females, 3/1 leukemias, 0/1 lymphoma, and 0/2 reticulosarcomas, and 0/2 myeloma cases. These small numbers will not permit statistical analysis, but they do not suggest any increased risk.

Among sites with apparent deviations, the respiratory system, including upper respiratory passages, shows numbers slightly over the expected, but in accordance with the sex ratio seen in most Western countries, and not beyond what may be expected from chance alone.

CONCLUSION

The case of the absence of carcinogenicity to man of phenobarbital is important in principle as well as in fact.

For decades the clinical observation of an association between cigarette smoking and bronchial carcinoma was subject to unfounded doubt, suspicion, and outright opposition, largely because the disease had no counterpart in mice. There seemed to be no end of statisticians craving for more documentation, all resulting in fateful delay of needed legislative initiative.

In recent years, so-called evidence to the carcinogenicity of the well-served anticonvulsant phenobarbital has been presented, based on mice predisposed to liver tumors, and rats responding in some experiments with benign growths. Had it not been for its merit, phenobarbital might well have been prohibited on the basis of such reports, without regard to their lack of conclusiveness in man. While such reports usually do not fail to mention the importance in human therapy of phenobarbital, they often fail to present the human evidence, if mentioned at all, with the lack of reservation bestowed upon earlier experiments.

The time may now have come for legislative authorities and advisory experimentalists as well to pay attention to cancer as a reality in clinical medicine. To protect man against the dangers to which we expose laboratory mice seems hardly worth the effort, and if evidence, as here presented, on 8,078 persons followed for one or two decades, should be of no avail in the discussion on the postulated carcinogenicity of phenobarbital, we may as well abandon cancer epidemiology.

REFERENCES

Clemmesen, C. Inanition und epilepsie. *Acta psych. neurol. suppl. 3,* 1932.

Clemmesen, J. Fuglasang-Frederiksen, & V. Plum, C. Are anticonvulsants oncogenic? *Lancet,* 1974(a), *1,* 705-707.

Clemmesen, J. Statistical studies in malignant neoplasms. *Acta path. microbiol. Scandin. suppl. resp.,* 1965, 1969, 1974b, 174; 209; 247.

Clemmesen, J. Incidence of neoplasms in a population on anticonvulsant drugs. In Richens & Woodford (Eds)., Anticonvulsant drugs and enzyme induction. Discussion by Sutherland. Elsevier, North Holland, 1976(a).

Clemmesen, J. Phenobarbitone, liver tumours and Thorotrast. *Lancet,* 1975, *1,* 37.

Clemmesen, J. Correlation of sites. Rep. Sympos. Origin of human cancer. Cold Spring Harbor, Sept 1976(b).

Clemmesen, J. On the etiology of some human cancers. *Journal National Cancer Institute,* 1951, *12,* 1-24.

Dorfman, R.F., & Warnecke, R. Lymphadenopathy simulating the malignant lymphomas. *Human Path.,* 1974, *5,* 519-550.

Faber, M. Follow-up of Danish Thorotrast cases. see 24. pp. 137-147. 1973.

Faurbye, A. Behandling af epilepsi med diphenylhydantoin. *Ugeskr. Læg.,* 1939, *101,* 1350-54.

Faurbye, A. 1942. Blodets reaktion ved epilepsi. Copenhagen Univ. Munksgaard, 1942.

Gams, R.A. Neal, J.A., & Conrad, F.G. Hydantoin-induced pseudo-pseudolymphomas. *Ann Intern. Med.,* 1968, *69,* 557-568.

Hendriksen, V. Spasmofili og epilepsi. (Thesis) Copenhagen Univ. Munksgaard, 1923.

Hyman, G.A., & Sommers, D. The development of Hodgkin's disease and lymphoma during anticonvulsant therapy, *Blood,* 1966, *28,* 416-427.

I.A.R.C. Monograph. On the evaluation of carcinogenic risk of chemicals to man, Vol. 13. Some miscellaneous pharmaceutical substances. I.A.R.C. Lyon, 1977.

Jørgensen, G.: Epilepsibehandling med mysoline. *Nord. Medicin,* 1954, *52,* 1400-1403.

_____. Is phenytoin carcinogenic? (Editorial) *Lancet,* 1971, *1,* 1071-1072.

_____. Are anticonvulsants teratogenic? (Editorial) *Lancet,* 1972, *2,* 839-843.

_____. Does this chemical cause cancer in Man? (Editorial) *Lancet,* 1974, *2,* 629-630.

Munch-Petersen, C.J. 1929. Spinalvæskens sukkerindhold. Copenhagen Univ. Munksgaard, 1929.

Nelson, M.M., & Forfar, F.J.M. *British Medical Journal,* 1971, *1,* 523.

Peraino, C., Fry, F.J., & Staffeldt, E. Reduction and enhancement by phenobarbital of hepatocarcinogenesis induced in the fat by 2-acetylaminoflourene, *Cancer Research,* 1971, *31,* 1506-1512.

Peraino, C., Fry, H.J.M., & Staffeldt, E. Enhancement of spontaneous hepatic tumorgenesis in C3H mice by dietary phenobarbital. *Journal National Cancer Institute,* 1973, *51,* 1349-1350.

Peraino, C., Fry, F.J.M., Staffeldt, E. & Christopher, J.P. 1975. Comparative enhancing effects of phenobarbital, amobarbital, diphenylhydantoin, and dichlorodiphenyl-trichloroethane on 2-acetylaminofluorene-induced hepatic tumorigenesis in the rat. *Cancer Research*, 1975, *35*, 2884-2890.

Ponomarkov, V., Tomatis, L., & Turusov, V. The effect of long-term administration of phenobarbitone in CF-1 mice. *Cancer Letters*, 1976, *1*, 165-172.

Faber, M. (Ed.), Proceedings of III International Meeting on Toxicity of Thorotrast. *Risø rep. no. 294 Danish Atomic Energy Comm. Roskilde*, 1973.

Rossi, L. Ravera, M., Repetti G. & Santi, L. The effect of long-term administration of DDT or phenobarbital-Na in Wistar rats. *International Journal of Cancer*, 1977, *19*, 179-185.

Saltzstein, S.L., & Ackerman, L.V. Lymphadenopathy induced by anticonvulsant drugs. *Cancer*, (Phil.), 1959, *12*, 164-182.

Schneiderman, M.A. Phenobarbitone and liver tumors. *Lancet*, 1974, *2*, 1085.

Schmähl, D. & Habs, M. Lifespan investigations of some immuno-stimulating, immuno-depressive and neurotropic substances in Sprague-Dawley rats. *Z. Krebsforschung*, 1976, *86*, 77-84.

Speider, B.D., & Meadow S.R. 1972. Maternal epilepsy and abnormalities of the fetus and newborn. *Lancet*, 1972, *2*, 839-843.

Teglbjærg, H.P. Stubbe. Epilepsi, en oversigt for practici. *Manedskr. praktisk Lægegern. og soc. med.*, 1957, 293-307.

Teglbjærg, H.P. Stubbe. Investigations on epilepsy and water metabolism. (Thesis) *Acta psych. neurolog.*, 1936, Suppl. 9.

Thorpe, E., & Walker, A.I.T. Does this chemical cause cancer in Man? The toxicology of dieldrin (HEOD) II. Comparative long-term oral toxicity studies in mice with dieldrin, DDT, phenobarbitone, β BHC, γ BHC. *Food & Cosmetics Toxicology*, 1973, *11*, 433-422.

Yde, A. Nyrefunktion ved epilepsi. Munksgaard. Copenhagen, 1938.

DR. WYNDER: I've always felt if you have one kind of animal evidence, and if the data on man happen to be available for many years, and if the data for man differ, man undoubtedly must win out. In other words, we have an instance here where the data by Dr. Clemmesen have suggested, and I haven't reviewed them in detail, but what he presented makes a good deal of sense to me, that even if a man takes phenobarbital for many years he is still free from liver cancer. And I would like to think, therefore, that in terms of regulatory forces this long-standing human evidence must win out over whatever evidence we have on mice or rats. As I pointed out the other day, the same approach applies to saccharin as well. Before making conclusions, I like to think that we will discuss the human evidence.

Remember I said to you earlier that there is only one triumph that we can count on, and that is that the incidence of cancer decreases in our lifetime; it so happens there's one example of this: cancer of the stomach. Cancer of the stomach has declined during the last 20 or 30 years, and some of my colleagues have said that we really don't know why it has declined. We really do not understand the mechanism. Now if I, for a moment, were the head of Public Health, I wouldn't really give a damn for the mechanism. After all, the key to public health is to *see* disease decline in our lifetime. It so happens I think there may be a mechanism related to ascorbic acid, and it's all in preventing the formation of nitrosamides, but even if that suggestion is wrong, the fact is that the United States today happens to be leading in one area; namely, that we have the lowest incidence of cancer of the stomach. It seems to me that this is a very interesting fact for which we should take credit, from the point of view of public health.

Now, toward the end I would like to ask one question to emphasize the point that I made; namely, what do we learn from animal experimentation as it relates to human epidemiology? And the first question I would like to ask relates to a point that was once asked of me by a member of the tobacco industry: "Why should we worry about smoking and lung cancer? After all, let us identify those smokers who smoke and obviously are immune."

It so happens that in the very first experiment that I did, we took some inbred mice and gave them a low dose of benzopyrene. Ten percent developed cancer but 90% did not, and I said to myself then, some 30 years ago, that if I knew the answer as to why these 90% in this inbred strain did *not* develop cancer, then we certainly would have a way of preventing cancer. Therefore, I would like to ask both Dr. Conney and Dr. James Miller, on the basis of their brilliant studies on the mechanism of carcinogenesis: Do we have an idea on how to identify the high risk patient or the patient that is a low risk based of available animal data? Thank you very much, and I appreciate your attention.

DR. CONNEY: Well, there are a few approaches for identifying individuals who have high risk. One is to use tissue culture studies in humans, that is, from different individuals, to look at the metabolism of carcinogens by their tissues.

Studies have been done in this area. Another approach in individuality in metabolic activation and detoxification would be if one could find safe drugs that are metabolized by the same enzymes that metabolically activate a carcinogen and study the metabolism of that drug in different individuals. One might be able to use the metabolism of the drug as an index of carcinogen metabolism among different individuals. These are two kinds of approaches that could be used to identify individuals in our population that have a metabolic profile which results in reactive metabolites that can result in the carcinogenic event. I think that there's more need for looking at individuality among individuals in terms of repair mechanisms. But there is also a great need for identifying those individuals who are at highest risk.

DR. MILLER: I really have nothing to add to Alan's comments on that particular point. I would like to point out something that Alan actually referred to this morning in his talk, a concept which we came to a number of years ago when the electrophile hypothesis seemed pretty evident to us. We were wondering about the possibility that, at the very low intakes of a variety of carcinogens—and we may all, as we know, be exposed to a wide variety—what happens to those electrophiles that are formed in metabolism?

We were struck with the idea that possibly in the cell there would be low levels of low molecular weight, noncritical nuclophiles that might help literally to soak up these small amounts of electrophiles, and this gave rise to the idea that, as you progressively lower the dose of a carcinogen, may be you get down to a level where suddenly the total amount of available electrophile would react with the information macromolecules that we think are more important. You might, theoretically, if you could do the experiment, see a rather drastic change in the slope of the dose-response curve at some range of a very low level of intake of a carcinogen.

I'm not saying that the noncritical nucleophiles would wipe out the critical ones completely, but they might actually drastically lower their level. So we attempted it, and we published this to see if we could reproduce this idea. We took AAF at the usual high levels, and we could get no effect on tumor incidence by feeding the animals rather high levels of common nucleophiles like guanidine, cystine, methionine, tyrosine, and so forth, but then we lowered the AAF level in the diet to .006% and, of course, as you normally find, it took a longer time for the first tumor to develop and the overall incidence was lower, but we actually did get a lessening of the induction time by feeding 2% methionine. That's kind of drastic and we haven't gone back to do any more. We were rather disappointed in the effect; we thought we might get a bigger effect, but I guess we would have to go to still lower levels of AAF with larger groups of animals, wait a longer time, and see whether externally-administered noncritical nucleophiles might help. But the idea, I think, needs more amplification.

DR. MAGEE: Before I start to lead this discussion, if that's the right term, I just wanted to make some comments on the remarks that David Clayson had made earlier in his very interesting presentation on the report of the British group on the oral contraceptives. I happen to be a member of that group, and there's nobody else here who was, so primarily what I want to say is that it wasn't quite so clear then as it was in the remarks that David made.

There was a lot of doubt at that time among many people about the significance of neoplasms or lumps in liver. At that time their significance was not nearly so clear as it now is. We didn't have the benefit of knowing about vinyl chloride. We hadn't seen Janet Baum's paper, because it came out about two years later. We hadn't had the benefit of Dr. Mays' excellent presentation today. We knew for many years, of course, that estrogens were carcinogenic, and what I want to say is illustrating the point that Dr. Mrak made at the very beginning of the meeting regarding the role of emotions in making up one's mind about these things.

Now, the issue of oral contraceptives is a very emotional one. People on this committee were aware of the importance of these chemicals, and particularly the importance of the population explosion going on, and there was sort of subconscious and conscious feeling that perhaps one must be very careful before one incriminates oral contraceptives too much. I think that concept may have been shared by people in the rest of the world, because the British group, I think, were the only people who initiated the study on the oral contraceptives. These are foreign chemicals that are given to human subjects, females, over a large fraction of their lifetime, at a dose level that's pharmacological and has an effect, because otherwise they are no good.

Note that no other regulatory agency that I know of did any work whatsoever on these compounds, so these results emerged and the details were published as Dr. Shellenberger said in his rather more sympathetic view of committee's opinion, and the data were all open, and yet there was remarkably little response after this. There was an editorial in the *British Medical Journal* written by Francis Roe mentioning some hepatomas. It was swept under the carpet with an unphraseable comment from my former director, but I'm not sure there were many more. Yet one would have thought, if it were so apparent, that quite a large number, even of the people in this room, might have been writing about it to the *New York Times,* as they now do. So what we conclude from this is that when a chemical is *really* wanted by people, regulatory agencies and scientists are less keen to see the evidence as clearly as they are in other cases—the case of saccharin, shall we say.

If oral contraceptives had been saccharin they wouldn't have had a chance, because several groups were determined to find saccharin carcinogenic. But the regulatory agencies were still reluctant to do anything about the oral contraceptives. We've seen this, as I can see, compelling evidence for the carcinogenic action of the oral contraceptives as Dr. Mays presented, but who's doing anything about it? Who's stopping it? Well, those are my comments.

DR. SHELLENBERGER: I want to continue with this oral contraceptive discussion that started in connection with the liver. Dr. Kraybill asked me two very interesting questions just before the afternoon session started. He said, "Do you have a daughter?" I said, "Yes, 18 years old." He said, "Well, what are you going to tell her about the birth control pills, the oral contraceptives?" and I said, "I don't know." And that's a very striking question and a hard one for me to answer. This then gets me into the other discussion we had at lunch.

I had the privilege of sitting with Dr. Mays and I asked him whether we are in a position now (thinking back to yesterday's discussion about risk-benefit and doing this within the scope of that editorial to be presented, by Dr. Wynder), to set up a risk-benefit analysis panel and committee. I wonder if this question of oral contraceptives (and so forth) wouldn't make a good subject for that initial discussion.

The risks—as we see it—are the endometrial cancer that has been discussed this afternoon by Dr. Peter Greenwald, as well as the item about malignant hepatomas that Dr. Mays mentioned this morning. On the benefit side, you have population control with ultimate means of contraception. But in addition you have, I would suspect, a decreased incidence of maternal deaths at births, either through intentional, supervised or unsupervised abortion, plus the natural death rate at birth. I think this might be a logical case to balance risk versus benefit, and I just throw that out for discussion.

DR. MAGEE: All I was going to say was I'm sorry if I upset your data.

I've done this before and I'm quite sure I'm going to do it again. But both of us know from experience in the United Kingdom how difficult it is to be on an advisory committee dealing with drugs. In the case in which you were concerned with humans, and the case in which I was concerned with animals, how easy it was for things to slip by or not to give mental impetus!

I think your argument this afternoon was very much on the lines of the risk-benefit assessment of these compounds. I hope that your risk-benefit assessment was correct, that these liver tumors are not very significant—300 out of 12 million or 20 million; it's a very low number indeed at this stage. If it gets higher, we are in trouble.

I think I would just say that I have commented in print before about unpleasant possibilities, but, as I said, we must hope that the grim thoughts that we sometimes have don't come to pass.

DR. WYNDER: I'd just like to reply to that, and there I agree with you absolutely. I am very worried because I don't know whether we are seeing just the tip of the iceberg with these benign hepatomas. From what I've heard from Dr. Mays' talk today, I'm more worried.

DR. COULSTON: First of all can I ask Dr. Clemmesen a question? Dr. Clemmesen, in view of the controversy that Dr. Schneiderman has engendered about this data, could you provide some really precise information on the pathological nature of those tumors and tell us something about the details of the amount of drug given to those patients? Question two is, in view of the discussion that we're now having on oral contraceptives, and the fact that benign hepatomas in rodents were the first lead to an understanding of benign hepatomas in young ladies, would you still stand by your statement that we should entirely ignore the induction of benign hepatomas in rodents as a lead to what we might find in humans?

DR. CLEMMESEN: Yes, indeed, there were eleven cases (we have the slides of most of them in my office), there may be one or two for which the slides have been lost, but for which we have the descriptions and the explanations. In November, 1938, there was a meeting of the Pathological Society of Great Britain and Ireland, and Sir Robert Muir got up and warned against the use of Thorotrast. He couldn't tell whether people would get cancers of the liver or cirrhosis, but they would quite often get one of them. When I went home, I mentioned this in a medical weekly in a review on cancer, and I shouldn't complain if people took it seriously at this hospital in Filadelfia. They took the warning and referred the responsibility of Thorotrast to the neurosurgeons; nevertheless, I had the definite feeling that they were so concerned about their patients that they contributed to this high number of case records.

I have slides, some of them have been published, and I have a sea of autopsy descriptions; since many of these pathologists have passed to a better world, the problem is whether one should use them and whether it's worth printing, but we do have the evidence. After all, how do you compare 800 or 900 rodents to 8,078 patients, of which we have quite a lot of more knowledge? I would disregard the rodents as just being rodents.

There was an international conference in '73, I think, and it appeared from the statements from all participants that you would see both hepatocarcinomas and cholangiocarcinomas, as well as some leukemias. Of course, I believe that in pathology that's the closest you can come to etiology; I don't believe in the story that one compound makes only one kind of tumor. There's usually some other organ or tissue affected. But they do belong to those types, and I have those here.

DR. SELIKOFF: I was delighted with Dr. Clemmesen's paper which raised the question about the relevance of the animal data with phenobarbital, because one of the problems in all animal studies is the fact that the investigators ignored the induction capability of phenobarb. And if there were carcinogens in either feed or water, the controls were not really controls. The controls should have been given some other inducer, perhaps polychlorinated biphenyl or something else, preferably an inducer that might *not* be a carcinogen. So there is a question in my mind about whether we *really* had controls and exposed animals.

On the other hand, I was delighted with Dr. Clemmesen's paper for another reason. If, indeed, there is no increased cancer incidence with phenobarb in humans, ignoring the animal data which I have some questions about, it tells us that—at least to the extent that the study has so far been carried—induction in man by phenobarb, at least, is not associated with an increased incidence of cancer.

This is a very valuable piece of evidence that Dr. Clemmesen has given us in this population study. I'm comfortable for another reason as well in that it tells us that phenobarb certainly in the short term doesn't cause any of the cancers. Dr. Clemmesen did what I think is superb. He didn't look for liver cancer, he looked for all kinds of cancers, which really is the proper way to do it, and he did it very, very well. However—and here's a big however, because it dogs us all the time, and to some extent I think that it even constrained Peter Greenwald in his studies on estrogen—there is the constraint of time.

Dr. Clemmesen looked at his people before 10 years and after 10 years. He was kind enough to tell me that of those classified as being more than 10 years, two-thirds were less than 20 years. So we had the vast majority of the subjects observed less than 20 years from the onset of taking phenobarb. Unless phenobarb causes early tumors, we're looking at empty data. I wonder if Dr. Hammond could tell us whether he could find the really powerful effect of smoking among those who have not yet reached 20 years from the onset of their smoking; whether he would see it in 20-year-old kids, 25-year-olds, and 30-year olds, even those who begin smoking at 8. I would strongly urge that Dr. Clemmesen continue this magnificent study of his on the unique population that he has under observation to tell us what is going to happen after 25, 35, 40 years or whatever, because the problem is an important one since phenobarb is an inducer, regardless of whether it causes cancer in animals.

Now I'm less comfortable, however, with Peter's presentation. He did the best he could, and in fact he did very well. He stimulated us; he certainly stimulated me. The question comes up: Can you compare gross economic data like sales of estrogen in dollars with incidence of uterine cancer year by year when we know darned well that that year doesn't mean anything. That constraint of time also bedevils all of the case control studies, because when they're reported as I saw in the bibliography in '73 and '74, it means they were written in '72 and '73. The work was done, and the cases were collected from '55 on. In order to have a number of cases in any series they may have been collected over the previous 10 years or maybe even more. Therefore, let us consider DES, or even birth control pills (which really began to hit a peak in '65); to include in series of cases, cases that were entered in the registries in 1955 or '60 or '65 or '70, makes you uncomfortable.

And this is the trouble with all case control studies and all registries. It was a constraint that (Greenwald) faced and however well he did it it was difficult to get around. I'm reminded of Richard Doll's current or recent studies with saccharin. When he used patients who had diabetes as an index of saccharin use, he did not know whether or not they took the tablets.

One of the things that happens in all series of cancers when you go back to them or in the registries is that the people who are dead are not available to be questioned about whether they were exposed, about whether they took saccharin, or whether they took DES, or whether they took anything else. So what he did was to take another group of diabetics and question them as to when and whether they used saccharin in Great Britain. Saccharin was used much more in Great Britain than in the U.S. because they had sugar rationing until 1952. Well, Doll found that only 10% of those who took saccharin (diabetics) took it for more than 25 years. So 90% did not take it, and it's, therefore, very difficult to get some judgment about what happens with drug-taking unless you really know the exposure. I come back over and over again, the way we all do, that there's hardly any question of exposure to drugs. It's a very difficult thing in prospective studies to obtain an accurate history of drug intake.

DR. GREENWALD: I'd like to respond to the questions about time, and I think some of the points are well taken. With DES, I think we validated the exposures well enough that it's not really a problem. With breast cancer, one of the key points was the same one that you made, that is, I don't believe we can draw conclusions from those case and control studies, because there hasn't been enough time for induction.

With endometrial cancer the time trends are crude. There's just one piece of evidence. If you look at the figure on page 10, you see that the interval between the marked increase of use in this country and the start of the steeper upswing is about 4-5 years, and that might raise some questions about whether it's causing it or whether it's accelerating it, or something of that sort. With the case control studies of endometrial cancer, there were more recent cases. Since the studies are positive, with exposure among cases being much greater, I don't see time as a problem. If the results were negative, you might be concerned that you would not be able to detect the result because of the time factor problem.

DR. SELIKOFF: When did they take the estrogen? Did they take it 2 years before they went to a doctor, because they were ill, or did they take it 30 years before?

DR. GREENWALD: All of these studies did have some information about duration. There isn't too much dose-response which gets into that. Five or more years use resulted in a much greater risk than less than 5 years. That's at the bottom of page 11. And Drs., Gray, Christopherson, and Hoover had probably the best data about that, when they showed that the longest duration had by far the greatest carcinogenic effect; that is, the greatest effect in inducing endometrial cancer.

DR. BUTLER: Going back for a moment to the phenobarb and possibly the contraceptive problem I, in fact, have done a two-year study of phenobarb in the rat and it was absolutely negative. I think if you look at others' data on phenobarb, it's highly doubtful whether they should be interpreted as being evidence that phenobarb is a carcinogen, because of the strain of rat they used. I won't get into the problem of how to interpret the mouse data, or I'll be here all day.

With the oral contraceptives I think Dr. Magee knows at least in private that I'm one of his critics; in public, at certain meetings as well. What is interesting about his findings is that mestranol was recognized as being a carcinogen for the rat in about 1961 and '62 and it didn't just produce benign tumors, it produced metastasizing hepatic carcinomas. These data were ignored for a variety of reasons, and as far as I know they have never been published. But one thing that has happened over recent years is that the dose levels of oral contraceptives have gotten smaller and smaller. Another thing that has happened is that one is using much more of the progestagens. People have been much more cautious in this because chlormadinone has come off the market due to the development of tumors in beagle dogs' breasts, and recently *megestrol* acetate was removed on the basis of six tumors in a 7-year study, and all four of these tumors had metastases.

I understand there's another antifertility agent which is under consideration at the moment and is likely to be removed. So I think people are being a little bit more cautious.

There are many other drugs one could consider in this respect which I think are of great interest. I think anabolic steroids were mentioned this morning. But the people that do interest me are the athletes that take these steroids, and I wonder if anybody is going to look at these people in the long term. I think this would be a most interesting group to study. There's a wide range of other drugs that are of concern, but I think possibly unnecessarily so. One example of this, the beta blockers, have come under a cloud recently. After all they've been used to treat arrhythmias and other rather serious illnesses; some of these may be carcinogens in animals. It's difficult to get these on the market without two-year carcinogenicity tests. In addition, there's a wide range of other drugs which are used prophylactically, like the antilipidemic agents. These are now known to be carcinogenic; some of them, but not all. These are going to be used for a long time, and the question is, should something be done? This is a very large problem and I'm sorry, in fact, that Dr. Shubik didn't give his paper on Flagyl. I'm not quite sure whether or not he considers Flagyl to be a carcinogen. As far as I can remember Flagyl increased statistically the incidences of leukemias and pulmonary adenomas. My view is that this would not be evidence of carcinogenicity, and this was a view taken by some regulatory authorities. Flagyl wasn't removed from the market, I would have thought, justifiably. It's been suggested there are feminists that want it taken off the market, and also it has now been used as the drug of choice by surgeons prophylactically for major bowel surgery. I don't know whether this is a fact in this country, but it is certainly the practice in Britain.

DR. CLEMMESEN: The histological diagnosis was 4 cases of cholangiosarcomas, 4 of endosarcomas, 2 characterized as adenocarcinomas, 1 only as malignant neoplasm, and 1 as primary, and 1 as having no histopathology. As to the others, we have been through the case records and can't give precise information, because they were just given one or two cc and part of the dosage would pass out of the vessels; as to that part of the evidence, in a number of cases it's possible histologically to demonstrate the presence of Thorotrast.

The experts realize that there's also a heavy risk to the wives of these people, because they have these enormous deposits in the liver of radioactive material.

Then, finally, with regard to the latent period or the time for development: now we have studied those we had before 10 years. One-third will have been exposed more than 20 years, and I think in six month's time we'll be able to give data for another five-year period, because at that time we'll have personal numbers on all of them and can work on that. But I would point out that we had a very good control in the positive control with Thorotrast, because we have, within 10 years, only a single case which really evolved later, and then we have data beyond 10 years, and it will be very easy to study the others.

DR. SHUBIK: We should publish it, and I think it's very important to do that. Send it to Dr. Clayson; he and I edit a journal together, and I'll persuade him to publish it.

DR. CLAYSON: May I comment on this and respond to Dr. Butler? I wasn't weasling my way out of it. While I don't mind repeating things that are already in print, Flagyl produces lymphomas and is not a terribly impressive compound.

And it produces lung adenomas in mice without any question. We didn't know that this had already been done twice by the manufacturers when we did it, because that was data in the files of the Food and Drug Administration. It was only after we had published it that we found that this was the case. That data, I believe, has not been spoken of widely. So everyone knows that Flagyl produces lung adenomas and lymphomas. The reason we tested it was because of its chemical structure—a nitro drug—and because the clinical reports in the literature indicated that a small number of blood dyscrasias had been observed with that drug. Additionally, it is, as you know, mutagenic. Therefore, it has all the characteristics, and it seemed to us to make the project of testing it worthwhile. There are a large number of other tests still underway, which I was not going to mention today because they're not finished.

There are suggestions, and no more than that, of possible additional effects, and I can't say any more than that at the present time. Flagyl is being tested transplacentally among other things since it is the panacea of pregnant ladies. What do I think about it? My view is that it is high time, and we've said this many times already, that an epidemiological study on the effect of Flagyl be instituted. One thing that has made me think that this meeting would be a very worthwhile operation was the suggestion that research of this kind should be done.

I think we know these things about this drug and in my view it is being used in much too large a doses for benign conditions, but I don't have any questions or doubt that Flagyl is an excellent drug for the treatment of a variety of parasitic infections. When it comes to amebiasis, there is no question about it at all; even in the case of some flagellates that are awfully difficult to treat. I think perhaps it's a justifiable treatment.

Other than that I think not enough caution is being exerted. Much too much energy is being spent trying to say that this means nothing, and to my mind that is a kind of objectless exercise. There is no question that this drug has adverse effects in animal systems, and these parallel in a sense some of the things already seen clinically. It hasn't produced any tumors in people, but I think we should set out to do a prospective study to see if there really is anything wrong with it. The additional animal studies which we are doing may case some further light on the subject.

DR. HAMMOND: When I look back at Peter Greenwald's page 10, Fig. 3, I'm astonished that people didn't get more excited. Several of us here remember some 30 years back when we saw an enormous rise in lung cancer. It was the most exciting thing in the whole field of cancer as far as etiology was concerned. If you look at Peter's Fig. 3, and then he has some added information that I will give you, this is a big if not more rapid rise, assuming the figures are correct.

Speaking of endometrial cancer, I should tell you something that Dr. Greenwald didn't mention; he wasn't bragging—a great problem we have had in time trends in uterine cancer is that the National Archives of Vital Statistics published data on cancer of the cervix, cancer of the corpus, and cancer of the uterus, site unspecified. This was around 40% of the total. People tried to proportion the other, and got a completely false notion about the division between the two. The New York Cancer Registry is the only one in this country under Peter's guidance. I should say Peter's the only one with a cancer registry where they have made a great effort to divide these cases into the two groups, and furthermore they have not thrown in the in situ carcinomas with the other cancers (which is completely legitimate), if you want to study figures over a long time.

Now the piece of information I will add to this is that the number of hysterectomies in this country, for reasons other than cancer, is simply phenomenonal. It's a medical scandal; there have been investigations about unnecessary operations, simply for the surgeon to get money out of it. This may be one of those cases in which absolutely unnecessary procedures saved a great many lives. Right now, the last time I got the data, well over 50% of women in New York State over the age of, I think, 50 had had hysterectomies. It must be very much higher now. There are 40,000 women affected in New York State where, as determined in 1959, '61, '63, '65, and '72, the rates are going up astronomically.

Figure 3 shows the incidence rate of endometrial cancer per 100,000 women. This is not the proper denominator. The incidence rate of endometrial cancer, per 100,000 uteri exposed to risk should be shown. I'm not joking. This is a case where you can't get cancer of an organ that doesn't exist. If you look at it with these adjusted figures I think you will find (I'll provide you with the data to adjust them Peter, had one part of the data) this is a more rapid and a more alarming increase that we saw when we met in Belgium some 30 years ago.

Now we said at that time that if the incidence of disease is going up rapidly this gives the best possible opportunity to look at the etiologic factors causing it. We've all heard today the evidence on estrogen as a factor. It may well be. But whatever it is, this is something that is just about as urgent as the lung cancer picture was some 30 years ago. We put more effort into that and everything else in cancer put together, as far as etiology is concerned. I think that's the real exciting thing in this meeting.

DR. LYON: Just as a follow-up on Dr. Hammond's comments: we just published in the *American Journal of Epidemiology,* using the U.S. data for hysterectomies and using a sample population model, a corrective factor for this. We estimate in the over-65 population about 40% hysterectomies in the U.S. The rate is for the years between 1965 and 1963, when it was increasing exponentially. It raises uterine cancer rates. We used the California registry data rather than Peter's data but it raised the California data from 1962 onward by peaking out at about 40%. Interestingly enough, it did not have any effect or had a very, very minimal effect, on cervical cancer. Some of you might want to take a look at this effect. Really, it would raise the level of Peter's rates.

DR. GREENWALD: On the cervical cancer, I have done this age group specifically with data from the same source, and hysterectomy accounts for a very large proportion of the total mortality in cervical cancer. Those figures you want on the population base, I can assure you, account for a large proportion.

DR. LYON: That's an excellent point and I think you're correct that with a rising incidence, if you correct the denominators there would be much more marked rise. We did the same thing for cervical cancer once and data on hysterectomy were a little rough, but it might account for about half of the fall in mortality. You know that in New York State about 80% or so of the in situs below age 40 are invasive. I don't have anything further to add.

I wasn't sure, and I didn't know if you had data on this, but we knew that hysterectomies were rising rapdily, from just talking to some obstetricians. We had thought that some of the indications were really for sterilization procedures, especially among the Catholic population, and I wondered if, with the more frequent use of tying tubes, that might tend to create a leveling effect on hysterectomy in the past few years, but is it still going up?

DR. GREENWALD: The last data we had was for the U.S. in 1973 and it had increased. It had doubled between 1968 and 1973, and from what I understand from Bunker it's still going up.

DR. LYON: I was very skeptical of this, skeptical that women weren't reporting this correctly. We took one test city, namely, Toledo, Ohio, and we looked back, we literally took a look in every surgery book showing every operation performed there dating back to 1945, and looked for any female genital operation whatsoever, if it was hysterectomy, what it was for, etc. What we got from that was virtually identical to what we got from the questionnaire for the general population sample. The population sample missed nothing and we had the same data from New York State based on annual figures, controls on socioeconomic class, and with controls on Black versus White, because the black people have very much higher rates.

DR. CLEMMESEN: We have the figures you're asking for. A rather low percentage of undefined uterine cancers, I think it's around 4% between 1943-47. We recently compared the figures with the Connecticut data, and it appears that in Connecticut they didn't have that small percentage of unspecified cases, but they had earlier a great number of carcinomas in situ and when we compared them with what we found in Copenhagen, the rates for cervical cancer had risen until we had screening programs introduced and then they dropped below the lowest value. But, to my surprise, we had two American visitors, who said that the corpus cancer must be increasing, and we looked up the data and found it was perfectly true; it has increased in Copenhagen, from 13 to 18 per 100,000 during the 20 years up to '67, and these increases are still going on. I don't think that the pill had been used as early in Denmark as in this country, but it did certainly show the same increase.

DR. COULSTON: Dr. Shubik made a very pertinent remark when he asked a question of Dr. Clemmesen, and I'm going to bring this discussion back to that if I can. It's absolutely delightful listening to the epidemiologists discuss this data, but the question Dr. Shubik raises is the point of this meeting. He said, knowing the animal data as we know it now with estrogens or DES, could you have predicted, or would you have used this data in part, at least, to determine the epidemiology, or vice versa? Would it have been something to tell an epidemiologist, "Go look in the liver for hepatomas?" Should Dr. Mays have been forewarned? Dr. Shubik is quite right in the way he tried to put it to Dr. Clemmesen and others have been touching on it.

Now what I'd like to see in the next, let's say ten minutes, is a very crucial discussion (knowing what we know and know now about the action of estrogens in rodents or in monkeys or in dogs), of whether this would have been enough of a clue from the animal researchers to have our colleagues in epidemiology do their thing, so to speak?

May I suggest to the discussion leaders, if we could stay on this point for a little bit, I think it would make not only me very happy, but also Dr. Shubik and others.

DR. HAMMOND: Well, I think the epidemiologists were warned 40 years ago to get a proper study of it epidemiologically. I think you have your answer. We were warned, and we did act on it.

DR. SELIKOFF: May I ask our laboratory colleagues a question instead? I don't think it's enough any more simply to warn the epidemiologists and for them to get a yes-no answer at some level of statistical significance. I've heard the term used here about risk and even benefit. It's hard enough to determine risk, it's even harder very often to determine benefit. What we're talking about is *level* of risk, so it's not enough any longer to get a yes or no answer. Can we then utilize laboratory experimental results to give some hint, some projection, some extrapolation on what might be the level of risk in humans? Now there are not many chemicals for which we have animal and human data. DES in one of the few. We have aflatoxin, and so forth. But very few. Can the laboratory people tell me whether there is any correlation between the experimental results with stilbestrol and the beginning of population-based risk data in humans that Peter reviewed with us and that others have published as well?

DR. SHELLENBERGER: I think as far as the mammary tumorgenesis end point is concerned, there was work in the mid-1930s, was there not? The mammary tumor end point?

DR. SELIKOFF: That started in the 1920s. I've never seen any later work done any better than that. I've recently reviewed the literature and they did a splendid job of it.

DR. SHELLENBERGER: Now about the cervical end point, the first report that I saw was Dunn's work in '63 which was well beyond the point before DES was used therapeutically. Now I don't know, based on the mammary tumor end point, that you would predict the cervical end point except that it's a target tissue and deliberately changes. Obviously, you knew the mammalian studies, the mouse uterotropic weight-gain assay which was known at that time.

The proliferation of weight increase is due to the 7-day assay. At that stage, which would have been the early 1950s, I don't know whether you could have seen the cervical end point. I stand to be corrected.

DR. COULSTON: But even with hindsight, can you tell me now whether the laboratory quantitative data on DES can project to within an order of magnitude what might happen in humans? The laboratory people can give us now important information. Are we going to ask the epidemiologist to give us the benefit-risk ratio which might take decades? Or are we going to extrapolate from the animal data to man right now?

DR. MAGEE: Not on estrogens, but I think you raised the question of aflatoxin, and I think this is going to be an example if we consider some of the Lyon data on the levels of aflatoxin that are being ingested by these people who have got this very high incidence of primary liver cancer. Here the laboratory cancer expert did lead the way and gave a fair indication to the epidemiologist where he should look and what he should study, and it seems to be working out very much as predicted.

DR. COULSTON: This is a fine example of what can be done. I still would like to know whether you can give us some quantitative judgment, otherwise we're going to be left with a yes or no answer, and for regulatory agencies they're going to have to utilize "no" answers for what they're going to do whenever there is any doubt as to safety.

DR. MILLER: I might just point out that there was a horrible outbreak of acute aflatoxicosis in West India about three years ago. It's in the literature, it occurred in over 200 villages where their only food in a very wet, rainy season was their maize, which they stored improperly and which became very heavily infested with *aspergillus flavis*. They had such high levels of intake. I can't recall the exact level, but in just a few weeks they got ascites and over 100 people died; their dogs died with the same condition. The survivors now are being watched. There are at least two papers in the Indian literature on this. So we might get a little data rather quickly.

DR. SHUBIK: I would like to skip that question for a minute but I'll come back to it. I'm contemplating it, and I think there are some answers, but what I would like to get back to is the question of some of these chemicals and drugs that we know to be carcinogenic in animals and what the epidemiologists think about doing follow-ups on these drugs. We discussed the one Dr. Butler brought up, Flagyl, which is very widely used. The other one is one that Dr. Clayson mentioned this morning, and that's griseofulvin which has been known since the first tests on it by Paget at ICI to be a compound that produces hepatomas. He produced hepatomas in mice, and it, of course, is also a toxic substance, producing porphyria and other adverse effects.

In recent data that we have, which is not yet published, it does seem as though griseofulvin induces tumors in the rat. It does this rather late in the dose-response relationships. There's no question as far as I'm concerned that it produces carcinoma of the thyroid in the rat as well as producing hepatomas in the mouse. It does nothing in the hamster as far as one can tell. Griseofulvin is used a great deal for all sorts of things, including athlete's foot, in very large doses, and for prolonged periods of time. I mentioned in my initial talk here that it had been given to the U.S. Army prophylactically in Vietnam in quite large doses. So it would seem to me that there must be a group there to be studied and followed up.

The third series deals with the question of niridazole on which Dr. Clayson presented the data and which has been given to literally millions of people with schistosomiasis. Niridazole is unequivocally carcinogenic in three species of animals, and we have been unable to find any data actually from any of those concerned with the original marketing of niridazole to tell us whether or not it had been adequately tested before being put on the market. The anti-schistosomal drugs, in any event, are terribly suspect all the way down the line, because by the very nature of the disease, they have to kill these parasites, and it's difficult to make one of them that doesn't have some sort of manifestation of toxicity. But in view of the serious nature of the disease, clearly here is one in which you balance your risks and benefits and you finish up saying that another drug, Hycanthone, certainly seems to be much less toxic.

I'd like to ask the epidemiologists if they would tell us whether or not the leads that we have are, in their view, amenable to follow up, worth following up, and what sort of things ought to be done to do this?

QUESTION: May I ask you about Flagyl, because we have various screening programs, and I have insisted that since trichomonas may produce scraping, which looks very much like a beginning precancerous condition, that it may be that trichomoniasis is preparing a precancerous condition; so whenever we have a case, we notice it, and then we treat the patient with Flagyl.

DR. SELIKOFF: May I try to answer Phil's question about whether is it possible to obtain epidemiological information on suspect drugs? Dr. Hammond and I were very interested in this a year or two ago with the reserpine problem, and we looked for epidemiological models so that we might explore this in a substantial way. Later on, we didn't place this very high in the order of priorities, because of new data with regard to reserpine. But we explored a cohort of pharmacies to see whether they kept their records, and how long they kept them, and we found that pharmacies love to keep their 30-year-old books of prescriptions in their windows to show how long they've been in business and how they keep their patients' records, and so forth. We then went through several thousand old prescriptions to find out whether we could detect prescriptions given for reserpine, whether the names were on the prescriptions, and whether the doctor's prescription had the form that he used so that we knew which doctor gave it.

We found that by and large these were available. However, in hospitals they were not. At least in my hospital the records were terrible. They were good in private practice but were not good in hospitals, perhaps because hospital patients are a very select group (they come in, they rest, they stay there a short time, and they never come back), and 20 years later nobody knows what happened to them.

Second, we were interested in whether the SV-40 virus which is carcinogenic in animals might also be carcinogenic in humans. We did know that it contaminated the yellow fever vaccine in World War II, and we explored whether the VA data could identify those who were given yellow fever vaccine and if their long-term experience would then give us some hint. Dr. Hammond even did something else which I thought was even more productive. The question came up of polio vaccine being contaminated and he had in his records in the cancer prevention study of the American Cancer Society a record of those who were given polio vaccine and those who were not given polio vaccine, and then he explored prospectively their cancer incidence, holding smoking constant. There are epidemiological techniques, they involve a great deal of work, but are right if the problem is important. I would think that we now have a new cohort; those who are in Vietnam will be able to tell you in 15 years whether griseofulvin is associated with an increased cancer risk. There are techniques, they can be used, we're delighted to have the hints that you're giving us.

DR. WYNDER: Well, we are currently involved in this; we have revised our drug questionnaire and let me just briefly review with you the problems involved in taking a drug history. I mentioned earlier the privacy act, and I just mentioned it to you because all of us have our problems and the privacy act alone has increased the cost of our studies in New York tremendously. Before you and others came in, as I indicated before, you've got to get permission each time, have got to get the permission of the patient, and have got to get this permission signed by witnesses.

That's number one. So now you've got the patient and now you're asking for drugs and drug recall; I don't have to tell you it is very, very poor. It's hard because we as physicians rarely tell the patient what we're giving him, and strangely enough the patient rarely asks. This, incidentally, doesn't only apply for drug therapy, it also applies for hysterectomies and other operations. I'm always amazed how many women don't know what's at the other end of the belly. So that's the second problem.

Now the patient gets a prescription and now we've got to make sure he takes the prescription. Many studies have been done in compliance, particularly in hypertension, and one is amazed how many patients, when they become symptom-free, will no longer take the prescription. This has to do with some psychological problems, because the patient figures if he takes the drug he's sick; if he doesn't take the drug and just has it in the medicine cabinet by definition, he's not sick. After we even have the information that the patient has said "Yes, the doctor gave me Flagyl, or whatever drug it is." I'm sure he took Flagyl as long he was itching, but if symptom-free, he would not take it.

So the first problem is that the patient who takes the drug is different from the patient who does not. Clearly, the epidemiology of Premarin will show that the patient who uses Premarin is different socioeconomically and in other ways from the control patient, and the patient who takes Flagyl may have different sexual habits from those who do not.

Now with all of those as negatives, nevertheless, we think it's important, and we are doing it, but I want you to know that it's costly and time consuming, and if any one of you who sits on funding and grant agencies wonders why it costs $122, or whatever, it costs, to get one good drug history, that's why.

DR. TRUHAUT: Thank you, Mr. Chairman. In listening to Prof. Selikoff, I have certainly the impression that I should read again recommendations made 12 years ago, that is in 1965, at an international symposium on carcinogenic hazards from drugs. This was published two years later in an ICC monograph, this meeting of 1965. It is exactly what you said, Prof. Selikoff, exactly.

DR. MOFIDI: I wanted to just add some information about the type of studies that are being carried out in Iran for the last 7 years on cancer. I'm sure all of you are familiar with the data, but anyhow this project which has been carried by the School of Public Health and MRC and NCI is intended to study the epidemiological aspect of a cancer which has high prevalence in one particular area of the northern part of the country, and every type of data from the human and environmental aspect has been assembled.

The original study gave a complete difference, at least a statistically significant difference, in the status of the area, where the cancer was prevalent versus the area where it was not. There was also a greater consumption of bread. Then, additional studies showed that various seeds have been added to the grain and types of mycotoxins have been now found there. Also a very important study now shows that they have a great concentration of toxins in certain families. Now studies are devised concerning the family case control study, and I'm just throwing this into the prospective epidemiology that you are trying to do. It should not consider only the etiological factors affecting the human population, but additional studies should be done about other factors as well.

DR. COULSTON: Well, since we are approaching the end I think it would be remiss, particularly for me, not to mention nonhuman primates. We've been listening to studies about rats and mice and hamsters and a little bit about dogs, and I think it's time we mentioned the monkey or the chimpanzee. In studies on the pill, as long ago as 1967, my colleagues found that a progestin-estrogen combination produced changes in the breast of monkeys and also produced changes in the liver which were tantamount to early nodular formation in the liver. This stopped the progress of this combination drug and it was reported to the Food and Drug Administration. It was information based upon that kind of study which was one of the reasons, if not the major reason, why the FDA initiated studies on rhesus monkeys. It was possible to see that these progestin-estrogens contributed a relatively small amount above what we would estimate the human use from natural, intrinsic production of these steroids. Now why was the monkey breast interesting?

The dog mammary organ has a duct system which is quite different from the human, and tends to plug itself up very easily, as the secondary ducts can become plugged and you get an inflammation and a swelling.

The female rhesus monkey and the chimpanzee have a duct system just like a woman, so if you're going to study mammary tumors or mammary changes it's obviously logical in my mind that we go in the direction of using a nonhuman primate at least. Concerning the question, Can the toxicologist predict? Of course he can; he does it every day. He has to make the decision whether to use a chemical for man as a drug, or whether to use a chemical as a food additive or a pesticide, and decide if it is safe for man. He's doing this all the time.

There are no mysterious ways to do this. He knows how and he can predict 70-80% of the time what the target organ of toxicity will be. And he can tell whether there will be blood changes, and so on. What he can't tell is whether the chemical is going to cause cancer, and this is the hangup of the toxicologist today. What I'm trying to point out is that it is possible for the toxicologist to answer the kind of question that Dr. Selikoff put to us, but the question in my mind is "Where is the dialogue between the epidemiologist and the toxicologist?" That is what I'd like to hear discussed for a moment.

DR. SHUBIK: I'd like to address a question on the subject of the pill, and ask the biochemists what they think about the possibility of the profound effect that most of the current pills have on metabolism of the liver. Mightn't we be missing other possible carcinogenic substances that might be present? It would seem to me there is ample evidence clinically that women on the pill can be shown to have depressed liver function. In fact, there are situations that I've heard of where internists that are friends of mine have told me that women with hepatitis who had left hospital were recovering very well, but then suddenly stopped recovering, and this coincided with the taking of the pill again.

It seemed to me that the pill had such a profound effect on metabolism that conceivably it really invalidates a great amount of the toxicology that is being done on rodents, say in the case of food additives. Surely a rodent administered a food additive in the normal state is not an animal which is applicable to the case of a lady who is taking the pill and who has had her liver metabolism and metabolizing enzymes so severely modified. I'm sure some of those here today, particularly Dr. Conney, might be able to comment on this and whether, in fact, they have looked at any of these steroids and steroidal combinations in the sort of context that we discussed today.

DR. CONNEY: Yes, the effect of the pill has been studied on drug metabolism and there is some inhibition in the metabolism of certain drugs, presumably by the monooxygenase system. There is some modification of the drug metabolizing system. Whether this results in more metabolic activation and less detoxification of environmental carcinogens, is an unanswerable question right now. I think that this is an important issue.

I'd be interested in knowing whether anyone has looked at the effect of the pill in a population of epileptics who are taking phenobarbital. There is evidence that phenobarbital enhances the metabolism of oral contraceptives in rats. One can inhibit the action of mestranol and also estradiol in rats by pretreating the animals with phenobarbital. In looking at some of the clinical literature, there's evidence that for women on the pill that are epileptics getting phenobarbital and diphenylhydantoin, the pill is less effective. There are more pregnancies in these women, so there's a suggestion that these drugs are also enhancing, perhaps, the metabolism of the pill in humans. Is there a difference in incidence of these liver problems in epileptics that are on phenobarbital and diphenylhydantoin and also the pill?

DR. MAGEE: Can I just make a comment on Dr. Shubik's question? There is an experimental model in carcinogenesis that may be relevant to this in that, if the metabolism of the carcinogen is depressed, in this case not by the pill but by dietary means or by a drug, you can profoundly influence the carcinogenic effect in other organs. You can increase the kidney cancer incidence from 20% to 100%, simply by depressing the metabolism of the carcinogen in the liver. So I would suggest that your idea is a very good one. If there is a profound effect on the liver it could be influencing the fate of other carcinogens and their effect on other organs.

DR. KENSLER: A recent doctoral study at M.I.T. demonstrated an excellent correlation, in fact, unbelievably good, for a whole series of hepatic carcinogens and their effects, irreversibly. At least, within the duration of the experiment, there were decreased corticoid receptors in the liver. I don't know how this will tie in, but the chemical carcinogens in a series tied into a corticoid receptor, suggest that something should be looked at in that area, and hopefully some people will.

Dr. Clayson, if I understood you this morning, you indicated that the use of immunosuppressives led to a very rapid appearance of human neoplasms, brain tumors, and so on, and I'm wondering if there is a population of people who are immunosuppressed who might be getting drugs, or do you have records of other exposures that would be worth looking at from the epidemiologic point of view in the hope that the time factor might be reduced?

DR. CLAYSON: I think, Dr. Kensler, that we are. In our animal studies we have great difficulty in knowing exactly what immunosuppression does. In the case of reticulum cell sarcomas, which I referred to this morning, we know nothing about the etiology, whether chemically-induced, or even whether they might be virally-induced. You've probably heard me talk about one tumor having a possible viral etiology, but the amount of work that is done on that one tumor, I think, has precluded going on and looking at a reasonable number. So the answer, to my mind, is at the moment, we don't know.

DR. KOLBYE: I'd like to inquire as to whether or not there's been any systematic investigation of the metabolism of estrogens and progestins, detoxification if you will, in relation to some of the known enzyme inducers or inhibitors to which many of the population are inadvertently exposed, sometimes in massive quantities. I'm thinking that Dr. Selikoff, I'm sure, will appreciate, for example, that in Michigan some people have had rather massive exposures to polybrominated biphenyls which are very active inducers, and I am aware that some of the antioxidants that are used in the food supply will have somewhat of an influence. But the real question that I think is highly relevant in relation to some of the earlier presentations is whether or not there are some critical interactions taking place that we should be aware of.

DR. SHELLENBERGER: In specific answer to the question: I don't think there's a lot of work being done on the metabolism of estrogens following hepatic stimulation. There is a little work going on but I don't think a heck of a lot at this point. On the other hand, there isn't a lot known about the metabolism of the estrogens. But I think it will come in the next few years.

DR. MAYS: In regard to Dr. Shubik's question about the different responses: It's been our impression that we can observe at least three responses of the liver to the oral contraceptives. We talked about only one of them this morning. We have a small group of patients, two or three, that were not included in our data to date in which rather than form nodules or tumors there is a diffuse portal fibrosis that occurs in the liver. Now these women seem to react to the oral contraceptives quite differently from the ones I talked about this morning in that the tumor-forming group of patients have normal liver function. In fact, the usual thing used to detect hepatocellular carcinoma is the absence of the α-fetoprotein, and the CEA are absent in these females.

But the second group of patient that we did, we do not include in this, because we don't know what to do with them yet. They simply have a diffused portal fibrosis, very much like nutritional cirrhosis or the early stages of the vinyl chloride liver. These females seem to act in a different way and they do have abnormal liver function tests. One 19-year-old woman noticed that each time she started the oral contraceptives, she turned yellow. She got married, went on her honeymoon to Florida, took the oral contraceptives, and had to go into Jacksonville Hospital because of jaundice. She stopped the oral contraceptives, and the jaundice subsided. She returned to Kentucky, decided to go back on the oral contraceptives, and again the jaundice came back and liver function studies were abnormal. So in this group of patients the liver function studies can be used to detect damage to the liver and it seems to be quite different from those patients who grow tumors.

Then there's a third group of patients which has a measurable inability to excrete bromsulfalein. And this is estimated by some authorities to be about 40% of the women taking the pill, who have these measurable deficiencies to excrete bromsulfalein. These are the patients who just have the jaundice associated with the pill intake. But I think we're seeing three different responses here rather than one single response.

DR. COULSTON: Thank you, Dr. Mays. The afternoon is wearing on rapidly, and I think we'll entertain one more question or comment at this point.

DR. HAMMOND: Dr. Shubik raised a question which I think is at the very heart of this meeting concerning human versus animal experiments. You mentioned specifically estrogen versus exposure to something else, in a test system. Now, it would seem to me that applies very much more broadly than just to that one exposure. To name others, smoking or asbestos inhalation, shouldn't you then have smoking in your experimental setup? I think what it really says is that you're asking the question in your animal experiment or in your epidemiological experiment, all other things being equal, does this affect the incidence of cancer? What are "all other things?" And if "all other things" that human beings are subjected to are missing from animal experiments, or vice versa, your correlation is not going to be very good.

What worries me about this, and I'll be as brief as I can, is not that we will overestimate and call too many things carcinogenic because of this in omitting them from the animal study; it's the other way around, which I think you've implied. We might miss some very potent carcinogenic agents for human beings, because the experimental animal didn't have that other factor to bring it out.

Now if we try to overcome this by, in each instance, testing our animals under this condition, that condition, and that other condition (high fat, low fat in the diet, you name it, those 100 substances which can be tested in a year in animal experiments), an estimate made yesterday, is going to be reduced to maybe five or ten, and this is a dilemma.

DR. COULSTON: Thank you, ladies and gentlemen, for a very stimulating discussion.

DR. SHUBIK: Good morning. I'm sorry, I forgot I was the chairman. I was waiting for somebody to do something. But that's just because I have so many interesting thoughts going round and round inside my head as a result of this meeting and all to do with cancer, because we haven't been allowed to think about anything else, actually.

This morning's program is going to start with Dr. Wynder talking about carcinogens or modifying factors as a key to cancer in man. I think that it's really a fine thing that we have Dr. Wynder starting off today, because he among all people in this business has really been a model of someone getting together epidemiology and chemical carcinogenesis. In the beginning of his career he started with the initial observations on cigarette smoking and cancer. I remember well meeting Dr. Wynder when he was beginning his mouse skin painting studies and recall his going straight to the laboratory to try and correlate the things that he had at that time.

He will keep this meeting really on track for sure. I hope that by the end of today we will really have gotten some positive and clear-cut ideas formulated and really can put together at least a few projects of the sort that we were aiming at, at the beginning of the meeting, where we will really get down to correlating animal and epidemiological studies. We hope that the epidemiologists will think of things that they might be doing that they wouldn't have thought of before we came here. Maybe the people working in the laboratory will equally react to some of the ideas that come from the epidemiologists. I have a few on my mind already, and I would be most surprised if anyone in this room had not learned something at this stage of this meeting. Dr. Wynder, would you like to carry on?

15. Approaches to Environmental Carcinogenesis

Ernst L. Wynder
The Division of Epidemiology
The Naylor Dana Institute for Disease Prevention
American Health Foundation, New York

Before discussing some specifics of environmental carcinogenesis, I would like to make a few general statements relative to cancer prevention.

First, cancer is not an inevitable consequence of living or of aging. Second, history has shown that diseases have never been eliminated through therapy alone; they have been eradicated through preventive measures and natural occurrences. Third, one does not need to know the precise mechanism of a disease in order to prevent it. And fourth, the most common causative factors affecting the greatest number of cancers are the ones which should receive our greatest attention, and not those that are exceedingly rare and affect a very small segment of our population. In environmental carcinogenesis we have too often stressed the uncommon occurrence and forgotten the commonplace.

With this as background, let me review briefly some of the major points in environmental carcinogenesis and present three examples of the interrelationship between epidemiology, laboratory experimentation, and public health.

As is well known, lung cancer continues to be the leading cause of cancer death in men (Fig. 1), a cause that has been well established. On the other hand, cancer of the stomach has significantly declined in the U.S., although the reason for this decline is not precisely understood. Naturally, we would all rather see a disease decline without knowing the mechanism than see a disease increase while being aware of the cause.

This work was supported in part by National Cancer Institute grant Nos. CA-17613, CA-12376, CA-17867, contracts NO1-CP-33208 and ECI-SHP-74-106 (under Prime Contract NOI-CP-55666), and in part by American Cancer Society grant Nos. R-88R and BC-56U.

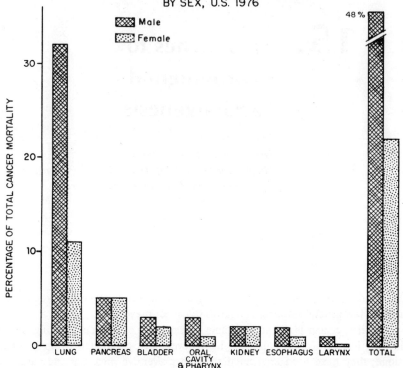

ESTIMATED TOBACCO-RELATED CANCER DEATHS
BY SEX, U.S. 1976

(SOURCE: ACS, FACTS & FIGURES, 1976)

FIGURE 1

Among the environmental factors that are associated with the development of cancer, tobacco stands out as accounting for about one-third of all male cancer deaths in this country. Occupational exposures are indeed an important factor as Dr. Selikoff has indicated, but there exists a strong association between smoking and various job categories, an interrelationship which must be recognized and controlled before attributing causation.

Diet is another major factor in the development of cancer. It is not as obvious as tobacco, but I hope to show you some convincing evidence of its important role.

Methods used to uncover the relationships between various exogenous factors and the development of cancer include (a) comparison of the incidence of disease in various countries with dietary practices, smoking, and drinking habits; (b) intracountry analyses to show differences in relation to geographic, socioeconomic gradients, sex, and religion; and (c) time trends and migrant studies. These techniques have permitted the conclusion that most cancers do

286

not have a genetic basis, but rather relate more to environmental influences. All of these techniques have been used by the American Health Foundation and independently by Sir Richard Doll to conclude that some 90% of all cancers are related to environmental factors, principally, factors that are part of our personal life-style: smoking, eating, and drinking.

TOBACCO AND CANCER

Now let me give you some specific examples, starting with tobacco. Over a quarter of a century ago, smoking was found to be an important etiologic factor in the development of cancer of the lung. When these data were presented to Dr. Graham, he said, "You know, now that we have found the truth, we have taken the first step." Little did I recognize then that 27 years later lung cancer would still be the leading cause of cancer deaths in most Western countries. It is a key disappointment to me to know, that in 1976-77, retrospective and several prospective studies have and continue to show the same relative risk for tobacco-related cancers (Fig. 2). Clearly, there is no question and no real need to study and demonstrate further that cigarette smoking is a major cause of cancer in man.

The question remains: What are we going to do about it? We know that successful smoking cessation results in decreased risk for tobacco-related diseases. Further, we know this decrease is related to dose as well as age. We have shown that the older you are, the longer it takes to reduce the risk to that of someone who never smoked (Fig. 3). The positive effect of smoking cessation is seen more quickly for coronary disease.

Three public health approaches may be taken with regard to tobacco use. The first is development of the less harmful cigarette or the managerial approach to preventive medicine. This approach changes the product at its source by reducing the tar levels as well as the makeup of cigarettes. Some may ask why so much time is spent by researchers on less harmful cigarettes, since that ought to be the job of the tobacco industry. The tobacco industry is not necessarily an expert in carcinogenesis and epidemiology, however, and the development of such cigarettes should continue to be the activity of nonindustry scientists.

For the past 20 years, Hoffmann and I have investigated the chemical and biological activity of tobacco and tobacco smoke. Hoffmann has identified initiators, promoters, and accelerators, and at present we have a good idea as to how tobacco carcinogenesis works on mouse skin and the larynx of the hamster.

The tar content of filter cigarettes and even of nonfilter cigarettes has decreased over the past years (Fig. 4). In the 1950s the average cigarette had 40 mg of tar. Today the average is 17 mg. Furthermore, on a gram-to-gram level, cigarettes of today are less carcinogenic than they were 20 years ago. Most probably, within 10 years the average tar level will be about 10 mg or less with a nicotine content of about 0.6 mg. Whether there will ever be a practical threshold at

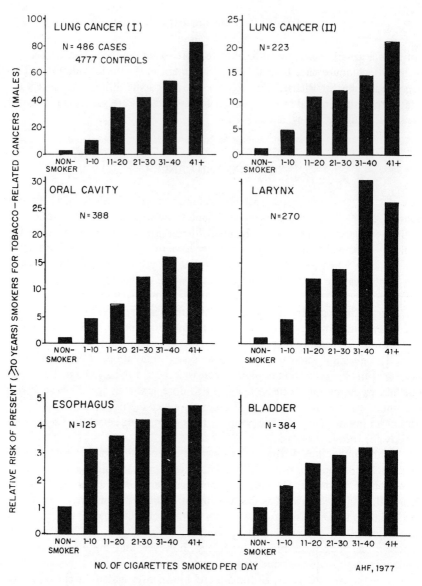

FIGURE 2

which moderate smoking would not lead to an increased risk is, of course, a question that remains to be answered.

How does this reflect in epidemiologic studies? We are currently monitoring the epidemiology of the less harmful cigarette and have found that filter cigarettes *do* have a lower risk than nonfilter cigarettes (Fig. 5). In the latest sample of more than 1,000 larynx and lung cancer cases we are showing a reduction in risk for lung and larynx cancer of about 25-30%. These data are similar to those found by Hammond in his prospective studies.

288

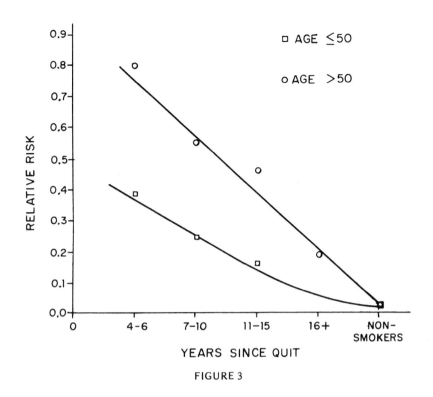

FIGURE 3

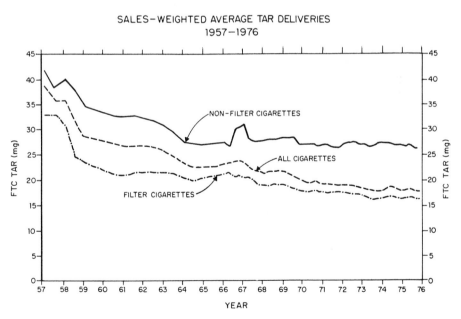

FIGURE 4

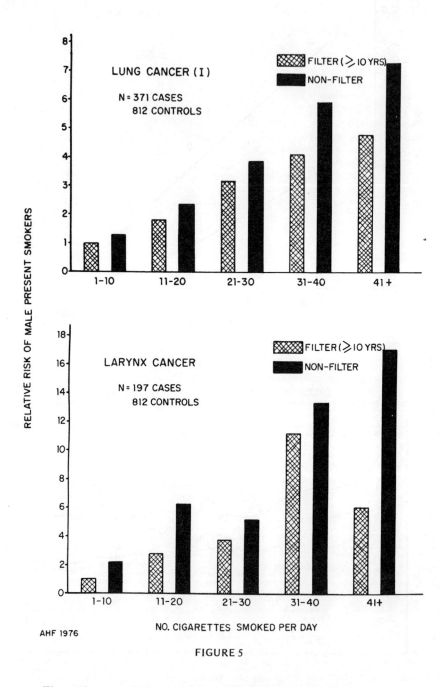

FIGURE 5

We need to recall that smokers with these cancers began their smoking habit with the old high tar, high carcinogenic cigarette. Thus, we cannot yet measure the risk associated with lifetime smoking of only low tar cigarettes.

290

DISTRIBUTION OF SMOKING HABITS OF MALE CONTROLS

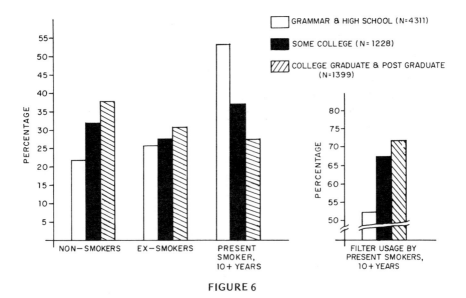

FIGURE 6

As is generally known, cigarette smoking habits are dependent on education and socioeconomic level (Fig. 6). Males seem to be especially affected by
the education factor in that well-educated males are more likely to be non- or
ex-smokers, or smokers of low tar cigarettes, than other groups. A similar trend
is occurring for women, although the differences are not so great. It is somewhat
reassuring to note that this shift in smoking habits is already being reflected in
lower rates of lung cancer among males. Twenty years from now, lung cancer
will appear even less often in the educated white-male group. This is similar to
what Doll has already shown for British physicians, whose lung cancer rate has
significantly declined during the period when lung cancer in the rest of the
British population has increased.

A second public health approach should concentrate on health education,
especially among our youth. So far we have done very little for our children. If
we say to children, "don't smoke," they tend not to listen because they do not
fully understand the consequences of the habit and they do not have the same
concept of age that we do. The American Health Foundation, therefore, has
developed a program called "Know Your Body," whose purpose is to make children aware of their bodies and how various factors affect them.

In this program we have screened over 3,000 children ages 10-14 and have
introduced the concept of risk factor identification. We have found that 40%
have at least one risk factor for coronary disease (Fig. 7), and that 12% of them
smoke cigarettes on a regular basis.

291

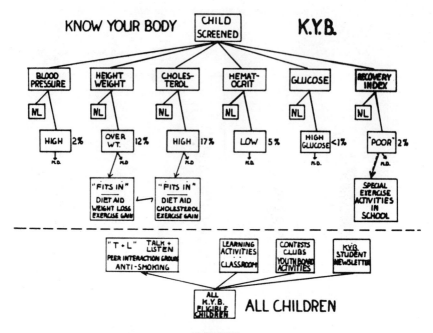

FIGURE 7

We are trying to affect adolescent behavior not by didatic teaching alone, but also by actually making children aware of, and responsible for, their own health. We go to the schools, take blood pressures and small samples of blood to determine cholesterol levels, as well as record smoking and exercise histories. We present these data in the form of a health passport and explain the meanings of the results to each child and parent. At the end of the first year of our study, these children are actively participating in groups to discuss risk factors and what can be done about them. We feel that this type of peer group involvement is essential if we are to make progress in our efforts to limit or curtail the early development of harmful habits.

We are trying out a similar program with adults and have included smoking cessation clinics as part of the preventive health package.

This interest in the more effective development and widespread use of smoking cessation programs is the third public health approach to tobacco usage. "Stop Smoking" clinics have proved to be cost-effective in many cases; but even so, very few physicians or hospitals are interested in smoking cessation efforts. We, as physicians, take great pride in trying to treat lung cancer patients, where our success has not been particularly encouraging, but when it comes to smoking cessation, we appear not to be interested. In a recent sample of one-year smoking cessation efforts, 44% of the participants had stopped smoking for an entire year. The success rate of such clinics is accomplished mainly, with the help of allied health professionals.

GENERAL PROBLEM AREAS

There are several problems related to preventive medicine. The first is public apathy. All of us think, "It cannot happen to us," in line with our "illusion of immortality." Second, there is the general physician disinterest. There is the fact that third party payments won't cover preventive programs. Hospital administrators say they cannot afford smoking cessation programs because Blue Cross won't pay for them.

Since the health insurance industry works on a cost plus principle, it is not in their interest for us to reduce disease. In public they may say, "Yes, we ought to reduce disease," but they don't put any major push behind that statement.

ALCOHOL CARCINOGENESIS

Alcohol abuse and the health consequences thereof are other areas where prevention is necessary. Alcohol has been shown to be a major promoter of cancer of the upper alimentary tract. This fact is borne out by a study we conducted at Memorial Hospital where 30-40% of the patients with head and neck cancer were found to be alcoholics.

Of particular interest is the mechanism of alcohol carcinogenesis. At the American Health Foundation, McCoy has recently isolated functional mitochrondria from the squamous epithelium of the cheek pouch of hamsters. We are proposing that one of the ways in which alcohol acts as a tumor promoter is via its effect on mitochondrial functions. A common denominator between alcoholism and Plummer-Vinson's Disease—riboflavin on the one hand, and iron on the other—is that each affects the respiratory enzyme system. Damage to this system may well initiate a cancer formation of the upper alimentary tract.

NUTRITIONAL CARCINOGENESIS

The last example relates to nutrition. As mentioned earlier, the relationship between nutrition and cancer etiology is not as obvious as that for tobacco and cancer, but increasing experimental evidence is strengthening the association.

Since what we eat affects every cell in our bodies, it seems feasible that a particular deficiency or an excess in nutrients could be injurious. In fact, in the 1950s Tannenbaum reported the results of his classical animal research in which he found that caloric and fat differences produced large scale differences in tumor yields.

Although food additives and food contaminants have been cited as being associated with various cancers, I would like to concentrate on one area in which I am the most interested: nutritional excesses.

Although we know that correlation does not necessarily mean causation, an important and significant correlation exists between fat consumption and cancer of the colon (Fig. 8). Of course, a correlation, in addition to being significant, must have a logical basis; and one need not be a brilliant scientist to suspect that what is eaten affects the stool. Since the stool is in contact with the colonic mucosa, it could thereby affect the mucosa.

Of particular interest are the differences between the U.S. and Japan with regard to colon cancer (Fig. 9). Among Japanese migrants to Hawaii and the continental U.S., colon cancer incidence increases. Migrant data give particular credence to the nutrition and cancer hypotheses.

One problem we have had with dietary studies, especially with retrospective studies, is getting meaningful dietary histories. Young at Cornell has shown that there is a 25% quantitative error in one's response to the question, "What did you eat yesterday?" Imagine the error when answering what one ate 30 years ago! Even the most sophisticated statistical manipulation will not make unreliable data any better or meaningful; and thus, we are faced with a very difficult situation in reference to dietary analyses.

LARGE BOWEL CANCER MORTALITY (1966-67) AND DIETARY FAT & OIL CONSUMPTION (1964-66)

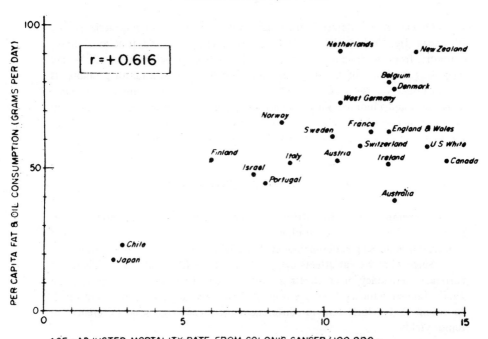

(FROM SEGI M., AND KURIHARA, M. 1972 AND F.A.O. 1970.)

FIGURE 8

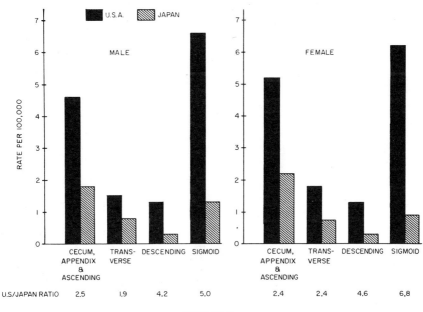

COLON CANCER MORTALITY BY SITE IN U.S.A. AND JAPAN
AGE 35-84, 1968

| U.S./JAPAN RATIO | 2.5 | 1.9 | 4.2 | 5.0 | 2.4 | 2.4 | 4.6 | 6.8 |

FIGURE 9

But Japan is an easier country to look at with regard to dietary habits, since their traditional diet has remained fairly stable for many years. Our study in Japan showed that patients with colon cancer ate a more Westernized diet, i.e., they had a higher intake of fat than did other Japanese.

An important area of epidemiology is metabolic epidemiology, which is especially useful when studying colon cancer etiology. Figures 10 and 11 show that groups with a high rate of colon cancer, such as Americans, excrete a significantly higher amount of neutral steroids and bile acids than groups with a low rate of colon cancer. In addition, patients with colon cancer have a higher output of neutral steroids and bile acids than do controls (Figs. 12 & 13). Certain fecal enzymes are also significantly higher in colon cancer patients than controls. In a number of other studies we have found that patients with familial polyposis, who are also at high risk for colon cancer, had a higher output of neutral steroids than controls but no difference in bile acids. Additionally, patients with ulcerative colitis, also known to have a high risk for colon cancer, excreted more neutral steroids and bile acids than controls.

Based on these studies, our current concept is that neutral steroids contain some type of carcinogens and that bile acids act as tumor promoters. In experimental studies we found that if rats are injected with MNNG and then painted with cholic and deoxycholic acid the tumor yield is increased (Fig. 14).

295

DAILY FECAL NEUTRAL STEROL EXCRETION OF VARIOUS POPULATION GROUPS

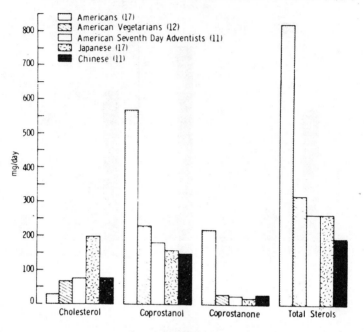

FIGURE 10

DAILY FECAL BILE ACID EXCRETION OF VARIOUS POPULATION GROUPS

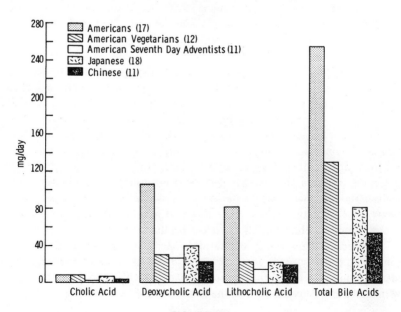

FIGURE 11

FECAL NEUTRAL STEROLS IN PATIENTS WITH COLON CANCER AND PATIENTS
AT HIGH RISK

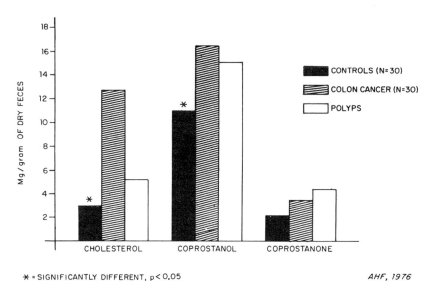

* = SIGNIFICANTLY DIFFERENT, p< 0.05   *AHF, 1976*

FIGURE 12

FECAL BILE ACIDS IN PATIENTS WITH COLON CANCER AND PATIENTS AT A HIGH RISK

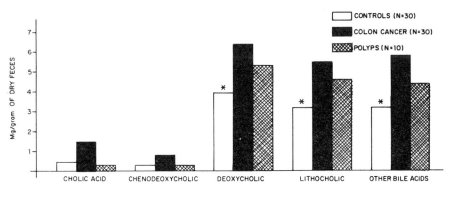

* = SIGNIFICANTLY DIFFERENT, p<0.05   *AHF, 1976*

FIGURE 13

Reddy has found cholestene triol, a derivative of cholesterol epoxide, in the stool. Whether this finding is significant is not yet known. Smith has proposed that oxidation products of cholesterol could be a factor. Wolf has suggested that reactive metabolites in cholesterol could play a role, and recently

297

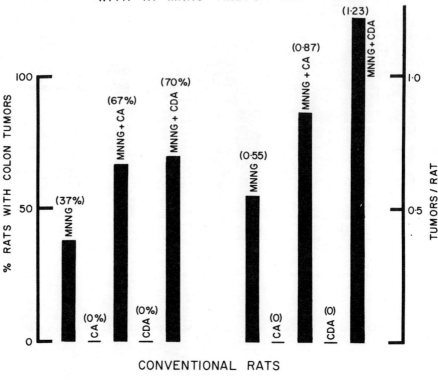

COLON TUMOR INCIDENCE IN CONVENTIONAL RATS TREATED WITH IR MNNG AND/OR BILE ACIDS

FIGURE 14

Bruce, in studying mutagenicity in stool, suggested that nitrosamines may be involved. Whatever the factor(s), dietary modification would be an important managerial preventive step.

One interesting feature in epidemiology are areas known as "outliers." For example, despite a high intake of meat, colon cancer rates are expected to be low in Utah. Another outlier is Finland, which has a high rate of coronary heart disease, a high fat intake, and yet, a low rate of colon cancer. Interestingly, the rate of breast cancer is also low in Finland. Most of the fat in the Finnish diet comes from dairy products—milk and butter—while the intake of meat is low.

This either means that meat has a carcinogenic effect or that dairy products are, in some way, protective. Both of these possibilities are being pursued.

Cancer of the breast has also been shown to have a positive correlation with fat intake. Differences in breast cancer rates between the U.S. and Japan are especially great in postmenopausal women (Fig. 15). In Japan, it is not only breast, but ovarian, endometrial, and prostatic cancer that have lower rates than

298

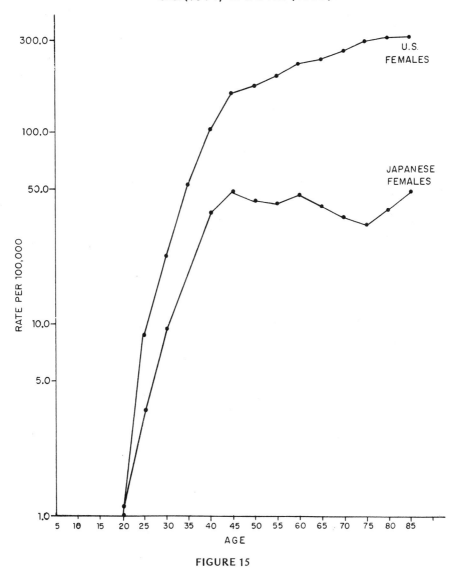

AGE-SPECIFIC INCIDENCE RATES FOR FEMALE BREAST CANCER,
U.S. (1971) & JAPAN (1973)

FIGURE 15

those in the U.S. These cancers all evidence an increase in rates when Japanese migrate to the U.S.

In a study of 785 breast cancer patients, we divided cases into pre-, peri-, and postmenopausal women to show a clear separation between pre- and post-

299

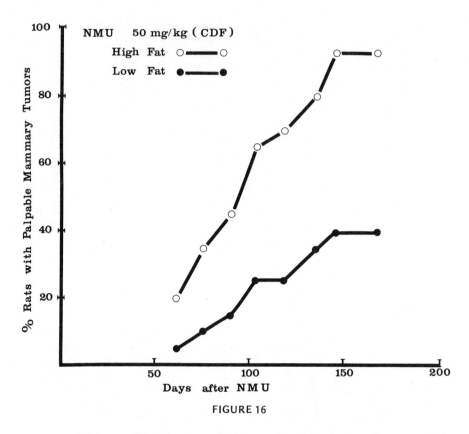

FIGURE 16

menopausal states. We found no difference for age or menarche, parity, or nursing; a moderate increase in risk for late age of first pregnancy was found for the pre- and perimenopausal group. In contrast to DeWaard, we found no significant differences between cases and controls for weight and height.

Our conclusions were that none of the variables studied could explain the great difference in cancer rates between American and Japanese women. We have suggested that environmental factor(s) contribute to the rate of disease. One of these factors could be fat intake. Animals given high and low fat diets were found to have different mammary tumor yields (Fig. 16). Moreover, there appears to be a correlation between high fat diets and prolactin levels, such that the prolactin/estrogen ratio is increased with increasing fat intake.

We studied the prolactin production of 4 female volunteers both before and after going on a vegetarian, low fat diet. After four weeks on that diet, their prolactin levels were significantly reduced (Fig. 17).

We have also been looking at cholesterol and hormone levels in breast fluid. Such studies could provide important leads because breast cancer is of ductal origin. In 10 women who could secrete an analyzable amount of fluid,

300

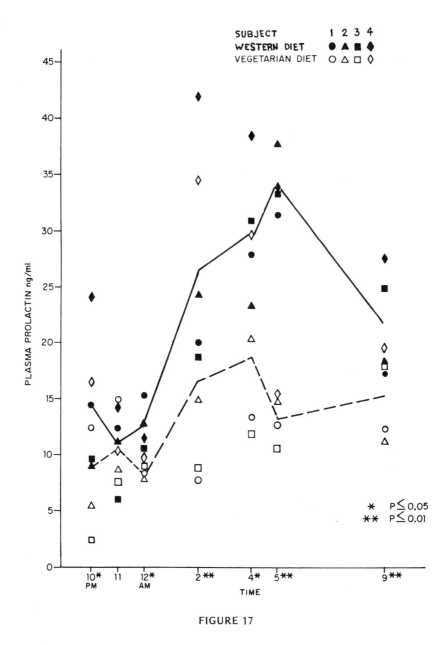

FIGURE 17

we found higher prolactin, estrogen, and triglyceride levels in fluid than in serum, although cholesterol levels were approximately the same as serum levels.

Since 1910, total fat intake in the U.S. has increased, while carbohydrate intake has decreased (Fig. 18). In the beginning of the century 32% of our

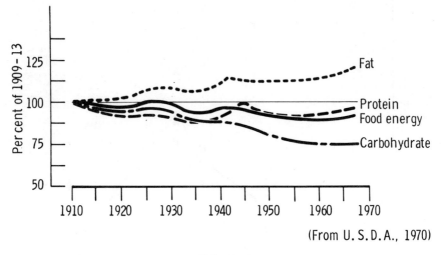

PER CAPITA CONSUMPTION OF ENERGY FOODS:
PROTEIN, FAT, AND CARBOHYDRATES (UNITED STATES, 1910-1970)

(From U.S.D.A., 1970)

FIGURE 18

calories came from fat and now over 40% are derived from fat. Judging from our disease rates, it appears that we do not have the metabolic capacity to deal with this amount or type of food.

Most of our fat intake as children comes from milk; as adults 40% of it comes from meat (Fig. 19). Studies have indicated that as early as one year of age, our children have elevated cholesterol levels. This astonishing fact must in part be related to large consumption of whole milk by our children.

Furthermore, the beef we eat today is quite different from that of 30 or 40 years ago. Today, most of our cattle are corn-fed, as opposed to grass-fed. Grass-fed cattle have 23% fat, while corn-fed have up to 50%. In addition, the fat content of beef is affected by its preparation. That is, fat is reduced as meat is cooked more thoroughly.

Figure 20 shows the type of prudent diet suggested by those in the field of coronary heart disease, suggesting that we should have a reduction in calories, in fat, and in cholesterol. Connor and Connor suggest a diet that is not more than 20% fat, with not more than 100 mg cholesterol.

In order to unravel the complicated interrelationships of various environmental factors, we should establish centers of environmental carcinogenesis (Fig. 21). In these centers epidemiologists, toxicologists, chemists, pathologists, biologists, and allied health professionals can work together to integrate their knowledge and experience.

FAT FROM FOOD EATEN IN ONE DAY
CONTRIBUTION OF FOOD GROUPS

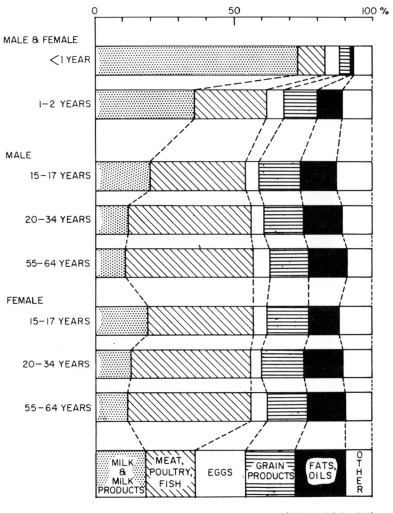

(FROM U.S.D.A., 1969)

FIGURE 19

303

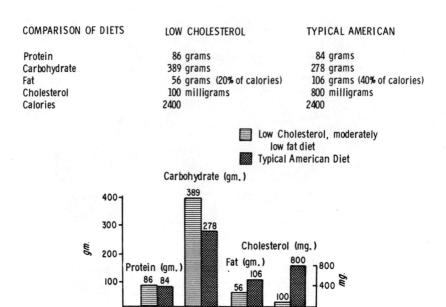

COMPARISON OF DIETS	LOW CHOLESTEROL	TYPICAL AMERICAN
Protein	86 grams	84 grams
Carbohydrate	389 grams	278 grams
Fat	56 grams (20% of calories)	106 grams (40% of calories)
Cholesterol	100 milligrams	800 milligrams
Calories	2400	2400

The composition of the low cholesterol, moderately low fat diet as compared to the composition of the American diet.

FIGURE 20

INTERDISCIPLINARY APPROACH TO CANCER PREVENTION

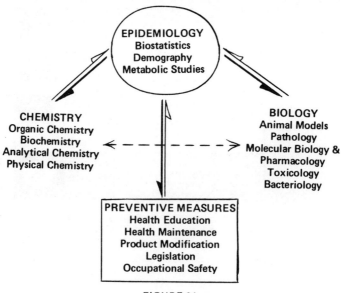

FIGURE 21

SUMMARY

In summary, I would like to end with these five suggestions:

1. We need to establish interdisciplinary centers for cancer prevention.
2. Specific funds should be earmarked for such centers by the National Cancer Program.
3. The activity of these centers should be integrated with centers for other disease entities, since many environmental factors affect more than one disease.
4. Priorities should be set for preventive activities by:
   a. considering the present mortality rates of various cancers;
   b. considering already identified causative factors;
   c. concentrating on studies based on greatest epidemiological and experimental leads; and
   d. providing a proper balance between fundamental and applied research.
5. Information and guidelines should be provided to the scientific community, to the public and mass media, to the executive branch and to Congress, to regulatory agencies, and to industry for their appropriate action.

If we are so organized, we can reach a day when what we know to be avoidable cancers and other diseases will no longer plague our society.

Discussion

DR. SHUBIK: Thank you, Ernst. I think that we will break with the tradition that has been established at this meeting in the last day or two, and take three or four questions. Dr. Kraybill.

DR. KRAYBILL: I think this is a very complex area, one I'm interested in, of course. In making some of these associations, you talk a lot about fat. I've had a strong feeling, of course, that fat is a reservoir and you have a lot of gunk in that fat. I think a good study would be to find out if the fat source is free of many of these contaminants versus fat that has all the contaminants, because this may influence your association.

The other thing is we've laid a lot of faults to the fat component of the diet, particularly in years past, on cholesterol, and now in many surveys we show that the carbohydrates play a role, particularly absorbable sugars and those that are highly sensitive.

You also had some data showing a decrease in carbohydrates. I wonder what the USDA data is implying here when you talk about carbohydrates and starches and things of that sort, because while the amounts of complex starches may have gone down (spaghettis, macaronies, and stuff like that), the absorbable sugar content has gone up. In the day of George Washington our daily intake of sucrose was about 15 g. per capita and now it's up to about 120 g., and some people take in 200-300 g. of absorbable sugar. So I think you can get some associations here, but one must delineate the role of some of these variants and what role they do play.

DR. WYNDER: Obviously, if we eat more of one food, we eat less of another. I think as far as carbohydrate is concerned, this principally reflects a reduction in the consumption of potatoes in this country; your point on fat, of course, is well taken. I regard and I define, for instance, fat as a modifying factor. Now you recall that I said that from the point of view of public health if we reduce a modifying factor and thereby reduce a disease, we are satisfied. We've got to find what the mechanism is. There are so many things fat can do. It can be a reservoir of hormones, as we know in obesity; I didn't mention it but obesity is clearly related to only two types of cancers, endometrial and female kidney, perhaps because it can be a reservoir for hormones. Then, of course, there are different kinds of fat—saturated and unsaturated—which our animal studies have shown both to have the same effect.

I've indicated that fats seemingly in animal experiments affect prolactin production. Fats certainly also affect the constituency and the makeup of cell membranes. And in this regard a point is, what is normal? I find this a very difficult area; next Friday I'm meeting with Dr. Rifkin from the National Heart and Lung Institute because we are convening a meeting to define normal serum cholesterol levels for the American people. The problem has been that we confuse "average" with "normal." The average physician who sees a patient with 220 or 240 mg says that's normal. Well, it is normal—it is less than 280; but clearly, as the Framingham study shows, it increases your risk for coronary disease. So my view of normalcy for cholesterol levels is between 100 and 140 mg %, and that becomes almost shocking. The reason I say it is normal is because, at that level, coronary death rates are very, very low. And it's very interesting, if you look at primitive populations, they as well as we are born with serum

306

cholesterol levels of 100, or blood pressures of 100/60. In primitive populations the blood pressure stays that way throughout life while in us it rises.

So the key point of debate is: What is normal for man? It is my considered view that the food that we take in today is abnormal in terms of fat, cholesterol, and total calories and sugars and other things. And the reason we don't quite see it is is that we are all part of the normal values.

DR. CONNEY: Dr. Wynder, in your human studies, on the relationship between fat and human cancers, isn't it true very often that whenever you have high fat you also have high protein? It's difficult to differentiate between changes of fat and changes of protein. I was wondering whether you might like to comment on the possibility that changes in protein may account for what you're seeing in humans.

DR. WYNDER: It is, of course, true that in human studies protein and fat go together, and you know Armstrong and Doll have done a study where they show a correlation between different food categories and cancer rates. There, the correlation is greater for fat than for protein, but obviously you can do this in animals. In animals we have shown that the breast cancer model responds specifically to fats, because we have kept protein constant, so in that model you can certainly do it. We are currently looking at these very interesting outliers, like Finland, where it would appear that the type of fat certainly is important. But in the animal model, clearly, we can demonstrate its effect rather than that of the protein.

DR. CLAYSON: I've been perhaps a little bit amazed at the way the fashion, particularly in the question of colon cancer, has changed over the past few years. It seems to me that Burkitt very recently was suggesting that fiber was important; it seems now we're into the fat phase. I think excessive eating in general might even be correlated, coming back to the Armstrong-Doll correlation studies, although fat came high up on the list. I think animal protein was high on the list, sugar was high on the list, positive correlations on a sort of an international basis and gross national product were high on the list. I would agree with you there is some factor here, but I think in view of these fairly wishy-washy sort of leads which we've got at the moment, we've got to look very, very carefully indeed at any animal experiments which may appear to confirm one factor or another.

I was unhappy—I know you haven't time to go into this in detail, Dr. Wynder—with the animal experiments in which you gave a carcinogen. You obtained rat mammary tumors for example, and you showed that a high fat and a low fat caused tumors. The one thing which came out clearly in Tannenbaum's work (admittedly in the mouse rather than the rat), was that the mammary tumor incidence was terribly sensitive to changes in body weight. One would like to know for example, whether your high-fat and low-fat diets, when given with various caloric levels, produced the same body weight? Were the pharmacokinetics, the pharmacodynamics of the agent which you gave the same, when you gave a high fat or a low fat diet? Or did you separate the time of administration of the carcinogen from the time of administration of the different diets, and so on? I think we've got to look at this experiment in terribly great detail before we really are sure that it is confirming what you want it to confirm.

DR. WYNDER: Well, first of all, may I say I never want an experiment to confirm what I want it to confirm. I want an experiment to be scientifically accurate and to affect what nature wants to tell us. You were perfectly correct that I did not have time to give you all the details, but we have published this. David (Clayson) is a very avid reader and I'm always amazed at how he understands and reads the literature. Well, you obviously missed our studies. After all, the one thing you must have learned from me over 25 years is that it's obvious I look at weight, and that this difference between high and low fat cannot be explained by weight. In fact, we have paid considerable attention to caloric intake and therefore, as you recall, I emphasized that in the human population, we specifically did not find a relation of weight to cancer of the breast. We had a lot of controversy on that with my friend DeWaard, who initially made a big to-do about weight and then height, and now he isn't quite sure. But in American data, we show nothing.

Second, you mentioned another one of our good friends, Denis Burkitt. Now Denis isn't here so he really cannot defend himself, but I have had a number of debates with him: in fact, in the *Journal of the National Cancer Institute* (Vol. 54, no. 1, 1975), they had two guest editorials, one by Burkitt on fiber and one by myself and Reddy on fat content.

Well, first of all, there is no worldwide correlation to fiber, as we have shown for fat. And second, it has been shown, let's say for coronary disease, that giving fiber does not reduce the risk of coronary disease, at least as shown by Connor.

It's again obvious that if you have a tremendous amount of fiber intake, you've got to take less fat. If you go to Africa, sure you've got a high amount of fiber intake, but their total fat intake is very low. This is not an area in which obviously you are familiar as with some of the others, but the fiber area has received a considerable industrial attention in this country, because there are many products relating to fiber that some manufacturer wants to sell. Consequently, the newspapers are full of reports of people who work in the area of fibers and are well supported by various industrial groups. If you are an avid reader of the *New York Times* and the *Ladies Home Journal* you really think that fibers are the "in" things. In my office I get mail from all kinds of people who say you've got to put your patients on fiber. It's quite a different thing with fat.

I can tell you there's a tremendous fat lobby in this country. I'm reminded that when we first started with smoking, everybody in the tobacco industry said smoke is nothing, it's fat and cholesterol, but not smoking. Recently I got a pamphlet from the American Meat Industry which said, "Look, it is certainly tobacco, and all this other stuff, but it is certainly not meat." So there's a tremendous lobby in this area which certainly wouldn't influence you, David, but would influence the general public.

I recognize this is a difficult area. The reason I'm mentioning it to you, and as our friend Higginson once said to me, "I really don't see diet as Wynder presents it," but I recall he said in a speech he gave in Lyon, that once before, in 1949 and 1950, Wynder was one of the few people in the world who talked about smoking and lung cancer, and nobody would believe him then. And I think perhaps lightning can strike twice in science.

I've given the nutritional concept of carcinogenesis a great deal of attention related to animals epidemiologically and metabolically, and it's my view that in the next 10 years we will find that next to tobacco, nutritional deficiencies, but particularly nutritional excesses, will be generally recognized as a major modifying factor. And let me again mention the word modifying; I didn't say carcinogenic.

DR. SHUBIK: Thank you very much, Ernst. Fred, do you wish to discuss this now, because I'd rather like to go on with the fiber-fat story. You know we always have to give rebuttal time in this particular debate.

DR. COULSTON: I will not expect an answer now, but later, perhaps. Ernie, you have presented this fat story so well and I presume you mean animal fat, not fats in general. Then if you don't mean animal fat, my question is very pertinent. The trend in recent years has been away from saturated fats to unsaturated oils and semisolid fats, and this certainly must have changed the statistics if your premise is correct.

DR. WYNDER: I specifically said that atherosclerosis, coronary disease, etc., specifically relate to saturated fats and that unsaturated fats have some benefit. But animal studies and those of Carroll clearly show that in the animal system, the effect of unsaturated fat is just as great as the saturated.

MRS. MRAK: My only comment is, you have to have a total number of calories, so that if you increase the fat you decrease something else; if you decrease the fat, you increase something else. You may find that what you increase and decrease in the fat may present a problem, too.

DR. WYNDER: Sometimes people say to us, "Well, if your concept is correct and you reduce colon cancer, will you now increase stomach cancer?" We think between the decreases in the incidence of stomach cancer and the excesses, in my view, of colon cancer there is a whole middle way. The diet that we have presented when supplemented by vitamins and minerals, I think, is that middle way. I hope that during the discussion we will be able to go over some of these points in further detail. I enjoyed particularly a discussion with my friend, Phil Shubik, and may I say, having heard yesterday a discussion on phenobarbital and some other drugs that may or may not relate to human liver cancer, this element of nutrition in cancer obviously has much greater possibilities, and has far greater importance, because it affects so many more of our major cancers. Therefore, we need to concentrate on it because if I'm right, it is time that we undertake some action. After all, the major cancers involved are those of the breast and colon and prostrate and not just the liver. Therefore, I think it's very important that we here who are the experts, Philippe, agree on some course of action so that we can make the proper decision for the public to follow.

DR. SHUBIK: Well, I think we've achieved our major objective because I did hear Ernst say, "If I am right," and that leaves an opening for a series of people to do additional experiments. The chief objective here is to keep us all employed and to make sure we do interesting experiments so that we can come back to these nice places. Dr. Kolbye, I think, is getting a little worried. He must think I am trying to suppress his paper and keep him off the program: there is actually no truth in that, so he is, in fact, welcome to start speaking now.

16. Confusion About Carcinogens in Food

Albert C. Kolbye, Jr.
Associate Director for Sciences
Bureau of Foods
Food and Drug Administration

My discussion will not deal with the usual approach to carcinogens in the food supply, which usually involves a list of substances demonstrated or suspected to induce cancer in test mammals, and the regulatory actions taken by FDA and other agencies in the name of protecting the public against cancer. Instead, I should like to explore the topic in greater depth to see whether or not more acceptable alternatives exist to improve our societal efforts to reduce the risk of cancer in humans.

Despite our many efforts, we still have not attained a constructive momentum of scientific energy applied in directions likely to produce meaningful results, as far as improving the wisdom of our societal policies is concerned.

Any single test factor in a so-called controlled lifetime feeding experiment may, in fact, result in a statistically significant increase in the incidence of tumors in the test animals as compared to controls, provided a critical convergence of relevant factors occurs in such a way to permit the expression of increased tumors in these animals. What we observe is the association between the exposure and the result; all too frequently we leap across a gap in logic and infer causation, and thus immediately label a substance as a carcinogen. In fact, the substance may or may not be carcinogenic.

We have seen situations where certain chemicals have been shown to induce cancer in test animals first and later observed to be associated with occupational exposures and cancer in man, and vice versa. In such cases, it is reasonable to infer some correlation between substantial exposures to test mammals, or to workers, and the incidence of cancer. Certainly, we have observed many rather drastic regulatory responses occurring as a result of statistically significant increases of tumors in test mammals. Such responses are usually in the direction of curtailing all exposures to any amounts of the substance in question and are based on the contention that "there is no such thing as a safe exposure to a carcinogen."

Mathematicians, seeing most biologists abdicate their responsibiliities, and sensing an opportunity to apply their own brand of logic, have created various extrapolation models based on radiobiological mechanisms of carcinogenesis in the assumption that the same mechanisms operate at all dose levels and carcinogenesis is just dependent on simple mathematics referring to the probability of the occurrence of critical hits. Then, extrapolating beyond mathematical observations, they induce some biologists to support their position by saying that radiation-induced carcinogenesis is broadly applicable to chemical carcinogenesis, which again involves a leap over a large gap in logic. The next assumption is that the same mechanisms that operate at substantial doses systematically incurred over a lifetime by test mammals will always operate in humans receiving sporadic low-level exposures to the substances in question.

Others argue that while the mechanisms may not be the same, we are not sure they are different, and, in any event, we are exposed to so many carcinogens that we shouldn't tolerate any exposure we don't have to, especially since interactions may occur in synergistic ways. Next, some mutageneticists say that of all the carcinogens we have studied, 90% are positive in certain bacterial systems with or without enzyme induction, and therefore any mutagen should be a suspect carcinogen. Others point out that such results would automatically require long-term tests for cancer in mammals. But critics contend that the mammalian systems may not be sensitive enough to detect all carcinogens and therefore negative results would not be very meaningful.

The obvious result is almost total chaos; the less obvious result is tantamount to a progressive disorder of society which will result in virtual paralysis, unless greater wisdom is applied to the overall problem to achieve constructive progress. Such progress is not likely when decision makers are faced with overreactions by politicians and a public in the grip of exaggerated fears of chemical carcinogens.

I doubt that I can add much wisdom to this confusion, but I should like to suggest several approaches.

With regard to cancer induction in humans occurring from exposures to food, we have reason to suspect that the content and quality of the basic diet can be an important factor. The high content of animal fat in the human dietary has been epidemiologically implicated as a substantial risk factor, but even highly unsaturated vegetable fats have come under some scrutiny. Variations in the type and content of protein in the diet have been demonstrated to affect the incidence of tumors in test mammals. Questions have been raised as to whether or not the presence of chemical residues deposited in animal fat has contributed to differences in the incidence of cancer observed when populations from different countries or migrant populations are compared. Fiber content has also been implicated epidemiologically.

Some epidemiological studies comparing the incidence of cancer in humans involve techniques for adjusting for differences in the age distributions of the populations, but do not satisfactorily deal with comparisons of cancer death rates in the context of all causes of death among age-specific cohorts of the populations involved. Many other differences exist besides those invoking dietary considerations, such as competitive causes of mortality. Controlling for many of these variable differences has frequently not been accomplished, nor are control techniques likely to be substantially improved in the near future.

Since the FDA regulates many substances in the food supply, including GRAS substances, direct and indirect additives, and residues of animal drugs, many consumer advocates invoke these as causes of human cancer and feel that they have been proved right every time a substance shows up positive in an animal test system. What they overlook is that certain other countries who claim to permit fewer "additives" have little or no regulatory control over many substances added to food, and, in fact, have little information about which chemicals are present in food as direct or indirect additives. Much higher human exposures to many more compounds are likely to occur in these countries than in the United States.

Prevention of cancer involves both educational and regulatory approaches, but where should we direct our efforts? Should we regulate all carcinogens in like fashion? Are all inducers more or less equal, so that a simple yes-no Delaney approach should be taken in all instances? That is the track we're on now and the question becomes, where we are going in the next decade with respect to cancer research and regulation of carcinogens? It is my belief that we must concentrate greater efforts to classify—even tentatively—the various types of inducers of cancer. To achieve this, we should combine research on mechanisms, including those influences that decrease resistance, both in animals and in man. This may require redirection and recombination of our efforts in toxicology and epidemiology.

We have no accurate idea of the totality of direct-acting, promoting, or modifying factors that influence the expression of cancer in humans as far as the natural components of the basic diet are concerned. We do have some hints about where to begin, but we lack perspective.

Nor are we likely to gain any accurate impression of the baseline load if we take the same roads in research that have followed Sutton's Law (pursuing the research fads that have the greatest funding), because it is far from popular—politically speaking—to even hint that natural foods could influence the expression of cancer in humans. It is far more fashionable to distort Higginson's approach and accuse man-made chemicals of causing most cancers in humans, and thus to indict chemical contaminants and additives.

A coordinated international program is needed in which competent scientists are persuaded to step outside their purely academic concerns and deal with the reality of political life and to start educating decision makers in the public arena as to the facts about cancer as best we know them today. That approach frightens many scientists. Unfortunately, many scaremongers prey on fears for vested interests, which sometimes include research funding or political power.

I see no way that all or even many substances can be fully assessed for chronic toxicity including cancer, and I have limited enthusiasm for carcinogenic bioassays as many are presently conducted. If we spend the money to do lifetime rodent studies, we should include several dose levels, not just two, and we should learn as much as possible from them, provided that information is relevant to the real world. It is paradoxical that we penalize the safer compounds in the sense of acute toxicity by insisting always on a maximum tolerated dose approach, even if such exposures are so large that they stagger the imagination, but in this respect, science has defaulted by not creating more logical alternatives.

I think we distort the β error concept and neglect inferences concerning potency when we go to the extreme of saying that we are testing too few animals per dose in relation to particular anticipated human exposures, and therefore we should test at highly exaggerated dose levels.

We will be forced, perhaps against better judgment, to shorter-term tests to set priorities. Since transformation systems are difficult to establish and then to replicate in independent laboratories, the Ames-type test becomes more attractive from a pragmatic viewpoint but not necessarily from a scientific viewpoint. The Ames test generally—albeit with exceptions—is very sensitive, perhaps even "hypersensitive."

Mutagenic strength is assayed in units that may have limited relevance to in vivo lifetime rodent assays which in themselves lack a standard definition, to my satisfaction at least, of a unit of potency. In rodent assays, we currently talk of dose-response in two dimensions, mg/kg BW in relation to response, and then look to the most sensitive rodent strains and the most critical comparisons among many statistical cells and incur a risk of false positives which is difficult to quantify. We ignore the concept of resistance (the third dimension), at least in direct relevance to effective dose, and thus by default compare carcinogenic strength among carcinogens as we would compare apples with oranges. Sometimes this crude comparison suffices; more frequently it helps little or not at all.

At the risk of sounding naive, I invite your attention to the equations concerning the relationship of electrical voltage to current times resistance. I invite you to invert that equation to solve for current and then to consider current as analogous to dosage and voltage as potency. I invite you to exercise your imagination and then look at the power equation transformations.

My point is that we need a standard or at least several standard units of measurement of carcinogenic potency. In order to obtain them, we need to grapple with the concept of biological resistance or its reciprocal, biological susceptibility, in quantitative terms. It may be that the Ames-type test will provide some measurement of "voltage," but only if we can determine the relevance of the degree of bacterial sensitivity—with and without enzyme induction—to mammalian sensitivity. I confess to failure in being able to grapple mentally with this, unless the degree of enzyme induction of the bacterial system has relevance to the degree of potential mammalian in vivo enzyme induction in quantifiable terms. Two other scientific problems related to the Ames type of approach concern whether the "stripped" bacterial cell wall has full quantifiable relevance to mammalian cells, and whether the bacterial DNA defense and repair mechanisms also have quantifiable relevance to mammalian cells. A major policy issue about requiring mutagenic testing is whether or not the false positive rate will be so high over the long term that some chemicals or foods will mistakenly be indicted as carcinogens, thus potentially creating even greater confusion. There are advocates who would like to expand the Delaney Clause to cover any mutagenically positive substance.

We are rapidly losing our ability to plan, as a society, the commitment of our resources in such a way as to maximize our effectiveness in protecting the public against real threats for cancer induction and yet to minimize needless disruption of all our human resources—national and international, public and private. Major efforts are underway to screen some compounds; yet we cannot anticipate the next substance to give a positive response. Nor do we know the technological consequences if we rush to judgment and impose a zero-tolerance philosophy as an automatic response to all uses of, and all potential human exposures to, the substance in question, no matter how small or sporadic. It is a difficult enough problem to make value judgments predicated on scientific data with respect to direct food additives which are intentionally and purposefully used in food, and for which the question is whether or not to permit the use. It is infinitely more difficult to make societal decisions related to environmental contaminants already present in food if questions concerning carcinogenic risk for man arise. In this situation, the question becomes much more complex: How much of the food supply should be banned from human consumption? If a "no detectable residue" approach is automatically adopted, the result would be to ban nearly all food. The phrase "zero tolerance" originated in setting pesticide tolerances for residues in food where the question was whether or not to permit usage of a pesticide on a food crop. A similar approach is involved with the Delaney Clause's application to food additives. The phrase "no detectable residue" emanates from the exception to the Delaney Clause which Congress enacted to permit usage of carcinogenic drugs in food-producing animals provided "no residues" were detectable by an analytical method approved by the secretary of Health, Education, and Welfare. Here the question is still one of permitting intentional use of the drug. However, to apply such a "no residue" approach blindly to substances such as aflatoxins, DDT, PCB's, or PBB's in all food commodities would be to invite major disruptions in our food supply, our diet, and our economy.

I should like to distinguish the words utility and validity in relation to the no-residue concept and mathematical extrapolation models such as that of Bryan-Mantel to determine the analytical sensitivity to be required to satisfy the "no detectable residue" requirements of the Food, Drug, and Cosmetic Act for specific carcinogenic drugs used in food-producing animals. These concepts have some utility to society in certain applications that are legally defined by Congress in the FD&C Act, but to generalize these concepts to all food situations is to court considerable confusion. Their scientific validity is very limited. Also, there is no magic by which we can completely or quickly eliminate certain residues in food from environmental contamination. The best we can do is to try to reduce critical human exposures as quickly as possible, without committing social suicide by other means.

We scientists working in fields related to carcinogenesis, toxicology, and epidemiology tend to be critical and to voice our opinions freely, sometimes forgetting that the lay public and press may distort the context of our statements. Anyone who has some differences of opinion from time to time with judgments that FDA, EPA, or any regulatory agency is required by law to make is urged to ask us why we made those judgments.

Those who are inclined to automatically take the "no residue" approach should spend a few moments getting the feel of quality control statistics and operating curve characteristics. Otherwise, they should be willing to take their share of the blame for the ensuing chaos.

I would also remind you that there is no right to cross-examine witnesses testifying before Congressional hearings dealing with cancer induction, so we in FDA are handicapped somewhat in defending ourselves against irresponsible witnesses.

I recommend some redirection and recombination of our efforts in toxicology and epidemiology to improve our identification and evaluation of the role of tumor promoters and modifiers of cancer induction. In my opinion, the factors that act as promoters or modifiers are likely to observe more classical dose-response relationships. These factors will require some degree of control on a public health basis including actions by regulatory agencies, but not necessarily always as drastic as current actions tend to be. Other problems with particular promoting or modifying factors may also be identified and these will require much more control than presently exercised by society. A more useful approach to cancer prevention may lie in controlling promoters or modifiers that act across a wide spectrum to activate carcinogens or increase susceptibility to cancer.

Discussion

DR. SHUBIK: I have rarely heard exasperation more elegantly expressed. I would like to ask Dr. Kolbye whether he has heard anything at this meeting so far that would allow him to proceed with competence to the area of judgment which he thinks will lessen his exasperation. And if he thinks this is so, in what way does he think that judgment should be undertaken?

DR. KOLBYE: I'd like to think about that and then have it come out in general discussion because it's an excellent question and demands some cerebration in putting together an answer.

DR. SHUBIK: We're going to have the cocktail party first, and now that we have Dr. Coulston back with us we can start. Dr. Lyon, would you like to take over? It's really very, very important that you stick with the facts, because-ing knowing what we should be doing about alcohol is something that is near and dear to quite a number of people here.

And for heaven's sake, don't scare us unnecessarily!

17. Alcohol and Cancer

J. L. Lyon

Alcohol has been used by human beings as a medicament since prehistoric times. It was used as a wound disinfectant by the Greeks and also constituted a form of treatment in the ancient world when taken internally for many diseases (Majno, 1975).

The ability to produce harmful effects when taken in large quantities has also been recorded since biblical times. But only in recent years has attention been focused on the chronic harmful effects of its use, and then, more on liver damage and its associated effects than on its potential carcinogenocity.

In the 1950s, case control studies, designed primarily to test the association of tobacco with malignancies of the oral cavity, larynx, and esophagus, obtained information about alcohol use (Wynder, Bross, & Day, 1956; Wynder, Bross, & Feldman, 1957; Wynder & Bross, 1961). Carcinogenic effects were identified, independent of tobacco. There appeared to be an independent association of alcohol use with cancers of the oral cavity, larynx, and esophagus.

These observations motivated a number of additional studies (Vincent & Marchetta, 1963; Keller & Terris, 1965; Martinez, 1969; Williams & Horm, 1977). The data from the original and subsequent studies are presented in Table 1. The original studies of Wynder et al. (1956-1961) and Williams (1977) all have used either hospital controls or selected controls with another type of cancer. There is often a confounding problem with alcohol in that tobacco or alcohol use may be related to other health problems that bring potential controls into the hospital, and thus such studies tend to underestimate the magnitudes of the relative risk.

319

TABLE 1
SUMMARY OF CASE CONTROL STUDIES ON ASSOCIATION OF ALCOHOL WITH CANCER

Author	Site	Number of cases		Number of controls	Odds ratio (Controlled for smoking)	
		Men	Women		Men	Women
Wynder, Bross, & Feldman (1957)	Oral cavity	543		207 hospital (other ca)	1.5-11.6	
Wynder & Bross (1961)	Esophagus	150		150 hospital (other ca)	2.5-6.4	
Martinez, (1969)	Oral cavity	170	51	1,200 hospital and neighbor-hood	4.2	6.0
	Esophagus	120	59		2.1-7.7	1.9-3.3
Williams, (1977)	Gum, mouth	57	27	6,170 (all other cancer cases interviewed)	3.7	1.5
	Pharynx	53	20		6.2	17.0
	Esophagus	49	23		1.4	8.1
	Larynx	106	13		2.3	0.8

Martinez' (1969) study used both hospital controls and a control drawn from the neighborhood where the case resided before diagnosis, to deal with this confounding problem. By matching cases and controls for tobacco consumption, Martinez was able to estimate the independent effect of alcohol as a potential carcinogen and found a strong independent effect. None of these studies was able to associate the type of alcohol, whether beer, wine, or spirits, with a carcinogenic effect. Wynder found that the amount of ethanol used correlated better than type of alcohol (Wynder, et al., 1956; Wynder et al., 1957; Wynder & Bross, 1961).

This lack of specificity between the types of alcohol is the second methodological problem in attributing carcinogenic potential to alcohol per se. Drinkers do not drink chemically pure ethanol, but rather alcohol in association with a number of other contaminants—some of which may have potential carcinogenic properties (Rothman, 1975). Unfortunately, other studies have not addressed this question in any detail.

The stimulus provided by the case control studies led to several cohort studies, wherein large numbers of individuals were followed for different time periods for subsequent cancer (Schmidt & DeLint, 1972; Pell & D'Alonzo, 1973; Hakulinen et al., 1974; Nicholls, Edwards, & Kyle, 1974; Monson & Lyon, 1975). Results of these cohort studies are presented in Table 2, with pertinent information about how the cohorts were identified, the length of follow-up, and the excess risk attributed to each cancer. Again, the association of excess alcohol ingestion with cancer of the oral cavity, esophagus, and larynx, appears consistent in all the studies, though there is some variability in the estimate of relative risk. None of the studies had sufficient data control for tobacco use in alcoholics.

A third line of evidence for the potential carcinogenic fact of alcohol comes from populations which have cultural or religious prohibitions on its use. Table 3 presents age-adjusted mortality rates for cancers of the oral cavity, esophagus, larynx, and lung from the Seventh-Day Adventists residing in California and from the Mormon population in Utah (Unpublished data, in possession of author). Comparable data for the U.S. population are also presented, and the relative risk for each population compared to the U.S. presented in the last column. Both the Mormon and the Seventh-day Adventist populations have prohibitions against the use of alcohol and tobacco. The Adventists remove people from Church records if they do not comply with this proscription, while the Mormon population does not and therefore is confounded with a number of alcohol users. Both populations have relative risks for these malignancies, significantly below the U.S. population at large. Again, the data are not adjusted for smoking.

Other factors undoubtedly play a role in producing cancer of the esophagus, since the highest rates in the world are reported among Moslem women living along the Caspian Littoral (Unpubl. data; Kmet & Mahboubi, 1972; Mahboubi; 1971; Mahboubi et al., 1973) who do not drink alcohol. Cancer of

TABLE 2
COHORT STUDIES

Author	Source and size of cohort	Time	Standardized mortality ratios				
			Oral cavity	Esophagus	Larynx	Lung	All Cancer
Schmidt & De Lint (1972)	Alcohol clinic (5,359 men; 1,119 women)	Avg. 7 yrs.	3.4	5.2	9.0	2.1	1.3
Pell & D'Alonzo (1973)	Alcoholic employees (842 men; 57 women)	3 yrs.	3/0[a]	1/1[a]	3/0[a]	2.5	3.7
Hakulinen (1974)	Alcohol abuser registry	Avg. 52 yrs.		1.7		2.0	
	Chronic alcohol registry		5.7	4.1	1.4	1.6	1.3
Nicholls, Edwards, & Kyle (1974)	Mental hospital admissions (678 men; 257 women)	10-15 yrs.	For all respiratory and upper GI:			1.7	1.8
Monson & Lyon (1975)	Mental hospital admissions (1,382 men)	41 yrs	3.3[b]	1.9[b]	3.8[b]	1.3[b]	

[a]Actual observed and expected values.
[b]Proportional mortality ratios.

TABLE 3

AVERAGE ANNUAL AGE-ADJUSTED MORTALITY RATES FOR CANCERS RELATED TO ALCOHOL AND TOBACCO (SEVENTH-DAY ADVENTISTS (1958-65), MORMONS (1968-72), AND U.S. WHITE (1965), AGE 35+)

	Sex	SDA Rate × 10^{-5}	Mormon Rate × 10^{-5}	U.S. Rate × 10^{-5}	Relative risk SDA/US	SDA/US
Oral cavity	M	0.7	3.9	13.5	0.08	0.29
	F	0.3	1.2	3.7	0.09	0.32
Esophagus	M	2.9	44.1	10.2	0.28	0.40
	F	0.6	0.6	2.7	0.22	0.22
Larynx	M	—	1.1	6.5	—	0.17
	F	—	0.8	0.7	—	1.00
Lung	M	5.4	54.5	117.4	0.05	0.46
	F	1.2	9.8	19.1	0.06	0.15

323

the esophagus has also been reported as occurring commonly in Africa and the suggestion made that it relates to a contaminant in native brewed beer (Mahboubi et al., 1973; Cook, 1971).

Within the population living in industrialized countries, it appears that alcohol has some role in the causation of cancers of the oral cavity, esophagus, and possibly larynx. The problem of confounding by the effect of smoking is a difficulty for almost all studies carried out, though Martinez' (1969) study offers the best evidence for an independent effect. It appears, from studies re-analyzed by Rothman and Keller (Rothman, 1974; Rothman & Keller, 1972), that the effect of tobacco with alcohol is a multiplicative one, and that individuals who are both heavy smokers and drinkers are about three times more likely to develop cancer of the oral cavity than would be expected from the individual relative risks for alcohol or tobacco use alone.

Cancer of the liver has also been attributed to the use of alcohol, though in only one of the cohort studies was there a significant excess of liver malignancies (Hakulinen et al., 1974), and this was in the order of 50% over expected. Evidence also comes from case control studies primarily dealing with cirrhotic patients (Parker, 1957; Lee, 1966; Leevy, Gellene, & Ning, 1964). The low frequency of this malignancy in all Western populations (2.2/100,000/year) Cutler & Young, 1975) means that a very large cohort would be required to detect a significant difference. Even if a large relative risk existed for cancer of the liver, it would be difficult to detect an increase using the cohort methodology.

No data are currently available concerning the effects of alcohol on carcinogenesis in females. While there is no reason to suppose that it would affect the same sites as in males, the liver damager often attendant with alcoholism may alter various steroid pathways and might modify the female risk factors for breast cancer. To date, few studies have been carried out on this topic.

Alcohol represents a major public health problem, but not from the standpoint of a carcinogen. Estimates have been made of the potential reduction in cancers if alcohol were totally eliminated from the human population, and in males, this would, at best, account for a 7% reduction and 2% in females (Rothman, 1975). Alcohol contrasted with other known carcinogens, such as tobacco, is not a serious public health threat as a carcinogen.

Additional research on this question, looking at kinds of alcohol, and trying to adjudge the effect of alcohol in certain types of steroid-dependent female malignancies seems warranted.

REFERENCES

Cook, P. Cancer of the esophagus in Africa, *Br.J.Cancer,* 1971, *25,:*853-880.
Cutler, S.J., & Young, J.L. (Eds). Third National Cancer Survey Incidence Data. National Cancer Institute Monograph 41, DHEW Publication No. (NIH) 75-787, 1975. Bethesda, Maryland.
Editorial: Esophageal carcinoma in Africa. *Lancet,* 1972, *1:*622.

Hakulinen, T., Lehtimaki, L., Lektonen, M., et al. Cancer morbidity among two male co-horts with increased alcohol consumption in Finland. *J.Natl. Cancer Inst.*, 1974, *52:*1711-1714.

Keller, A.Z., & Terris, M. The association of alcohol and tobacco with cancer of the mouth and pharynx. *Am.J.Public Health*, 1965, *55:*1578-1585.

Kmet, J., & Mahboubi, E. Esophageal cancer in the Caspian Littoral of Iran: Initial studies. *Science*, 1972, *175* 846-853.

Lee, F.I. Cirrhosis and hepatoma in alcoholics *Gut*, 1966, *7* 77-85.

Leevy, C.M., Gellene, R., & Ning, M. Primary liver cancer in cirrhosis of the Alcoholic. *Ann.N.Y.Acad.Sci.*, 1964, *114* 1026-1040.

Mahboubi, E. Epidemiologic study of esophageal cancer in Iran. *Int. Surg.*, 1971, *56* 68-71.

Mahboubi, E., Kmet, J., Cook, P.J., et al. Oesophageal cancer study in the Caspian Littoral of Iran: The Caspian Center Registry. *Br.J.Cancer*, 1973, *28* 197-214.

Majno, G. *The Healing Hand*, Harvard Univ. Press, Cambridge Mass., 1975, pp 186-188.

Martinez, I. Factors associated with cancer of the esophagus, mouth and pharynx in Puerto Rico. *J.Natl.Cancer Inst.*, 1969, *42* 1059-1094.

Monson, R.R., & Lyon, J.L. Proportional mortality among alcoholics. *Cancer*, 1975, *36* 1077-1079.

Nicholls, P., Edwards, G., & Kyle, E. Alcoholics admitted to four hospitals in England. *Q.J. Stud.Alcohol*, 1974, *35* 841-855.

Parker, R.G.F. The incidence of primary heaptic carcinoma in cirrhosis. *Proc.R.Soc.Med.*, 1957, *50* 145-147.

Pell, S., & D'Alonzo, C.A. A five-year mortality study of alcoholics. *J.Occup.Med.*, 1973, *15*, 120-125.

Rothman, K.J., & Keller, A.Z. The effect of joint exposure to alcohol and tobacco on risk of cancer of the mouth and pharynx. *J. Chron.Dis.*, 1972, *25* 711-716.

Rothman, K.J. Persons at High Rick of Cancer, Academic Press, 1975. pp. 139-150.

Rothman, K.J. Synergy and antagonism in cause-effect reltionships. *Am.J.Epidemiol.*, 1974, *99* 385-388.

Schmidt, W., & de Lint, J. Causes of death of alcholics. *Q.J.Stud.Alcohol*, 1972, *33* 171-185.

Vincent, R.G., & Marchetta, F. The relationship of the use of tobacco and alcohol to cancer of the oral cavity, pharynx, or larynx. *Am.J.Surg.*, 1963, *106*, 501-505.

Williams, R.R., & Horm, J.W. Association of cancer sites with tobacco and alcohol consumption and socioeconomic status of patients: Interview study from the Third National Cancer Survey. *J.Natl.Cancer Inst.*, 1977, *58* 525-547.

Wynder, E.L., Bross, I.J., & Day, E. Epidemiological approach to the etiology of cancer of the larynx. *J.A.M.A.*, 1956, *160* 1384-1391.

Wynder, E.L., Bross, I.J., & Feldman, R. A study of etiological factors in cancer of the mouth. *Cancer*, 1957, *10* 1300-1323.

Wynder, E.L., & Bross, I.J. A study of etiological factors in cancer of the esophagus. *Cancer*, 1961, *14* 389-413.

Discussion

DR. SHUBIK: Obviously, Dr. Lyon, you've been fortunate enough not to become familiar with the problem of adding caramel color to beer. This is, in fact, a major problem at the moment in the British beer industry, among other things. I understand, looking at the slides, that the relative risk rate has not been adjusted for cigarette smoking, and that when it is adjusted, Dr. Wynder tells me, it comes out to be 1. And so I assume that on that basis, there are some beneficial effects from alcohol. Since there are these higher incidences of certain cancers, there must be some cancers for which the incidence is decreased. Could you tell us which those are, Dr. Lyon?

DR. LYON: As I was commenting to Phil as he was looking for standardization, I said, "We are delighted to see that he has been promoted to a lay epidemiologist, who has recognized this." What I did say is that when you standardize for smoking the difference of alcohol to lung would disappear, while that to larynx and perhaps the esophagus would remain. I think that Dr. Lyon gave a very fine overview. I'd just like to stress that he didn't mention the word "congeners" which had come up in the literature, as to whether or not they would prove to be carcinogenic.

It's our view that it's alcohol per se rather than an ingredient in the alcohol. One interesting aspect that came up recently was that we found the same correlation to extrinsic larynx cancer as to vocal cords. In other words, direct contact is not required, and it's for that reason that we think it is, in fact, related to deficiencies related to alcoholism. The final point is, of course, we were talking about small numbers. Compared to some of the things we discussed yesterday; these are major numbers.

DR. SHUBIK: You didn't really answer the question I posed as to which cancers are cured by alcohol. One might observe in correlating animals and man in this regard that animals are really quite sensible and love alcohol and you can feed rats alcohol until the cows come home. You may remember Dr. Harcourt's experiments in which his rats lapped up alcohol for their lifetimes, I regret to say, with no adverse effects. I think, perhaps, some of the other esters, and so forth, in the alcohol might indeed be important in view of the story.

DR. CLEMMESEN: I happened to run into an experiment on animals many years ago in which alcohol was injected into the rectum of mice, and this resulted in metastasizing carcinoma. When I returned from England I said to the worker, "Well, sir, they don't think much of your experiment." He said "Well, my only argument is that you should not take your alcohol that way."

But thinking over the epidemiological evidence with tongue cancers, 29 times as frequent among laborers, waitresses, etc., as among the clergy, etc., would that not fit in with the assumption that alcohol merely acts as a solvent? Perhaps these intestines may have obtained some carcinogen which would be dissolved with the alcohol and the same thing might apply to the tobacco.

DR. HAMMOND: This doesn't pertain to cancer, but it may be related to it. I made a study in which I matched the amount of cigarette smoking and alcohol use. Now, there's one group of people just plainly missing. I don't know where you got the heavy drinkers who were nonsmokers. I had practically none in my experiments. One part of the puzzle is just plainly missing. But there were plenty of smokers who claimed not to be drinkers.

Now I don't know their lifetime history; maybe they were reformed drinkers for all I know. I can only report this, that in those who claimed not to be drinkers, there was a big association with cirrhosis of the liver and amount of smoking. With the smokers and drinkers, the two interacted. Finally, it was very much like you see for esophageal cancer and mouth cancer. But this appears to apply to cirrhosis of the liver as well, and I think too much attention has been given to the alcohol part and not enough to the smoking part in that disease.

DR. LYON: There have been Dr. Wynder's studies on this. There were studies by Rothman and Keller that were really reanalysis of data that Keller collected through the VA system—a third, large study that adjusted for variables was done by Martinez down in Puerto Rico. All of them have made attempts to adjust for the problems of the joint exposure to both malignancies. Martinez did it by matching the factor and was able to get about 300 individuals, where he did match out the effect of tobacco for alcohol. All of them have come to the same conclusion: alcohol itself had a relative risk in the order of 3-5 for the three cancers I've mentioned. We didn't find that. You didn't actually compute that. The Rothman study and the Rothman-Keller study and Martinez I think, concluded that.

DR. WYNDER: From the larynx paper and rat cancer, we find that there are very few people who are very heavy drinkers but do not smoke. We have enough samples, and furthermore the data by Rothman and Keller are based upon very few cases. We reached the conclusion that alcohol by itself has no carcinogenic effect. But it is a powerful promoter, and what you say about cirrhosis is absolutely right.

DR. HAMMOND: I mentioned this for another reason, too. When I talked about cirrhosis what I had in mind was cancer, indirectly, because from everything I've heard, it is that cancer is interacting from the chemical carcinogen; the liver may be involved. If you have liver disease, then the alcohol combined with smoking might have an effect here. This is why I mentioned it.

DR. MOFIDI: I think here we have a good example of what Dr. Wynder has said about the need for comparative epidemiology in various countries. In fact, in our country I mentioned yesterday we know that there is no alcohol consumption in the Caspian area, so there must be additional factors to be studied. I guess what Dr. Shubik mentioned concerning the ingredient or impurities also has been shown in the study in Britain and France that alcohol which may be produced illegally may contain enormous amounts of carcinogens. I assume that one may really look here at disturbances at the cellular level which may be caused by so many different factors and then from there taking a causative agent and working down to the cellular level. In other words, I would say that one has to start thinking differently and taking the inhibition of growth mechanisms or the DNA repair mechanism and see what are the latest studies which may create that. They may be numerous and then work backward.

DR. LYON: I did want to comment on Dr. Mofidi's point that, indeed, an area on the Caspian Sea does have the highest incidence of esophcgeal cancer in the world. It is an area of apparently nonalcohol-consuming Moslems, and this presents again a factor to be considered. In the United States you can argue that alcohol is associated with cancer. In what, form, I think, is very much open to question, including metabolic derangements and major displacement of calories with excessive consumption of this agent.

One other factor I didn't mention, because it isn't relative to carcinogenesis: there are two other syndromes associated with alcohol. One is apparently the syndrome of children born to alcoholic mothers in which there is definitely some derangement which you can characterize by facial and body change. There seems to be some mutagenic effect. This has taken us a long time to sort out, but there have been several papers published recently on this effect. The other is that the latest *New England Journal of Medicine* has a very interesting paper by Friedman and others out of the Permanente group out in California. Using their data system and taking into account all of the variables they had on this huge cohort of about 80,000 people, alcohol was apparently found to be associated with a slight, but statistically significant, elevation of diastolic and systolic blood pressure.

We had some observation data on the Utah Mormon population, where we found a significant difference in deaths from hypertensive heart disease. We were hesitant even to report it because we thought it was an artifact. Seeing this data today I'm a little more comfortable that there may be an effect. If it is, indeed, associated, it could be a major public health finding.

DR. BUTLER: I'm puzzled about your observations on the liver; you said there was no increase.

DR. LYON: No, what I said was that in these cohort studies, liver cancer was such a rarity that we didn't find enough cases for reliability. This is the problem with rare malignancies in a small cohort. The data associating cirrhosis with hepatomas came from a followup on cirrhotics.

DR. MAGEE: It's been said twice during the meeting that primary liver cancer is very rare in human beings. Now I know what this means; it applies in the United States and Western countries, but we often forget that it is a prominent form of cancer in some human beings. Here is one of the best examples in relating laboratory investigation and epidemiology.

18. New and Old Methods

Irving J. Selikoff
Mt. Sinai School of Medicine
New York

I'm very pleased that the title of my presentation was listed as "Old *and* New Methods," not *or,* because most of what I'll discuss is really methods that are descendants of the classical descriptions of analytical and descriptive epidemiology. These go all the way back to infectious disease epidemiology: the classic population and demographic studies in Great Britain during 1970, and then by the pioneers in this country, such as E. B. Wilson, Wilhelm Frost, and others. In the last 30 years there have been new opportunities and new responsibilities, and with these have come concomitant developments and extensions of epidemiological approaches. These have included methods particularly suitable for the difficult problems of cancer. Rather than list epidemiological methods I thought it best to consider these problems and how we have been approaching them to obtain the needed information. The problems as I see them can be listed as perhaps five in number.

First, there is the particularly difficult question of clinical latency: the time constraint. This is the so-called 20-year rule with many exceptions; among them, of course, there is the chloronaphazin bladder cancer, some of which developed in as little as 2½ years, and we know well of the leukemias at Hiroshima that peaked in 1952. I understand we're having a second peak of this now, but by and large the problem of clinical latency is inherent in almost everything we do.

Second, there is the whole question of quantitation. Unlike other areas of toxicity, most cancers are not too common in large human populations, since few reach 1% or 2% of deaths. If we see a 7% incidence in males (male smokers,

329

for example), we consider that very high, and therefore one of the difficult questions is to find reliable correlations in small numbers.

Third, there is the very difficult question of biased selectivity, not only the competitive risk: people dying of malaria at age 30 certainly don't live to die of cancer at age 55. Also, there is the question of availability for selection. I'm reminded that a year ago at another meeting in Florida someone asked a very astute question, about a discovery he had made, namely, that none of the reported cases of angiosarcoma of the liver were to be found in blacks; this was very interesting metabolic observation, except for the fact that when most vinyl chloride polymerization workers went to work for the first time in the 1940s and 1950s, blacks weren't hired in chemical plants. And so in the 1960s and 1970s, they haven't been dying of angiosarcoma.

Fourth, there is the whole question of selectivity within groups. Why do some people in a group develop cancer while others do not?

And fifth, how can we generalize to society at large? This is really our basic responsibility.

I will consider these five problems, how we're approaching them in terms of epidemiological methodology, and then finally I will go into some ideas that we may have, and touch on some epidemiological horizons.

First, with regard to the critical question of clinical latency. Here a major epidemiological advance has been made by the much more widespread use, not of the prospective epidemiological method alone, but by what Dr. Hammond calls the "retrospective-prospective" technique. This means identifying a cohort without bias at a point in time in the past, and then following the group forward as if one had been with them at that point in time in the past, and continuing from there. This serves to telescope the situation. For example, with regard to asbestos, where we have a good deal of this difficulty in clinical latency the question came up: How can we find data that would be useful in a relatively short time? What was done was to make a list of every single asbestos worker in New York City on January 1, 1943, from union records. Incidentally, union records are superb. Industry just doesn't have good records for far back enough in the past.

Yesterday Vaun Newill was complaining to me that at Exxon he's trying to establish some cohorts as of 1950, and the records just aren't available. On the other hand, unions which started out as death benefit societies *have* to keep good records. Which widow gets the $500 or the $1,000? Also, their records say which worker has seniority, so that when business gets slow they can say who gets laid off and who doesn't. Those records are very accurately kept.

It's amusing sometimes when I go to a union office with Dr. Hammond. He's very uneasy and he keeps looking around; I know what he's looking for. He's looking for the door to the basement, because in the cellar is where the records we want are kept. That is, all the senority lists, and so forth. On January 1, 1943, there were 632 men in New York City in this particular union, and these people were traced—every single one of them—by the mortuary fund records, to 1963. And it was found that total deaths were increased in an important way with 203 expected and 255 observed. The excess of 52 was due almost entirely to cancer, with 6 or 7 deaths of cancer of the lung and pleura anticipated and 45 observed, and there was also a modest increase in gastrointestinal cancer.

My purpose here is to emphasize the long period of observation that is needed, because for the first 5 years there was no increase in the death rate, with 40 deaths expected, and 28 observed. Even in the second 10 years, 50 deaths were expected and 54 were observed.. This was the so-called "healthy worker effect." Any group that's employed for the first 5 years and sometimes even 10 years tends to have a better experience than the population at large.

By the end of 1974, in this group of 632 people in which 305 deaths were expected, 451 were observed, and the excess was almost entirely due to cancer, with 52 expected, and 200 actually found. By looking at the total mortality picture you can actually work out which cancers are associated with this increase: these individuals have lung cancer, these have mesothelioma, and these have gastrointestinal cancer. This, then, was an example of the use of a retrospective-prospective epidemiological approach.

This approach allows us to telescope 20 years of experience to within 20 months. We have used the same technique for the United States and Canada. On January 1, 1967, there were 18,000 men in this particular union in the U.S. and Canada, and we've observed them since. Here I will show you how we overcame one of the important difficulties of looking at the 20 years' experience, which is that you can overlook cancers which may occur in *less* than 20 years.

This problem can be solved by looking at a larger cohort, thereby including what would ordinarily turn out to be so-called empty data. Among these 17,800 men, by 1976 there should have been 1,483 deaths; actually there were 2,000, and again where 281 deaths of cancer were anticipated, 867 were found, with the usual causes that I mentioned before.

But now we were able to decide whether we were overlooking something and avoid this trap into which we could have fallen had the time sequences been the same as with chloronaphazin. For example, in this group of 17,800 men there were many who had been exposed for less than 10 years, and certainly less than 20 years.

Observing that over the 9-year period, covering some 100,000 person-years of observation, we found virtually nothing: there was no statistically significant increase in lung cancer in less than 15 years from onset. So we knew that there had to be a long period of clinical latency.

This is also true for mesothelioma, where in these 17,800 men we had 150,000 person-years of observation; there were no mesotheliomas of the pleura, and no mesotheliomas of the peritoneum were to be found in less than 15 years from onset of exposure.

This means that we are able, by utilizing the retrospective-prospective approach, to meet this difficulty (which ordinarily would occur with the problem of clinical latency), and still have a prospective study.

The problem can be illustrated in many other ways. I think Dr. Zapp will agree with me that this has been one of the difficulties in Salem County (N.J.) with the work at DuPont, with the clinical latency dating back to before 1931, but still reflected in bladder cancers that have been seen during the 1960s and 1970s.

Finally, I would call attention to the importance of time from another point of view, and that is the relationship between dose and time of induction of tumors.

So that is the first technique that we have used to meet the problem. With regard to the question of a quantitative response, a major epidemiological advance and really a great technological discovery was how to use populations of very large size.

We accept this as if it were something that would be easy enough, but it had never been done until less than 20 years ago. I wanted to point out that the laboratory people had warned us about the induction period that in skin cancer, as we decreased the dose of benzo(a)pyrene, the time of induction increased. This was also true with other chemicals (Druckrey's work): when the daily dose was decreased, the time of induction was increased.

With regard to the use of population size study, the classic work is Dr. Hammond's, and that is one of the real epidemiologic discoveries of our age. In 1959 he successfully registered over one million people in one third of the counties of the United States (all over the country), and these people answered all kinds of questions: How old was you father when he died? How much did he smoke? How much fried food do you eat? How many hours a day do you sleep? etc.

Then he used the classic technique, showing the interrelationships of matched-pair analysis. Among these one million people there were 440,000 men, and he matched them for various suggestions that had been made with regard to the cause of lung cancer. This cancer is more likely to occur when people are nervous, when they drink a good deal, or when they are exposed to dust, or may depend on their particular religion, and so forth.

By matching them for all of these factors except for one—that is, cigarette smoking—Hammond was able to obtain the critical data that we needed. People matched in every way except for smoking had much more lung cancer and other cancers if they smoked than if they did not. So the use of very large populations became a reality, and we hope that it will be continued.

I have another example that Dr. Hammond and I have worked on. Here we were dealing with a chemical carcinogen, that is, benzo(a)pyrene. There has been a great deal of concern throughout our country about the fact that there are microgram levels of benzo(a)pyrene per m^3 in city air.

This has been with us for 200 years, since the days of Percival Pott. To look at this we took routine samples of pitch and asphalt from some fairly different sites around the country (California to New York). These and the exposures were analyzed, and some of the pitches were found to have as much as 1% benzo(a)pyrene. An extraordinary material.

Again, using large populations, we went to the Roofers' Union and they gave us a list of all of their members. There were 6,000 or so who were members as of January 1, 1960, and who had been in the union for at least 10 years, most of them for 20 or 30 years. So they had had been exposed for decades to the material, some of which contained as much as 1% benzo(a)pyrene.

We were able to follow this group. It's hard to follow 100% with very large cohorts, but you can come pretty close to it. Also we had these men wear masks with filters so that we could, by estimating the amount of benzo(a)pyrene on the filter, measure how much benzo(a)pyrene would have been inhaled had the men not been wearing the mask during their work.

We studied many of the different kinds of work which are involved in roofing operations, and by measuring the amount of benzo(a)pyrene on the masks we were able to get some sense of the daily exposure. We calculated that many of these men had inhaled benzo(a)pyrene at levels equivalent to somewhere around 700 cigarettes a day.

These are the experiences based upon some 60,000 person years of observation. For periods of less than 20 years for the pulmonary site of exposure, there was no significant increase in cancer. After the 20-year point, 216 cancer deaths were expected, but 315 were observed. Now we were able to bring to light the data that we needed; that is, not only that skin cancer occurred with benzo(a)pyrene, but there were some increases in other organs as well. There were very big increases in the mortality rates. With this, we were able to demonstrate how nowadays large populations can be used as a method in epidemiological research.

The second problem was the question of dose-response. This was fairly easy in the laboratory, but now we were able by some subtleness of epidemiological approach to get some sense of dose-response as well.

For example, Dr. Hammond's study involved about 6 million-person years of observation, and the dose-response was clear. By using large populations one can also begin to get some dose-response information for human disease.

This can also be done by the use of occupational groups. Here, for example, is an old manufacturing plant in an eastern U.S. city, rescued from the wrecker's hammer by the Navy in 1940, and given over to the manufacturer of asbestos insulation.

From 1941 to 1945, 933 men worked in this plant, some for a day or a week or a month, and some for 13 years, until the plant closed in 1954. The usual deaths were found by 1975: the usual distribution of lung cancer, mesothelial, intestinal cancer, and so forth.

Of interest to us was the dose-response. Dose, as you remember, is concentration X time. At least, this applies if the time doesn't go too long, when time itself can have an important influence. We had groups of people exposed for from less than a month, to as much as 5 years, and for even those exposed for less than a month there was an increase in lung cancer death rates.

But the larger the dose (that is, time)—they all worked in the same plant, in the same years, in the same city, with the same machinery, with the same fiber, and making the same product—with all the other things constant except the dose, with a great deal of exposure, the lung cancer incidence was considerably greater than with the low doses. Now it is possible, using appropriate epidemiological methods, to work our dose-response relationships for human cancer as well.

Before I come to the question of bias and selectivity, I would say that we had very good confirmation from the laboratory where elegant studies by J. C. Wagner have shown that the inhalation of asbestos by rats is definitely characterized by a dose-response relationship. One day of exposure is enough to produce disease, but increasing the time will give even more disease.

Now, with regard to bias and selectivity: How can we use our epidemiological approaches to minimize this? First and foremost, there are the techniques of cohort studies and cohort analysis, i.e., where you type the entire group and look at the entire experience. However, there is no perfect cohort, because really you have to go back to the day everyone is born, but cohorts can still be reasonably good.

So, by this method we are able to develop information concerning dose-response. Regarding selection within groups, we may ask, why do some people develop cancer and not others? We are even beginning to be able to utilize some epidemiological approaches for this. This is the question on which we are attempting to get answers. Here's what has been done. Again we had a very good lead from the laboratory from the classic studies of Bittner who, starting in the 1920s and continuing for two decades at least, was able to show in his susceptible strains of mice that it still required, to get maximum cancer response, hormonal stimulation with estrogens, and what he then called "milk factor," but which many people now consider to be probably a virus. So the question of multiple factor interaction has been with us for a long time.

It can also apply to humans, with appropriate epidemiological study. For example, when the asbestos workers in New York were examined in 1963, each was asked about his smoking habits. Eighty-seven had no history of cigarette smoking, but 283 did. By 1967, using smoking-specific data from the American Cancer Society's cancer prevention study, it was calculated that statistically, not quite one death was expected among the nonsmokers, but not one occurred. When these people died, their lungs were full of asbestos. They died of asbestosis or other diseases, they did not die of lung cancer. On the other hand, of the 283 with a history of cigarette smoking there should have been three deaths from lung cancer; instead, 24 occurred. So if death occurred from smoking alone, only three would have died of lung cancer. It wasn't the asbestos alone since none died of lung cancer; rather, it was the combination of the two. These data were sparse; we have attempted to expand them, and it can be done. When the 17,800 men were registered, it was found that approximately 2,000 had no history of cigarette smoking and 9,500 had. By 1976, among the 2,000 men with a history of regular cigarette smoking, there were 52 expected deaths from lung cancer with 285 observed. Now these expected rates, unlike the others that I've shown, are not smoking-specific yet. Dr. Hammond and I are reviewing this now with smoking-specific data. Of the 2,000 individuals who have never smoked we have seen only 6 deaths from lung cancer. Now that might be slightly more than in other nonsmokers, but it certainly is not a major public health problem. Among the 600 men who only smoked pipes or cigars, covering over 5,000 person-years of observation, we have only seen two deaths from lung cancer despite all the asbestos in their lungs.

To show the sensitivity of the epidemiological technique we have looked at the relationship of cigarette smoking to mesothelioma. There was no difference whatsoever that we could find. For the people with a history of cigarette smoking (and this is outside the full 81,000 person-years of observation), there were only 0.38 deaths/1,000 years from pleural mesothelioma. For the nonsmokers the rate was 0.39/1000; that is, no difference at all. The multiple factor interaction of asbestos and cigarette smoking is quite specific for lung cancer; it is not generally across-the-board for cancer. That's how sensitive the method can be.

I would also call attention to the interaction between uranium mining and cigarette smoking and lung cancer on the Colorado plateau, and to the fact that individuals with a greater tendency to develop leukemia following the Hiroshima exposure have a still three times greater incidence if they also worked with benzene *after* Hiroshima.

The question of selection within groups also depends upon dose. Dr. Hammond and I are looking at the data very carefully with additional experience, but they're of interest and I would like to show them to you. You will remember that in the factory group some people worked for a month and some for 13 years. Regarding the sensitivity of the method; this is a new study, I don't think it's been published yet, and so I thought you might want to see it so you can sort out things.

A very interesting study was done at the Royal Technological Institute in Stockholm by Dr. Olin, a young physician stationed at the engineering school. Swedish people are quite progressive, and his job is to teach engineers something about environmental problems and occupational problems so these factors will be considered in the engineers' practice. While he was there he thought he might do a little research, and in cooperation with the emeritus professor of chemistry, he made a list of all graduates in chemical engineering of the Institute from 1930-1950, and he traced them to 1973.

He was able to trace almost all of them because they all kept corresponding with their professor. Dr. Olin found that there was, based on small numbers, an increased amount of cancer among these chemical engineers. He broke the group of 500 into two parts: 400 continued in chemical engineering per se and 100 went into management. All the excess in cancer occurred in the chemical engineers who continued at the bench. He had a perfect control group made up of those who graduated at the same time and who didn't continue to work in the chemical laboratories.

To get back to the induction period and the question of dose: for those heavily exposed in the asbestos factory, there was a great deal of lung cancer. Not only was there a great deal, but it occurred at an earlier date. It occurred at 15 years after onset of exposure. On the other hand, in those who were exposed a month or less, there wasn't very much lung cancer. There was a slight excess, but it didn't appear until 30 years after onset of exposure. So, the epidemiological method is even sufficiently sensitive to give us information concerning dose-induction period relationships. These are very useful approaches. Well, then how do we begin to utilize epidemiological methods to obtain information concerning generalization to the community at large?

One of the epidemiological approaches has been to use populations exposed to the same agent under different conditions, where we can get some sense of differences in the kinds of exposure. And for this we have been using this unusual tumor, mesothelioma. For those of you who are not acquainted with this extraordinary tumor, we can say that it is invariably fatal. Our first hint in this regard was a brilliant demonstration by J. C. Wagner of the fact that he saw 47 cases of mesothelioma in a 5-year period. These were all in the northwestern portion of Cape province (South Africa), a place where there are many small asbestos mines and mills. In a very astute observation he visited the relatives and found that in 45 out of the 47 there had been, 30 years earlier, the opportunity for contact with asbestos. Now they didn't for the most part work in these mines or mills; they lived on the roads along which the donkey carts were taking the bags of ore to the mills.

With this observation available, M. L. Newhouse, a very good epidemiologist at the London School of Hygiene, looked at the 76 cases in the files of London Hospital. About 31 had worked with asbestos, and that comes as no surprise. But of the 45 who had not, 9 had simply lived in the household of an asbestos worker. These were women who had washed their husbands' clothes when they came home from work. Of the 36 who had neither worked with asbestos nor lived with someone who worked with asbestos, 11 had lived within one-half mile of one of the asbestos plants in London. So, we have been able to utilize groups exposed in other than occupational circumstances. For example, we have taken dust measurements in houses of asbestos workers. When you take a sample of the dust, you can get, at least within an order of magnitude, some idea of exposures within households.

What we are doing now is establishing a cohort of all wives and children who lived with the factory workers from 1941 to 1945. We're using the cohort approach to get quantitative information concerning the spectrum of asbestos-associated cancers. Of the first 626 we examined (this is work now in progress), one-third had abnormal x-rays. In the usual things that you see, the pleural changes, calcification, parenchymal fibrosis, and so forth, it made no difference whether they were wives, sons, daughters, etc.

We are now, or will soon be able with a cohort approach to see the experience of a human population group exposed other than very heavily. Another observation has recently been made at the Devonport dockyard in England by P. G. Harries. In 1968 he reported 5 cases of mesothelioma. This was no surprise in itself, but what was surprising was that not one patient was an asbestos worker. These cases included a boilermaker, a pipe fitter, a laborer, and a ship welder. Take one look at ships and you know the reason why. A worker installing asbestos insulation has around him 100 other workers of all kinds; he's the Typhoid Mary in the group.

As you can see, here in the United States, one out of 500 shipyard workers is an asbestos worker. Four hundred and ninety-nine are in the other trades, but they're all exposed to the same dust, except intermittently and not as intimately.

By 1973, Dr. Harries had 55 cases of mesothelioma in the Devonport dockyard, but only 2 were asbestos workers. And so we are looking now at, in a cohort fashion, the experiences of shipyard workers other than those involved with asbestos. So we can titrate, in a sense, the cancer experience, taking into account the long period of clinical latency, the degree of exposure, and so forth. There have come into our lexicon now, such epidemiological phrases as "family contact disease," "neighborhood disease," and for the shipyards, the construction industry, and so forth, "bystanders' disease."

From a public health viewpoint the epidemiological methods, again derived from Dr. Hammond's basic work, have been extended to the utilization of something we knew from infectious disease epidemiology: what happens with the reduction of exposure, i.e., the effective removal from exposure. We knew that this occurred, because in the migrant studies there was not only a great deal of variation from one area to another, but the changes occurred when people moved from one country to another.

Dr. Hammond published evidence some years ago, that when people stopped smoking and were observed for periods up to 10 years, the risk of cancer went down. In terms of numbers, nothing occurred certainly for the first year (the first year after stopping smoking has higher rates and that's because people who cough blood generally tend to stop smoking), but after 5 years' cessation a very significant decrease occurred. Removal from exposure could be defined in proper epidemiological terms on a "present years at risk" level.

In terms of public health significance, I would call attention to a missed opportunity. This is angiosarcoma of the liver, but we should have been forewarned, because here a biologically active material was involved. In 1967 we already knew of the acro-osteolysis that would occur among vinyl chloride-exposed workers and of a liver fibrosis of a very special kind. There is a pseudoclubbing, a shortening of the fingers, and hepatic fibrosis. We are able not to begin to develop some horizons, and some priorities based upon the techniques we have available.

First, I would point out, in these horizons, the interaction between the laboratory and the epidemiological studies. Epidemiological studies are sensitive, effective, and accurate, and they do give human data. Second, there is the question of our looking at agents which are chronically active. There is a need for earlier identification of those agents which will eventually prove carcinogenic. We have to begin to learn how to use morbidity data, rather than depend so heavily on mortality data.

Then there is the question of selection within high risk groups. This involves using other techniques, including immunological and chromosomal changes (especially in prospective studies), as well as the selection of these problems which deserve our most immediate attention.

First, and here I speak to industry, there are many groups which have already had 20 years of exposure and their experience is available to us for the asking. For example, in Hudson Falls, New York, there are some 2,000 people who have been heavily exposed to polychlorinated biphenyls for 25 years. If we're worried what PCB's will do in the Hudson River, we can certainly look at what happened to the workers at Hudson Falls.

The same thing applies to nitrosamines. There are now populations that have been exposed for 15 to 20 years. Dr. Shubik mentioned yesterday the importance of getting some additional information on Flagyl and griseofulvin. We can certainly look at the first workers who manufactured these products and also the first people who took them. In this regard we've had an immediate problem about "first people;" it was alluded to by Dr. Kolbye earlier this morning, and that was in Michigan.

This is the hyperkeratosis that is seen in cows with polybrominated biphenyls. In the hoof of the cow this is sometimes very disabling; the hyperkeratosis is so bad that the cows just literally can't walk. They stay in their stalls and die. It's a pathetic sight; they trip all over themselves. The question naturally arises, what happens to people? Here is a biologically active material that is a very powerful inducer, and so forth.

We have undertaken a survey in Kent County, Michigan, and several months ago we examined over 1,000 Michigan farmers and their families and have established considerable baseline material. Here are the first people known to be exposed to polybrominated biphenyls. As a result of the contamination of the food chain, virtually everyone in Michigan now has PBB's in his tissues, at greater or lower levels.

What will happen to them we simply don't know. When we examined these people in Michigan, we, of course, needed a control group, and that is very difficult to get. Last month we went to Wisconsin, in the Marshfield area, the center of dairy farming in this country, and we examined 250 people altogether (150 adults); the various symptoms that were seen in Michigan were not seen in Wisconsin.

The amount of PBB in their blood has been measured; these are our first 267 results and you can see the levels. Most of them have low levels, but a few have high levels of PBB's in the ppm range. We also used the tricks we've learned. We went to the company that made PBB and examined 55 workers in that company. We found that they have more PBB in their tissues than the farmers do. The farmers got it by ingestion, while the workers got it partly by inhalation and partly by ingestion.

But even here, we can see how the available techniques can be utilized. There were 12 workers who were actually producing PBB and there were 27 who were in the same plant, but who worked in other locations. The levels are considerably higher in the people who were actually at the production line, although the others have measurable levels.

Finally, with regard to priorities, the question of protection of the newborn becomes important. It has been known now for some time that PBB's, like other fat soluble chlorinated hydrocarbons, readily appear in the breast milk. And in Michigan, especially in the lower part, virtually all (about 90%) women who have breast milk and are breast-feeding have PBB's in their milk and the kids are getting it. Also, in the upper peninsula, around Sault Ste. Marie, approximately 50% of women have PBB's in their breast milk. It has been calculated that in any year in Michigan some 20,000 women breast-feed. The only hint we have of what's going to happen with breast-feeding is from PCB's, where Allan Conney, in his very elegant studies, fed PCB's to monkeys and then allowed them to breast-feed the newborn. The newborn get chloracne, as well as weight loss, and sometimes they die.

We have no knowledge whatsoever if this is going to happen with polybrominated biphenyls, but again the importance of protection of the newborn must be stressed.

Discussion

DR. SHUBIK: In view of the time we have, I think we can accept only one or two specific questions. They must be directed very specifically to the point; otherwise we're going to be late.

QUESTION: I would like to ask you, have you worked out the distribution curves for the latent periods? These would be most useful to have so that we can find cases as soon as they appear.

DR. SELIKOFF: For asbestos this has been done. One slide that I passed over gave some information for vinyl chloride, but we only have some 50-60 angiosarcomas with vinyl chloride. There are too few data yet to develop curves. We do have them for asbestos, and I agree with you that for all of the human studies where carcinogens have been defined for human populations these are available and should be obtained.

DR. SHUBIK: Thank you very much.

19. Animal Models for the Study of Tobacco Carcinogenesis

C.J. Kensler, S.P. Battista, and P.S. Thayer
Arthur D. Little, Inc.
Cambridge, Massachusetts

The subject assigned to us is the use of animal models to study tobacco carcinogenesis. To sum it up, we really don't have a satisfactory animal model although several appear to provide useful information for some facets of the problem. As indicated in Fig. 1, we are dealing with a very complicated situation; we have the agent(s) that compose smoke, defense mechanisms, and a variety of cells at risk with different degrees of susceptibility influenced by genetic and other factors. The cells at risk in man may also be influenced by other environmental factors; e.g., exposures to asbestos, air pollution, nutritional deficiencies, etc. In cigarette smoke there are initiators for tumor induction in experimental animals, particularly the polycyclic hydrocarbons and small quantities of other animal carcinogens such as nitrosamines and some radioactive elements. There are also promoters (cocarcinogens), mutagens and defense system inhibitors. The latter include agents that inhibit the mucociliary apparatus, macrophage activity, immune response, and biochemical effects; for example, the level of activity of such enzymes as aryl hydrocarbon hydroxylase (AHH), and, finally, transport problems such as absorption and distribution of smoke components from the lung and gastrointestinal tract and the availability of substrates for a host of metabolic pathways.

If one examines the role of initiators, one must consider aromatic polycyclic hydrocarbons as important. However, the fact that roofers exposed to coal tar tolerate amounts (mgs/day) of aromatic polycyclic hydrocarbons for up to 20 years with relatively small increased risk of lung cancer (Hammond et al., 1976) would indicate that perhaps these compounds are not as important to the smoker (μgs/day) as most people are inclined to believe.

341

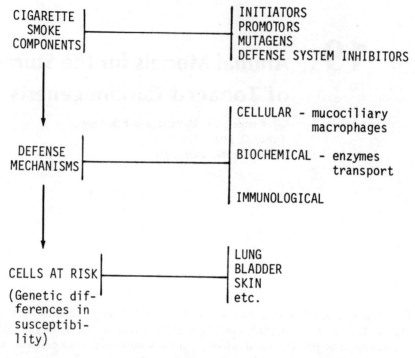

CIGARETTE SMOKE COMPONENTS ——— INITIATORS / PROMOTORS / MUTAGENS / DEFENSE SYSTEM INHIBITORS

DEFENSE MECHANISMS ——— CELLULAR - mucociliary macrophages / BIOCHEMICAL - enzymes transport / IMMUNOLOGICAL

CELLS AT RISK (Genetic differences in susceptibility) ——— LUNG BLADDER SKIN etc.

FIGURE 1
Factors that influence or modify carcinogenic responses to tobacco smoke.

Bentley and Burgan (1960) reported that nitrates (e.g., $Cu(NO_3)_2$), added to tobacco, reduced polycyclic hydrocarbons. Wynder (Wynder & Hoffman, 1961; Wynder et al., 1968) and members of our lab have shown that nitrates added to tobacco of cigarettes can reduce the skin cancer incidence—at least for the mouse, and of tumor incidence, for hamsters by inhalation (Dontenwill et al., 1973). We also know there are bacterial mutagens present, and if you apply the Ames test to cigarette smoke condensate, as Ames' laboratory did (Kier et al., 1974), you find that mutagenic activity in the condensate of nitrate-treated cigarettes is not reduced, but higher. In other words, the results in the Ames test are the reverse of those observed in the in vivo test on the skin of the mouse.

In the case of defense system inhibitors, Drs. Battista, Thayer, and I have studied this problem and concluded that the active components in smoke are primarily hydrogen cyanide, acrolein, and related aldehydes. Immune responses, and cytotoxicity to alveolar macrophages, lymphocytes, etc., are also important, but there are other factors than cyanides and aldehydes involved. With respect to the biochemical mechanisms, aryl hydrocarbon hydroxylase, which Dr. Conney discussed the other day, is an example of an enzyme that can be induced by cigarette smoke in the fetus as well as the smoking mother. Kellermann et al. (1973) suggested that perhaps we can identify the high risk individuals among the smoking population by finding those individuals in which the enzyme is readily induced. Kellermann's preliminary data were certainly encouraging in this respect. In our laboratories we carried out experiments in which mice were skin-painted for 24 months. We used several hundred animals, and only about 50% of the animals developed tumors, so we had a population that was painted with condensate of which some developed cancer and some didn't. This appeared to be a good opportunity to study the relationship between AHH levels and inducibility in susceptible and nonsusceptible mice. Unfortunately, our data for the skin of the mouse indicated that there wasn't any difference in levels between these two populations with respect to this enzyme, either in terms of the base level or its induced level. Recent publications (Trell et al., 1976; Paigen et al., 1977; McLemore et al., 1977) on this subject showed that there were no differences with respect to this phenomenon between patients with lung cancer and the appropriate controls. So one might conclude that the skin of the mouse gave us a decent prediction for man for that particular phenomenon.

As an inhalation model would be most appropriate, it is desirable to consider the distribution of lung cancer types associated with smoking. For smokers and nonsmokers as shown in Table 1, the data show that the major type of cancer in nonsmokers is the adenocarcinoma and for smokers it is squamous cell carcinomas. For the sake of comparison we have also tabulated data on the incidence of epithelial cancer in laboratory animals exposed to smoke and smoke condensate. Table 2 summarizes the results for mouse, rabbit, rat, hamster and

TABLE 1
DISTRIBUTION BY TYPE OF LUNG CANCERS IN A
COMPOSITE SERIES OF NONSMOKERS AND A
REPRESENTATIVE HOSPITAL SERIES[a]

	Incidence (%)			
	Nonsmokers		All patients[b]	
Type of cancer	Men	Women	Men	Women
Squamous cell carcinomas	14	12	47	22
Oat cell carcinoma	4	4	17	11
Bronchiolar carcinoma	—	5	8	23
Adenocarcinoma	57	54	10	20
Large cell anaplastic carcinoma	8	8	17	19
Carcinoid	14	16	0.6	4
Other specific types	—	<1	1	2
Undifferentiated[c]	4	2	—	—
Total no. of cases	51	274	1903	315

[a]Adapted from Berg (1970).

[b]Representative hospital series.

[c]Includes oat cell carcinoma and large cell anaplastic carcinoma (Harris, 1973).

TABLE 2

RESULTS OF INHALATION STUDIES WITH CIGARETTE SMOKE

Species	Strain	Approx. observation/ treatment (years)	Lung tumors		References (senior authors)
			Epidermoid/small cell	Adenoma bron. alveolar/ adenocarcinoma	
Mouse	A	1.2	No	Yes[a]	Essenberg (1952)
	Hybrid DBA/020	2	No	Yes[a]	Mühlbock (1955)
	Inbred	0.5	No	No	Scala (1955)
	A/JAX	1	No	Yes[a]	Essenberg (1956)
	CF$_1$	0.6	No	Yes	Leuchtenberger (1958)
	CF$_1$	1.6	No	Yes[a] (related to age)	Leuchtenberger (1960)
	Inbred	2	Yes (2/60)	Yes[a]	Otto (1963)
	C57B	2.5	Yes (1/200?)	Yes	Harris (1967)
	dd	1	No	Yes	Naito (1968)
	C57B	1.2	No	No	Wynder (1968)
	dd	1.5	No	Yes	Yoshida (1970)
	Snell	2	No	Yes[a]	Leuchtenberger (1974)
	C57B	2	No	No	Leuchtenberger (1974)
Rabbit	N. Zealand	5.5	No	No	Holland (1963)
Rat	IC and Wistar	2	Yes (4/68)	Yes	Guerin (1959)
	Buffalo	0.2	No	Yes[a]	Mori (1964)
	Wistar (SPF)	2.8	Yes $\dfrac{(1 + 3?)}{406}$	Yes (4/489)	Davis (1975 a or b)

TABLE 2 (continued)

| Species | Strain | Approx. observation/treatment (years) | Lung tumors | | References (senior authors) |
			Epidermoid/small cell	Adenoma bron. alveolar/adenocarcinoma	
Hamster	Syrian	2	No	No	Dontenwill (1966)
	Syrian	2	No	Yes[a]	Dontenwill (1973), 1974 (larynx cancer 10.6%)
	Inbred	2	No	No	Homburger (1974) (early cancer-larynx) a. 15.16 - 19% b. 87.20 - 4%
	a. Bio 15.16				
	b. Bio 87.20				
	Syrian	0.5	No	Yes[c]	Karbe (1974)
	Syrian	1	No	No	Kobayashi (1974)
	Syrian	1	No	No	Resnik-Schüller (1975)
	Syrian	2.3	No	Yes	Wehner (1974)
Dog	mongrel	3.2	Yes (1/10 i.s.[c])	No	Rockey (1966)
	Beagle	1.2	No	No	Auerbach (1967)
	Beagle	2.5	Yes (2/62)[b]	Yes(30/74[b])[c]	Auerbach (1970)

[a]More than 5% of controls had tumors.

[b]Nonfilter cigarettes.

[c]i.s. in situ.

dog—all exposed to smoke by inhalation. The overall incidence of epidermoid tumors was very low in contrast to the human situation. In the case of the mouse there were only three reported, two of 60 by Otto (1963) and 1 of 200 by Harris (1967). In general, there were few epithelial carcinomas and many adenocarcinomas. For the rat and hamster the same situation exists. For the dog, Rockey (1966) reported a carcinoma in situ in 1 of 10 and Auerbach (1970), 2 of 62 animals. In the former case the lesion was noninvasive if in situ, while in the latter study the two lesions were described as "invasive." Nettesheim (personal communication), in inhalation experiments in rats given cigarette smoke, determined the retained dose using cigarettes labeled with a long chain hydrocarbon (dotriacontane) that was carried along with smoke into the lung. He found that 3 mg of total particulate matter per rat per day was retained in the lower respiratory tract. His results showed no incidence of squamous cell carcinoma in those animals even though a few doses of methylcholanthrene did produce these cancers.

Another approach that has been used to determine the carcinogenicity of tobacco smoke is based on application of smoke condensate or fractions of smoke condensate to one part of the lung or another. The results of such studies are shown in Table 3. The only studies that showed a reasonably high incidence of epidermoid tumors, useful for bioassay purposes, were the ones reported by Stanton (1972) and, to a much lesser extent, those reported by Blacklock (1961) and Rockey (1962, 1966). It should be pointed out that Rockey reported one invasive carcinoma and five in situ carcinomas in his condensate experiments, which covered several years. The one invasive carcinoma was in a dog killed eleven days after the start of the experiment; thus, it is doubtful that this cancer is related to the treatment.

More promising methods are those that permit localized application of a condensate or carcinogen to the same area of the respiratory tract repeatedly, as are shown in Table 4. For rodents, Schreiber et al. (1975) used a special catheter for instillation of the carcinogen into the trachea. Kendrick et al. (1974) applied the carcinogen to tracheal grafts implanted subcutaneously in another animal or recipient. Stanton et al. (1972) developed a technique for implanting in the lung beeswax pellets containing condensate or carcinogen that results in a reasonable incidence of squamous tumors.

Using the beagle, Dr. Battista has been exploring the possibility of developing a model in which it would be possible to achieve local application of condensate or native smoke to bronchi using catheters or bronchoscopes. Okita et al. (1974) have used the bronchoscope to inject carcinogens. The technique is also applicable for injecting multiple doses of smoke condensate as a means of estimating carcinogenic potency, since it involves administration of the agent directly onto the respiratory epithelium.

In addition to the dog, a second model that allows exposure of the lung to smoke without first passing it through the nose is the bird. We found that its

TABLE 3

RESULTS OF STUDIES WITH CIGARETTE SMOKE CONDENSATE

| Species | Strain | Approximate observation/ treatment (years) | Exposure mode | Lung tumors | | References (senior authors) |
				Epidermoid/ small cell	Adenoma bron. alveolar/ adenocarcinoma	
Rat	C. Beatty	1.4	Inject "tar" in oil into lung	No	—	Blacklock (1957)
	C. Beatty	2	Inject "tar"	Yes (1/72) (6/72?)	—	Blacklock (1961)
	Os. Mendel (SPF)	2.3	a. inject into lung; wax pellet contain. "tar"	a. Yes (14/36)	—	Stanton (1972
			b. Hex. So. Fract.	b. Yes $(16/69)^a$		
	Fisher	0.7	treat. tracheal graft	No	—	Kendrick (1974)
	Wistar (SPF)	2.5	a. intratrach. instillation	a. No	No	Davis (1975)
			b. Fract. "p" (polycyclics)	b. Yes $\dfrac{(1+4?)}{54}$	No	
Hamster	Syrian	1	tracheal instill (s)	No	No	Della Porta (1958)
Dogs	mongrel	5	bronchial instill. via bronchoscope	Yes $\dfrac{(1+5 \text{ i.s.}^b)}{130}$	No	Rockey (1962, 1966)

^{a}2nd-year deaths.
^{b}In situ.

347

TABLE 4
MORE PROMISING BIOASSAY METHODS
FOR CARCINOGENICITY OF THE LUNG

1. Methods that permit direct application of carcinogen (condensate) to the bronchus or trachea (less desirable)
   a. Rodents
      (1) Schreiber (1975): special catheters to exposed trachea
      (2) Kendrick (1974): tracheal grafts
      (3) Stanton (1972): wax pellet implant in lung
   b. Canine
      (1) Battista (unpublished): bronchoscope used for topical application of agent to bronchus
      (2) Okita (1974): bronchoscope used to inject agent into bronchus
      (3) Battista (1973): instill or infuse agent on bronchus via implanted catheter

2. Methods that permit inhalation of aerosols (smoke)

   Most of the present inhalation methods are acceptable as bioassays for potent carcinogens but, because of toxicity, are unacceptable for native cigarette smoke.

anatomy is ideally suited for chronic smoke exposure since the larynx is easily exposed and it can be isolated from the upper airways merely by opening the bird's beak. We felt that the direct exposure of the tracheal and bronchial tree to concentrated cigarette smoke would provide a very effective means of studying carcinogenicity of cigarette smoke. We exposed groups of white leghorn hens (SPF) for 3 1/2 years. One group received smoke from two (1R1) cigarettes/day, five days a week; a second group received ten doses of diethyl nitrosamine (DEN) at two-week intervals, and a third group received both smoke and DEN. We also included another group within each of these treatments that consisted of animals that had multiple denudations of the tracheal epithelium, in order to expose cells in a stage of rapid proliferation and under conditions of impaired mucociliary clearance. Previously, we found that we could mechanically remove the tracheal epithelium and that the epithelium is regenerated in about 14 days; so in addition to exposing normal epithelium, proliferating tissues were also exposed to a known carcinogen (DEN) and to daily exposures of cigarette smoke which was delivered directly to the trachea and lung. Again, for the purposes of bioassay our results showed that we did not get much in the way of malignancies, as shown in Table 5. For smoke, over the 3 1/2 year exposure, we have an incidence of 7-10% for animals that died or were sacrificed. The data from the denuded trachea animals were no different from the non-denuded trachea birds, contrary to our expectations. An additional observation from this study is that the combination of DEN and cigarette smoke didn't increase the incidence of malignancies, indicating a lack of promotion or synergism between the two agents.

TABLE 5

SUMMARY OF THE INCIDENCE OF MALIGNANT LUNG TUMORS IN ANIMALS
THAT DIED OR WERE SACRIFICED DURING THE STUDY

Treatment time (years)	Year #1			Year #2			Year #3.5			Total		
	No. animals	No. tumors	% animals with tumors	No. animals	No. tumors	% animals with tumors	No. animals	No. tumors	% animals with tumors	No. animals	No. tumors	% animals with tumors
Died												
Controls	12	0	0	7	0	0	7	0	0	26	0	0
DEN	32	0	0	6	2a	33	3	2a	67	41	4	10
Smoked	16	1b	16	6	1a	16	7	0	0	27	2	7
Sacrificed												
Controls	17	1	6	29	0	0	24	0	0	70	1	1
DEN	14	3	21	25	6d	24	24	0	0	63	9	14
Smoked	6	0	0	8	3a	38	12	0	0	26	3	12
Smoked + DEN	4	1	25	4	0	0	8	0	0	16	1	6
Total 1st, 2nd, and 3.5 years (Died and Sacrificed)												
Controls										96	1	1
DEN										104	13	13
Smoked										53	5	9
Smoked + DEN										26	2	8

aOne lung tumor, possibly metastatic from liver.

bProbably metastatic from kidney.

cOne borderline malignancy.

dIncludes one carcinoma in situ.

349

Any consideration of carcinogenicity of cigarette smoke must involve some attention to the smoke generating and exposure system. Since the subject has been reviewed recently in detail by Guerin, Maddox, and Stokely (1975), the following discussion will be limited to the beagle smoking system developed by Cahan and Kirman (1968) and used by Auerbach et al. (1970), since it is the one that has provided the highest incidence of malignancies. The original system used a smoking machine initially to acclimate the animals to smoke; then the machine was removed and the animals smoked by placing a lit cigarette into a cigarette holder connected to the tracheostomy tube. Thus, each time the animal inhaled, it puffed the cigarette. One advantage to the original system is that high doses of fresh smoke were delivered directly into the animal's lung via the trachea. The disadvantages are that the size of the dose and the nature of the puff were uncontrolled and the latter, to a large extent, was determined by the laboratory attendant. It is evident that heavy doses of CO, CO_2, etc., in smoke result in progressively greater and greater hyperventilation as the cigarette is consumed and it, in turn, produces deeper and deeper inhalation unless the puffing is terminated by intervention of the technician. Failure of the attendant to terminate the exposure at a reasonable dose can easily result in extreme stress due to severe hypoxia.

In an attempt to limit the puff volume and frequency to values more like those of a human smoker, a system has been developed in our laboratory that would mechanically take a 35 ml puff of smoke from the cigarette and deliver it to a 40 ml smoke-holding tube once every 30 or 60 seconds. One end of this tube is connected to the smoking machine and the other to the animal's tracheostomy tube. A one-way valve on the smoker allows air to enter the tube and displace the smoke during inhalation. It also prevents purging of the smoke from the smoke-holding tube during exhalation, as well as loss during delivery of the puffs of smoke from the smoking machine. A more recent modification of the exposure system has been made by Hazleton (unpublished) that involved the addition of an inflatable cuff on the tracheostomy tube. The cuff is inflated prior to smoking in order to occlude the distal portion of the trachea. This modification minimized the exposure of the upper airways which contain receptors that are sensitive to the irritant effects of smoke and permits more normal breathing as well as reduces the amount of smoke dilution from air inhaled through the posterior pharynx. Studies that utilize this system of mechanical puffing and direct inhalation of smoke are now in progress and results are forthcoming.

As referred to earlier, we have also been interested in developing a large animal bioassay system for carcinogenicity that provides the following:

1. ability to provide direct exposure of the bronchi, the target tissue of interest, for estimating carcinogenic potency of the tobacco products;
2. facility for direct viewing of the exposed and surrounding tissue for tumor formation during the course of treatment;

3. facility for tissue biopsy for sampling changes in cell populations;
4. elimination of the need for extensive autopsy procedures since the site of application and lesion formation is known a priori;
5. exposure to high doses locally with minimum systemic toxicity; and
6. lower costs, since fewer animals and cigarettes would be needed.

To achieve the above, it is evident that success is dependent upon techniques for achieving accessibility to the desired bronchi. Two approaches have been used, bronchoscopy and intdwelling catheters. We have had animals whose bronchi have been treated topically via biopsy channel of the bronchoscope with 3-methylcholanthrene (known carcinogens) as well as with cigarette smoke condensate for over one year. Using intdwelling catheters lodged in bronchi of beagles, we have also instilled the materials continuously over two- to three-hour periods. To date, we have observed bronchial hyperplasia and metaplasia within several months, but as yet no malignant tumors. A slight modification of the catheter technique is now being developed to provide a means of exposing selected segments of bronchi to doses of cigarette smoke that would otherwise be lethal if inhaled in conventional chambers or via tracheostomies. The proposed system (shown schematically in Fig. 2), consists of two catheters implanted in two adjacent bronchi. Smoke is introduced under pressure into one bronchus and evacuated under reduced pressure from the other. A timer/synchronizer is used to phase the time of puff generation so that the smoke introduction occurs at FRC and amount of smoke inhaled into the deeper parts of the lungs is minimized. Preliminary experiments indicate that such a system is feasible.

None of the inhalation models have permitted the evaluation of the role of promoters although the production of tumors on mouse skin by smoke condensate is probably the result of the presence of initiators and promoters. The important promoting agents in smoke have not been identified, although phenol and catechol possess this property, but they are not present in cigarette smoke in sufficiently high concentrations to account for this effect.

The long time-requirements for assaying smoke condensate for carcinogenic activity on the skin of the mouse, or in the even less satisfactory inhalation experiments where the final incidences of malignancy have been too low for meaningful bioassay purposes, emphasize the need for short-term assays. The measurement of short-term (one week) effects on mouse skin sebaceous glands and epidermal thickening has provided useful information on the activity in smoke condensate in Wynder's, Bock's, and our laboratories. An example of the relative activity of cigarette smoke and some promoters and initiators is presented in Fig. 3. An example of the results observed when an active fraction is further fractionized by chromatography is presented in Fig. 4. A comparison long-term skin-painting experiment indicated that the fractions containing the sebaceous gland suppressing activity were those which resulted in higher incidence of mouse skin tumors.

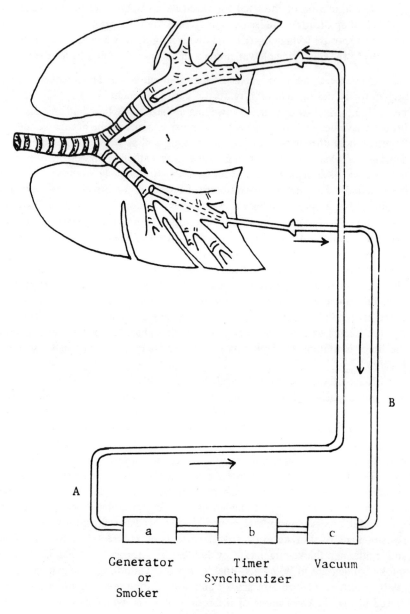

FIGURE 2
Modified catheter technique.

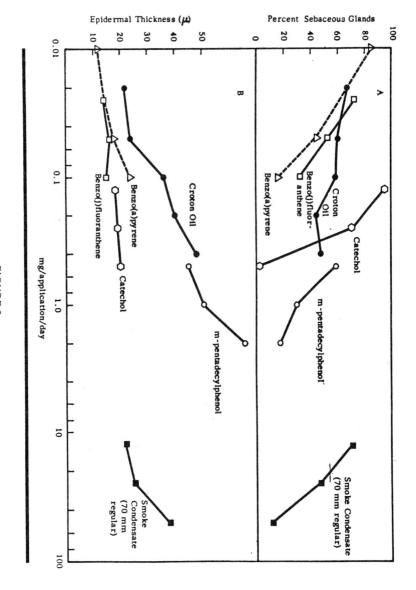

FIGURE 3

Activity of materials of different potencies in sebaceous gland (A) and epidermal thickness (B) assays.

353

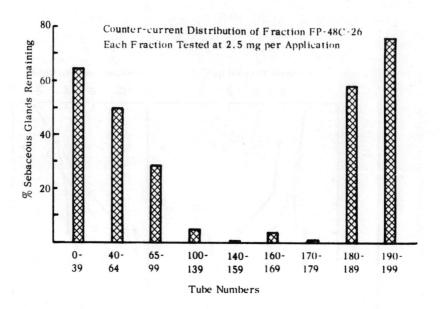

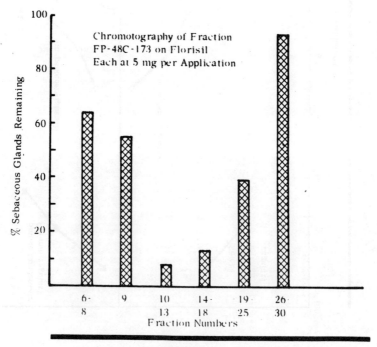

FIGURE 4

In summary, despite the numerous studies on cigarette smoke, we still don't know the active carcinogenic agents for man or the relative importance, if any, of initiators versus promoters. Under these circumstances the prudent thing to do is to lower the exposure to potentially harmful agents in cigarette smoke by particulate or selective filtration, dilution, and additives in the tobacco column to reduce the intrinsic activity.

In addition, the search for cigarettes that yield smoke with lower specific activity for mouse skin and in inhalation experiments as exemplified by the National Cancer Institute's Tobacco Working Group program shows promise. As the final indication of success in these endeavors will be a decreased incidence of lung cancer in man, it is obvious that it will be some time before the true merits of potentially beneficial changes in cigarette smoke composition will be apparent.

REFERENCES

Auerbach, P., Hammond, E.C., Kirman, D., Garfinkel, L., & Stout, A.P. Histologic changes in bronchial tubes of cigarette-smoking dogs. *Cancer,* 1967, *20,* 2055-2066.

Auerbach, O., Hammond, E.C., Kirman, D., & Garfinkel, L. Effects of cigarette smoking on dogs. II. Pulmonary neoplasms. *Arch. Environ. Health,* 1970, *21,* 754-768.

Battista, S.P., Steber, W.D., Green, M., & Kensler, C.J. Technique for implanting lower airway catheters chronically in dogs. In order to expose and record pulmonary function. *Arch. Environ. Health,* 1973, *27,* 334-339.

Bentley, H.R., & Burgan, J.G. Polynuclear hydrocarbon in tobacco and tobacco smoke. III. The inhibition of the formation of 3,4-benzopyrene in cigarette smoke. *Analyst,* 1960, *85,* 727-730.

Blacklock, J.W.S. The production of lung tumours in rats by 3:4 benzopyrene, methylcholanthrene and the condensate from cigarette smoke. *Br. J. Cancer,* 1957, *11,* 181-191.

Blacklock, J.W.S. An experimental study of the pathological effects of cigarette condensate in the lungs with special reference to carcinogenesis. *Br. J. Cancer,* 1961, *15,* 745-762.

Cahan, W.G., & Kirman, D. An effective system and procedure for cigarette smoking by dogs. *J. Surg. Res.,* 1968, *8,* 567-575.

Davis, B.R. Whitehead, J.K., Gill, M.E., Lee, P.N., Butterworth, A.D., & Roe, F.J.C. Response of rat lung to tobacco smoke condensate or fractions derived from it administered repeatedly by intratracheal instillation. *Br. J. Cancer,* 1975(a), *31,* 453-461.

Davis, B.R., Whitehead, J.K., Gill, M.E., Lee, P.N., Butterworth, A.D., & Roe, F.J.C. Response of rat lung to inhaled tobacco smoke with or without prior exposure to 3,4-benzopyrene (BP) given by intratracheal instillation. *Br. J. Cancer,* 1975(b), *31,* 469-484.

Della Porta, G., Kolb, L., & Shubik, P. Induction of tracheobronchial carcinomas in the Syrian Golden Hamster. *Cancer Res.,* 1958, *18,* 592-597.

Dontenwill, W.P., & Wiebecke, B. Tracheal and pulmonary alterations following the inhalation of cigarette smoke by the Golden Hamster. In L. Severi, (Ed.). *Lung tumors in animals.* Perugia, Italy: Division of Cancer Research, University of Perugia, June, 1966. Pp. 519-526.

Dontenwill, W.P., Chevalier, H.J., Harke, H.P., Lafrenz, U., Reckzeh, G., Scheider, B. Investigations on the effects of chronic cigarette smoke inhalation in Syrian Golden Hamster. *J. Nat. Cancer Inst.,* 1973, *51,* 1781-1832.

Dontenwill, W.P. Tumorigenic effect of chronic cigarette smoke inhalation on Syrian Golden Hamster. In E. Karbe & J.F. Park (Eds.), *Experimental lung cancer.* Berlin: Springer-Verlag, 1974. P. 331.

Essenberg, J.M. Cigarette smoke and the incidence of primary neoplasm of the lungs of albino mice. *Science,* 1952, *116,* 561-562.

Essenberg, J.M., Leavitt, A.M., & Gaffney, E. The effect of arsenic in tobacco on primary de cigarette. *Bull. Assoc. Franc. Étude Cancer,* 1959, *46*(2), 295-309.

Guérin, M.R., Maddox, W.L., & Stokely, J.R. Tobacco smoke inhalation exposure: concepts de cigarette. *Bull. Assoc. Franc Étude Cancer,* 1959, *46*(2), 295-309.

Guerin, M.R., Maddox, W.L., & Stokely, J.R. Tobacco smoke inhalation exposure: concepts and devices. Proc. of the Tobacco Smoke Inhalation Workshop: Experimental Methods In Smoking and Health Res. DHEW Publication No. (NIH) 75-906, 1975.

Hammond, E.C., Selikoff, I.J., Lowther, P.L., & Seidman, H. Inhalation of benzopyrene and cancer in man. *Annals N.Y. Acad. Sci.,* 1976, *271,* 116-124.

Harris, C.C. The epidemiology of different histologic types of bronchogenic carcinoma. *Cancer Chemotherapy Reports, Part 3,* 1973, *4,* (2), 59-61.

Harris, R.J.C., & Negroni, G. Production of lung carcinomas in C57BL mice exposed to a cigarette smoke and air mixture. *Br. Med. J.,* 1967, *4*(5580), 637-641.

Hoffman, D., & Wynder, E.L. Reduction of tumorigenicity of cigarette smoke by addition of sodium nitrate to tobacco. *Cancer Res.,* 1967, *27,* 172-174.

Holland, R.H., Kozlowski, D.J., & Booker, L. The effect of cigarette smoke on the respiratory system of the rabbit. *Cancer,* 1963, *16*(1) 612-615.

Homburger, F., Bernfeld, P., & Russfield, A.B. Cigarette smoke inhalation studies in inbred Syrian Hamsters. In E. Karbe & J.F. Park (Eds.), *Experimental lung cancer.* Berlin: Springer-Verlag, 1974. Pp. 320-330.

Karbe, E., & Koster, K. Carcinogenicity of inhaled cigarette smoke in the MMU-treated hamster larynx. In E. Karbe & J.F. Park, (Eds.), *Experimental lung cancer: Carcinogenesis and bioassays.* pp 369-382, Springer-Berlin: Springer-Verlag, 1974. Pp. 369-382.

Kellerman, G.., Shaw, C.R., & Luyten-Kellerman, M. Aryl hydrocarbon hydroxylase inducibility and bronchogenic carcinoma. *New Eng. J. Med.,* 1973, *289,* 934-937.

Kendrick, J., Nettesheim, P., & Hammons, A.S. Tumor induction in tracheal grafts: A new experimental model for respiratory carcinogenesis studies. *J. Nat. Cancer Inst.,* 1974, *52*(4) 1317-1320.

Kier, L.D., Yamasaki, E., & Ames, B.N. Detection of mutagenic activity in cigarette smoke condensates. *Proc. Nat. Acad. Sci.,* 1974, *71,* 4159-4163.

Kobayashi, N., Hoffmann, D., & Wynder, E.L. A study of tobacco carcinogenesis XII. Epithelial changes induced in the upper respiratory tracts of Syrian Golden Hamsters by cigarette smoke. *J. Nat. Cancer Inst.,* 1974, *53*(4), 1083-1089.

Leuchtenberger, C., Leuchtenberger, R., & Doolin, P.F. A correlated histological, cytological and cytochemical study of the tracheobronchial tree and lungs of mice exposed to cigarette smoke. *Cancer,* 1958, *11,* 490-506.

Leuchtenberger, R., Leuchtenberger, C., Zebrun, & W., Shaffer, P. A correlated histological, cytological and cytochemical study of the tracheobronchial tree and lungs of mice exposed to cigarette smoke. *Cancer,* 1960, *13*(4) 956-958.

Leuchtenberger, C., & Leuchtenberger, R. Differential response of Snell's and C57 black mice to chronic inhalation of cigarette smoke. Pulmonary carcinogenesis and vascular alterations in lung and heart. *Oncology,* 1974, *29,* 122-138.

McLemore, T.L., Martin, R.R., Busbee, D.L., et al. Aryl bydrocarbon hydroxylase activity in pulmonary macrophages and lymphocytes from lung cancer and noncancer patients. *Cancer Res., 1977, 37*, 1175-1181.

Mori, K. Acceleration of experimental lung cancers in rats by inhalation of cigarette smoke. *Gann, 1964, 55*, 175-181.

Mühlbock, P. Carcinogene werking van sicarettenrook bij muizen. (Carcinogenic action of cigarette smoke in mice). *Nederlands Tijdschrift voor Geneeskunde, 1955, 99*(31), 2276-2178.

Naito, M. A study of the pulmonary neoplasm of mice after prolonged exposure to cigarette smoke. (In Japanese) *J. Kyoto Prefect. Med. Univ., 1968, 77*, 694-702.

Okita, M., Cohen, A.H., & Benfield, J.R. Localized submucosal bronchial injections of carcinogens in dogs. In E. Karbe & J.F. Park (Eds.), *Experimental lung cancer.* Berlin: Springer-Verlag, 1974. Pp. 102-114.

Otto, H. Experimentelle Untersuchungen an Mausen met passiver Zigarettenrauchbeatmung. (Experimental investigations on mice through passive inhalation of cigarette smoke). *Frankfurter Zeitschrift für Pathologie, 1963, 73*, 10-23.

Paigen, B., Gurtoo, H.L., Minowada, J., et al. Questionable relation of aryl hydrocarbon hydroxylase to lung cancer risk. *New Eng. J. Med., 1977, 297*, 346-350.

Reznik-Schuller, H., Reznik, G., & Mohr, U. Effects of cigarette smoke on the bronchial epithelium of Syrian Hamsters: Ultrastructural studies. *J. Nat. Cancer Inst., 1975, 55*(2), 353-355.

Rockey, E.E., Speer, F.D., Ahn, K.J., Thompson, S.A., & Hirose, T. The effect of cigarette smoke condensate on the bronchial mucosa of dogs. *Cancer, 1962, 15*, 1100-1116.

Rockey, E.E., & Speer, F.D. The ill effects of cigarette smoking in dogs. *International Surgery, 1966, 46*, 520-530.

Scala, C., & Vicari, F. Inalazione sperimentale di fumo di tobacco nei topolini bianchi. *Riv. Pat. Clin., 1955, 10*, 673-684.

Schreiber, H., Schreiber, K., & Martin, D.H. Experimental tumor induction in a circumscribed region of the hamster trachea: Correlation of histology and exfoliative cytology. *J. Nat. Cancer Inst., 1975, 54*(1), 187-197.

Stanton, M.F., Miller, E., Wrench, C., & Blackwell, R. Experimental induction of epidermoid carcinoma in the lungs of rats by cigarette smoke condensate. *J. Nat. Cancer Inst., 1972, 49*, 867-877.

Trell, E., Korsgaard, R., Hood, B., et al. Aryl hydrocarbon hydroxylase inducibility and laryngeal carcinomas. *Lancet, 1976, 2*, 140.

Wehner, A.P., Busch, R.H., & Olson, R.J. Effect of chronic exposure to cigarette smoke on tumor incidence in the Syrian Golden Hamsters. In E. Karbe & J.F. Park (Ed.), *Experimental lung cancer.* Berlin: Springer-Verlag, 1974. Pp. 360-368.

Wynder, E.L., & Hoffmann, D. Present status of laboratory studies on carcinogenesis. *Acta Pathol. Microbiol. Scand., 1961, 52*, 119-132.

Wynder, E.L., Taguchi, K.T., Baden, V., & Hoffmann, D. Tobacco carcinogenesis. IX. Effect of cigarette smoke on respiratory tract of mice after passive inhalation. *Cancer, 1968, 21*, 134-153.

Yoshida, H., Yoko, S., Takeshita, Y., Okumura, K., Aoji, O., Masaki, K., Takahata, J., Ide, M., Naito, M., Shindo, T., Abe, N., Ave, A., & Fujii, M. An experimental study on the pulmonary neoplasm of mice after exposure to cigarette smoke. *Jap. J. Med., 1970, 9*, 293-294.

20. Tobacco Epidemiology— A Simulated Animal Experiment

E. Cuyler Hammond
Lawrence Garfinkel
Department of Epidemiologic and Statistical Research
American Cancer Society

Animal experiments are often undertaken to simulate (or predict) what might happen to human beings under certain specified conditions. For this meeting, we decided to use epidemiological data to simulate what might happen in an animal experiment. The general subjects are:

(1) Lung cancer death rates by attained age in relation to inhalation of an agent which increases the risk of dying of that disease, and
(2) Competitive risks.

EXPERIMENTAL MODEL

Our model is a simple little experiment designed to test the hypothesis that outbred male animals of a certain species are more likely to die of lung cancer if they intermittently inhale Z mg of Substance X per day than if they are not exposed to Substance X.

Equipment is designed in such a way that Substance X, mixed with air, is admitted into exposure chambers for 3 minutes and then replaced by pure air; this is repeated 20 times a day. The concentration is such that an animal placed in a chamber inhales Z mg of Substance X per day. According to plan, N animals, all of exactly the same age at the start, are to be put in these chambers daily until all have died. Under these conditions, total dosage up to any particular day is Z mg times the number of days from start of exposure.

Control animals are to be put in similar chambers daily but without exposure to Substance X.

Unfortunately, as so often happens in real life, the supply house, instead of delivering N animals all of exactly the same age, delivers a far larger number animals of various ages. Faced with this, our investigator accepts only N animals, these being the youngest available. Still, some of these are older than others. So, in an attempt to keep total cumulative dosage as close to uniform as possible, he alters some of his exposure chambers to deliver slightly more or less of Substance X per day. This is not ideal, but is the best he can do under the circumstances.

During the first several months, very few animals die and hardly any die of lung cancer. For this reason, the investigator chooses to report results starting with the age at which lung cancer death rates become appreciable. (It would be better to report results starting with the number of animals alive at the start of the experiment).

EPIDEMIOLOGICAL DATA

The epidemiological data available for our simulated experiment came from a prospective study which was started nearly 18 years ago and is still in progress.

Between October 1, 1959 and March 15, 1960, 1,078,000 men and women in 25 states answered rather lengthy questionnaires about themselves. They were traced annually through September 30, 1965, surviving subjects being requested to answer brief repeat questionnaires in 1961, 1963, and 1965. Subjects enrolled in 22 of the original 25 states were traced again in 1971 and 1972 and, in the latter year, were requested to answer a final questionnaire.

Because of interest in the occurrence of cancer in "long-lived people," it was decided to continue to trace the oldest subjects periodically until almost all of them had died. These were arbitrarily defined as men born in 1887 or later (age 72 or older in 1959) and women born in 1885 or later (age 74 or older in 1959).

Some of the cigarette smokers said that they were not currently smoking cigarettes at the time they answered a repeat questionnaire. Many of these alternated between smoking and not smoking from the time of one questionnaire to the time of the next. However, if twice in a row they said they they were not currently smoking cigarettes, they generally did not resume the habit at a later date, and for purposes of analysis we made the assumption that this was always the case. In analysis, ex-cigarette smokers (so defined) were excluded from further "exposure to risk" after 8 years had elapsed from the date when they presumably gave up the habit for good. A total of some 51,540 such subjects was originally enrolled in the 22 states. We have now traced 99.4% of them through January 1, 1975. Several had lived to see their 106th birthday; none had as yet seen their 107th.

ANALYSIS OF DATA

This report is confined to male subjects originally enrolled in 22 states. The starting date is July 1, 1960 (i.e., about 6.5 months after the mean date of enrollment; about 6 weeks after the last subject was enrolled). The ending dates are June 30, 1972 for men born after 1887 and June 30, 1975 for men born 1887 or earlier.

For the unexposed "control" group we used nonsmokers defined as men who, at the start of the study, said that they had never smoked regularly. For the exposed group, we chose men who at the start of the study said that they were currently smoking cigarettes regularly, had never smoked pipes or cigars regularly, and who fell into one of the following four groups:

1. *Began to smoke cigarettes when they were under 20 years old.* The majority of these subjects smoked 20 to 39 cigarettes per day and inhaled the smoke at least to a moderate degree. This was by far the largest of the four groups.
2. *Began to smoke cigarettes when they were 20 to 24 years old and, at start of study, said that they smoked over 9 cigarettes a day and/or inhaled the smoke at least to a moderate degree.* This was the second largest of the four groups.
3. *Began to smoke cigarettes when they were 25 to 29 years old and at start of study said that they (a) smoked 20+ cigarettes a day and/or inhaled the smoke deeply: or (b) smoked 10 to 19 cigarettes a day and inhaled to at least to a moderate degree.* This group was much smaller than the second group.
4. *Began to smoke cigarettes when they were 30 to 34 years old and at start of study said that they smoked 20+ cigarettes a day and inhaled at least to a moderate degree.* This was a very small group.

As revealed by repeat questionnaires, some of these cigarette smokers (as defined above) gave up the habit during the course of study. These were excluded from analysis after approximately eight years had elapsed since the date they had quit smoking.

RESULTS

For each single year of attained age, we calculated the observed value of p_x, that is, the number of men alive at exact age $(x + 1)$ divided by the number of men alive at exact age x. Using the usual life table procedure, we then chain multiplied the "p_x's" to calculate the proportion of men alive at age 40 who would still be living at each birthday, thereafter assuming a stationary population with age-specific death rates as observed.

Figure 1 shows the resulting curves for cigarette smokers (as defined above) and for nonsmokers. The point for each single year of age has been plotted here with no smoothing of the data. The only exception to this is for cigarette smokers over the age of 97 where p_x's had to be estimated because of lack of information.

The area under each curve is proportional to the total person-years of exposure to risk of cancer (or any other disease) from age 40 onward. The total person-years at risk is far greater for nonsmokers than for cigarette smokers for the simple reason that, as a group, they live longer. This is due partly to their much lower lung cancer death rates but mainly due to their lower death rates from various other diseases.

Figure 2 shows the death rates per 100,000 man-years of cigarette smokers and nonsmokers. Plotted here are the mean rates for successive 5-year attained age groups, standardized to the single year of age distribution in the stationary population of each of the two groups of subjects, respectively. Since very few of the cigarette smokers in our study lived past the age of 95, their death rate for age group 95 to 100 has been omitted from this chart because of lack of statistical stability.

PERCENT OF MEN SURVIVING – AGE 40 TO AGE X

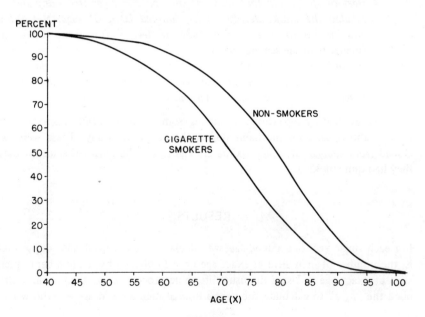

FIGURE 1

DEATH RATE PER 100,000 MAN YEARS
CIGARETTE SMOKERS AND NON-SMOKERS

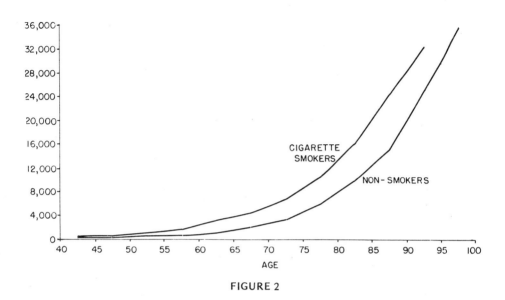

FIGURE 2

The shape of the curves is roughly exponential up to about age group 80 to 85 in the case of cigarette smokers and up to age group 85 to 90 in the case of the nonsmokers. After that the rates are lower than would be expected from extrapolation of an exponential curve. This is probably due to selective mortality with advancing age.

The effects of selective mortality are illustrated in Fig. 3. The middle line on the chart represents death rates at successive ages in a mixed population which, at age 40, was composed half of cigarette smokers and half of nonsmokers. At first, the death rate of the combined population is midway between the death rates of the two component populations. Since the cigarette smokers die off more rapidly than the nonsmokers, at each succeeding age, the surviving population has a lower proportion of cigarette smokers and a corresponding higher proportion of nonsmokers. Therefore, with advancing age, the death rates become closer and closer to the rates for nonsmokers.

Actually, all populations are mixed in respect to genetic factors or environmental factors, or both. If this were not so, barring accidents, all individuals would die at the same age.

For purposes of this analysis, we counted a death as being due to lung cancer if, under international rules, lung cancer would be classified as either the underlying or a contributing cause of death. Figure 4 shows lung cancer death

DEATH RATE PER 100,000 MAN YEARS
CIGARETTE SMOKERS AND NON-SMOKERS

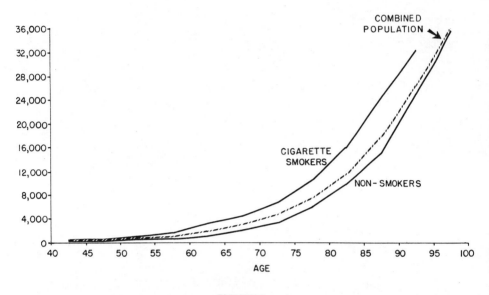

FIGURE 3

rates of cigarette smokers and nonsmokers plotted at successive 5-year attained age groups up to age group 90 to 95. A rather exaggerated scale is used for the ordinate in order to show both lines on the same chart. Asterisks on the chart signify points which are extremely unstable statistically.

The rates for both groups increase with advancing age—more sharply in smokers than the nonsmokers—up to a certain age. However, the rate for cigarette smokers seems to reach a peak somewhere between age 75 and 80 and then declines. Possibly, this is due to statistical sampling error or some artifact in the data. We are more inclined to think that the decline is real and is due to selective mortality.

Mortality ratios for successive age groups are shown in Fig. 5. These mortality ratios were calculated by dividing the death rate of the cigarette smokers by the corresponding rate for the nonsmokers. The ratios for total death are reasonably stable statistically; those for lung cancer are rather unstable, extremely so for the points marked with asterisks. The mortality ratios for lung cancer rise up to age groups 70-74 and decline steeply after age group 75-79. Those for total deaths decline after age group 60-64.

Mortality ratios, while useful and meaningful can give a misleading impression if viewed alone. Figure 6 shows the mortality differences—that is, the death rate of the cigarette smokers minus the death rate of nonsmokers by 5-year age

LUNG CANCER DEATH RATES PER 100,000 MAN YEARS
CIGARETTE SMOKERS AND NON-SMOKERS

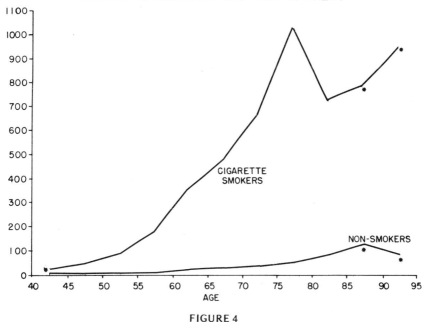

FIGURE 4

MORTALITY RATIOS CIGARETTE SMOKERS VS NON-SMOKERS

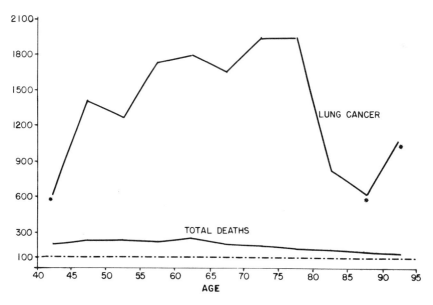

FIGURE 5

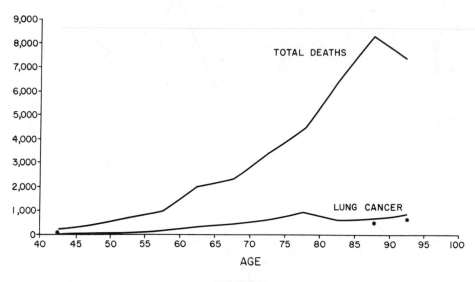

MORTALITY DIFFERENCE
DEATH RATE OF CIGARETTE SMOKERS
MINUS DEATH RATE OF NON-SMOKERS

TOTAL DEATHS

LUNG CANCER

AGE

FIGURE 6

groups. First, note the curve for all causes of death combined. While the mortality ratio goes down with advancing age (Fig. 5), the mortality difference goes up with advancing age (Fig. 6). For lung cancer, the mortality difference goes up steeply, reaches a peak at age group 75 to 80 and then appears to go down.

Now, let us turn back to the object of the animal experiment which we took as our model. Slightly reworded, it was: to test the hypothesis that outbred male animals of a certain species are more likely to die of lung cancer if they inhale a specified agent daily than if they are not exposed to that agent.

In our simulated animal experiment, the agent inhaled was cigarette smoke. The findings are summarized in Table 1. Up to the beginning of each 5-year age group, the cumulative number of lung cancer deaths was far greater in cigarette smokers than in nonsmokers. The final totals were: 8,200 lung cancer deaths per 100,000 cigarette smokers alive at age 40 (i.e., 8.20%) and 1,010 per 100,000 nonsmokers alive at age 40 (i.e., 0.96%). This is a ratio of 8.12:1. Other findings in this respect will be discussed a little later on.

A far more important finding was that the proportion of subjects living up to any particular age was considerably greater for nonsmokers than for cigarette smokers. This was only partly due to the fact that fewer nonsmokers than cigarette smokers die of lung cancer.

366

TABLE 1
NUMBER LIVING AT EACH 5-YEAR AGE GROUP AND CUMULATIVE NUMBER AND PERCENT OF LUNG CANCER DEATHS OF 100,000 CIGARETTE SMOKERS AND 100,000 NONSMOKERS ALIVE AT AGE 40

Age	Cigarette smokers			Nonsmokers		
		Cumulative no. of lung cancer deaths			Cumulative no. of lung cancer deaths	
	Number living	No.	% of total	Number living	No.	% of total
40	100,000	0	0	100,000	0	0
45	97,830	149	1.8	98,973	25	2.5
50	94,505	376	4.6	97,693	41	4.1
55	89,264	786	9.6	95,643	76	7.5
60	81,762	1,557	19.0	92,168	125	12.4
65	70,810	2,743	33.5	86,397	217	21.5
70	56,497	4,280	52.2	77,489	338	33.5
75	39,781	5,831	71.1	64,971	461	45.6
80	23,316	7,354	89.7	47,784	611	60.5
85	10,159	7,904	96.4	29,120	781	77.3
90	2,884	8,114	99.0	12,731	910	90.1
95	403	8,180[a]	99.8	3,434	940[a]	93.1
100	63[a]	8,195[a]	99.9	597	960[a]	95.1
105	12[a]	8,200[a]	100.0	113	1,010[a]	100.0

[a]Extrapolation.

SECOND SIMULATED EXPERIMENT

Now let us carry out a simulated animal experiment with hypothetical cigarettes. These cigarettes are unique. They produce age-specific lung cancer death rates identical to those produced by ordinary cigarettes; but they produce no other effects upon the smoker. Death rates from all causes other than lung cancer are identical to the non-lung cancer death rates of nonsmokers. This of course, alters the situation in respect to the competitive risk of dying of lung cancer or dying of some other cause.

This simulated experiment was carried out as follows: for each single year of attained age, the difference between the lung death rate of the ordinary cigarette smokers and the nonsmokers was added to the death rate of the nonsmokers. These new death rates were then converted into q_x's by dividing each death rate by one plus half of the death rate. (This is simply the reverse of estimating the death rate from the value of q_x). The survivorship curve was calculated as before from the p_x's where $p_x = 1 - q_x$.

367

In consequence of the above, the eventual number of deaths from lung cancer is greater for smokers of the hypothetical cigarettes than for smokers of ordinary cigarettes (see Table 2). The figures are 11,490 lung cancer deaths per 100,000 hypothetical cigarette smokers alive at age 40 versus 8,200 for ordinary cigarette smokers, a ratio of 1.40:1.

TERMINATION OF AN EXPERIMENT

In an actual experiment, we not only want to know whether exposure to an agent under test increases the risk of dying of cancer of a specified site; we also want some estimate of the degree of the increased risk.

We have seen that this depends upon whether the effect of the exposure is limited to increased death rates from cancer of the specified site or whether it extends to other causes of death as well. As shown, in Table 10, it also depends upon whether or not the experiment is continued until all of the exposed and all of the unexposed animals have died.

TABLE 2

NUMBER LIVING AT EACH 5-YEAR AGE GROUP
AND CUMULATIVE NUMBER AND PERCENT
OF LUNG CANCER DEATHS OF 100,000
CIGARETTE SMOKERS AND 100,000
HYPOTHETICAL SMOKERS ALIVE AT AGE 40

	Cigarette smokers			Nonsmokers		
		Cumulative no. of lung cancer deaths			Cumulative no. of lung cancer deaths	
Age	Number living	No.	% of total	Number living	No.	% of total
40	100,000	0	0	100,000	0	0
45	97,830	149	1.8	98,853	150	1.3
50	94,505	376	4.6	97,372	381	3.3
55	89,264	786	9.6	94,960	809	7.0
60	81,762	1,557	19.0	90,797	1,644	14.3
65	70,810	2.743	33.5	83,971	3,000	26.1
70	56,497	4,280	52.2	73,971	4,889	42.6
75	39,781	5,831	71.1	60,244	7,029	61.2
80	23,316	7,354	89.9	42,506	9,491	82.6
85	10,159	7,904	96.4	25,169	10,589	92.2
90	2,884	8,114	99.0	10,867	11,167	97.2
95	403	8,180[a]	99.5	2,865	11,401[a]	99.3
100	63[a]	8,195[a]	99.9	499[a]	11,480[a]	99.9
105	12[a]	8,200[a]	100.0	94[a]	11,490[a]	100.0

[a]Extrapolation

The most usual measure of degree of risk is the mortality ratio computed by dividing the total number of (lung) cancer deaths occurring in the exposed animals by the total number of (lung) cancer deaths occurring in the unexposed animals.

In order to save time and money, some investigators discontinue an experiment before all of the animals have died. Now let us suppose that our simulated experiments had been discontinued when somewhat over half (52.2%) of the nonsmokers had died. At that point 76.7% of the cigarette smokers and 57.5% of the hypothetical cigarette smokers had died (see Table 3). At the same point, 0.61% of the nonsmokers, 7.35% of the ordinary cigarette smokers and 9.49% of the hypothetical cigarette smokers had died of lung cancer. The lung cancer mortality ratios were then 1.00 for the nonsmokers, 12.05 for the cigarette smokers, and 15.56 for the hypothetical cigarette smokers.

Next, let us suppose that the simulated experiments were continued until 96.7% of the nonsmokers had died. (This occurred at age 95.) At that point, 0.94% of the nonsmokers, 8.18% of the cigarette smokers, and 11.41% of the hypothetical cigarette smokers had died of lung cancer. The mortality ratios were then 1.00, 8.70, and 12.14 for the three groups, respectively.

TABLE 3

PERCENT OF ALL CAUSES AND OF LUNG CANCER AT AGE 80
AND OVER AMONG NONSMOKERS, CIGARETTE SMOKERS,
AND HYPOTHETICAL CIGARETTE SMOKERS

Age X	Nonsmokers % dead before Age X		Cigarette smokers % dead before Age X		Hypothetical Cigarette smokers % dead before Age X	
	All causes	Lung cancer	All causes	Lung cancer	All causes	Lung cancer
40	0	0	0	0	0	0
80	52.2	0.61	76.7	7.35	57.5	9.49
81	56.1	0.68	79.6	7.52	6.12	9.80
82	59.9	0.71	82.2	7.55	64.6	9.95
83	63.5	0.74	85.1	7.73	68.1	10.21
84	67.2	0.75	87.7	7.86	71.6	10.49
85	70.9	0.78	89.8	7.90	74.8	10.59
86	76.6	0.80	92.0	7.99	78.1	10.79
87	78.2	0.84	93.7	8.05	81.3	10.96
88	81.5	0.87	95.0	8.07	84.1	11.02
89	84.6	0.90	96.1	8.11	86.8	11.17
90	87.3	0.91	97.1	8.11	89.1	11.17
95	96.6	0.94	99.6	8.18	97.1	11.41

It is seen from this that the eventual lung cancer mortality ratio for the cigarette smokers would have been overestimated if the experiment had been discontinued before almost all of the subjects had died.

We conclude that an animal experiment, with the stated purpose as described, should not be discontinued until *all* of the animals have died.

You may ask why we discontinued our simulated experiment before that point had been reached. It was simply because we are of the same species as our subjects and older than many of them. We will never see the day when the last remaining one of them dies.

DISCUSSION

Just as animal experiments are carried out to gain insight into the etiology of cancer in man, we carried out two simulated animal experiments (using human beings as subjects) to gain a better insight into the design and interpretation of results of animal experiments with factors which may increase the risk of cancer.

The number of cancers of a particular site or type which eventually occurs in any cohort of animals or (human beings), followed until all have died, depends both upon age-specific death rates for cancer of that site and upon the number of animal-weeks (or person-years) of exposure to risk during each successive interval of time along the survivorship curve. A survivorship curve depends upon age-specific death rates from all causes of death combined. For exposed animals, it is dependent upon the effect of exposure on the total age-specific death rates, not just upon age-specific death rates for cancer of a particular site or type.

There are at least some agents which increase death rates from cancer of more than one site. Therefore, we must admit the possibility that this may be so for any previously untested agent under investigation. If it be so, then this will reduce the total number animal-months of exposure to risk of developing cancer of any one specified site.

We found in our simulated experiments that lung cancer death rates of cigarette smokers increase rapidly with age up to a certain point and then diminish. This may be so for cancers of other sites under some conditions of exposure to various agents other than cigarette smoke. We suspect that whether death rates from cancer of any particular site continue to increase with age or decline after a certain age depends upon dosage and varies with cancer of different sites.

For all of these reasons, we are of the opinion that in animal experiments of the type under consideration: (1) the animals should be retained until every one of them dies; and (2) that judgment of the major results in respect to cancer should be made on the basis of the total number that die of cancer rather than on the basis of the number that die of cancer of any single site or type. Further details such of the distribution of cancers by site, type and age at first appearance are, of course, of considerable interest.

The most difficult problem to cope with is the problem of competitive risk of death from causes other than cancer. Obviously, if a certain high dosage of an agent under investigation kills most of the animals within a few weeks, there is little chance that any of them will die of cancer. For this reason, the usual procedure is to carry out a preliminary experiment to determine the dosage just below which few, if any, animals die within a short time. One group of animals is then exposed to the agent at that dosage while other groups are exposed at lower dosages. Very low dosages are seldom tested because of the large number of animals required to do so.

If a certain moderately low dosage of a previously untested agent is capable of producing cancer, then, until proof is available to the contrary, we must accept the possibility that the same dosage is capable of causing death from causes other than cancer. This could have a considerable effect upon the outcome of an experiment when degree of risk of cancer is judged in terms of mortality ratios. Unfortunately, with small numbers of animals at the start (i.g., less than 100 in each group) so few remain alive at old ages that the long-term effects of exposure may not be apparent. We know of no way to overcome this problem except to use a much larger number of animals.

Discussion

DR. SHUBIK: Thank you. Are there any specific questions addressed to Dr. Hammond's extremely interesting paper?

DR. COULSTON: You know, Dr. Hammond, you have raised what is I think the heart of this meeting. In my lifespan I probably have done at least a 500 two-year animal studies alone, and I can recognize from the things I heard from Dr. Wynder and Dr. Selikoff, and now from you, that we've been doing it all wrong. Let me make a few points.

What we're interested in usually, let's say in the usual two-year rat study, is the rate of the body weight gain and the biochemistry and pathology. We worry about how many animals we have left before the statistical analysis. We count the live ones and the dead ones. We are told by many people that when you get down to 10 or 20% of animals left in the experiment you should terminate the study because you don't have enough animals left to make any statistical evaluation.

As you pointed out, there's a lot more than statistics involved here. It's a question of getting down to the final animal, which is the way I would like to do it, at least to where all the controls may be gone but a few of the animals are struggling on. You pointed out the many parameters that are missing in our usual chronic toxicity test and certainly even in our carcinogenicity test. I think that one of the points that Dr. Clayson should make in the summary tomorrow is a reevaluation of our standard procedures in animal testing to come more to grips with the real world of epidemiology as presented by you three gentlemen. I can see many ways now to improve our so-called long-term animal toxicity studies. I would like tomorrow perhaps to have suggestions from anybody that we can incorporate into the final statement. But I thank you all very much.

DR. SHUBIK: Thank you. I'd like to hear from some of the animal scientists in this room who run these long-term tests. Am I right? Most of the animal people here are now humanized. Dr. Kensler has volunteered to be an animal person.

DR. KENSLER: Actually I wanted to ask Dr. Hammond a question and not praise the animal at the moment. He didn't say that the reason why lung cancer was going up was because stomach cancer was going down, by this numbers game. I wonder why he didn't?

DR. HAMMOND: I think I implied it. I had already gone over my time. One of the reasons why lung cancer, total deaths, I didn't say death rate, had no effect upon death rate, is that the total number of lung cancers is going up while gastric cancer is going down. Now if you really want to see everybody die of cancer, just find a magic pill which prevents stroke, which prevents coronaries, and which prevents cirrhosis of the liver, you will hugely increase the eventual number of people who die of cancer. That doesn't increase their death rate, but they'll live a great deal longer.

DR. COULSTON: That's still one per customer. I think the points that you've made are valid in a sense, but when toxicologists and pharmacologists are trying to compare various materials for potency they pick an end point which is measurable with more or less precision, and they do their dose-response curves and they get the relative potency. Now this gives them an answer in terms of the specific end point, which hopefully is related to the disease or whatever it is they're trying to treat. I think if you reduce the indicence of lung cancer as you go, fine, people are going to die of something else. That is an achievement. A less harmful cigarette would be an achievement.

DR. HAMMOND: A less harmful cigarette is less harmful in terms of coronary disease and this would be a huge achievement, but then more people would die from cancer.

You can do a relative mortality study; the percent of people who die of this, that, and the other thing in a hospital. They started a study at Los Angeles General Hospital a few years ago and they came to the conclusion that Mexicans, principally wetbacks, were practically immune to cancer. So few of them had cancer in the hospital. When you look into it you found they had a very high rate of tuberculosis and that is the reason there were so few cancer cases. Relative mortality does not tell you the answer. It is the change in life expectancy, the average time of test which shows the effect, as far as what most people are most interested in.

Now another thing of some interest, of course, is whether or not death is accompanied by disability and pain. If you're talking about disability you'd better speak of emphysema, and some of those diseases, as well as strokes. If you're talking about pain, cancer is very high on the list. If you're talking about what shortens the life of American men more so than others, talk about coronary disease. Each of these things is valid but I have to tell you this, Charlie (Kensler); you said what you're interested to know is the degree in a toxicological study of the effects, whatever the effect is you're looking for. As far as the effect upon a particular disease is concerned, the degree you get measurement is going to depend upon when you cut off your experiment, and that is arbitrary.

DR. COULSTON: Mr. Chairman, what is coming to the fore in my mind is something that we used to try to do, particularly with higher animals like dogs and monkeys, namely, look at the animals from the point of view that doctors and physicians like yourself look at people. We've gotten away from that now. We look at animals, they die, they live, we weigh them, we do some blood counts, we do some pathology at the end, but we don't know whether they're debilitated in the sense, especially rats and mice, that can occur with individual monkeys or chimpanzees. You can treat these larger animals just like human beings and you can study them like human beings because there are less of them than rats. You can even teach them to tell you whether they're in pain or not—literally communicate with you—because you recognize when they're in pain. It's hard to tell whether or not a rat's in pain, although even there you possibly can. What I'm driving at, and I wish Bill Upholt or Al Kolbye would get into this, is that we're perhaps asking the wrong questions, particularly of our chronic toxicity studies. I'm leaving cancer out of this for the moment. I mean that we're not treating the animals as individuals, we're treating them as mass groups and doing the statistics on the mass groups, rather than studying the individual signs of illness of one kind or another. I would hope that the regulatory people would begin to recognize this now, and if that could come out of this meeting I'd be very happy.

We should go back to the old days when we looked at animals as individuals as one would look at a patient in a hospital. I'd rather have fewer animals and do this, than have a larger number of animals and just play the statistics game and miss the point. Parenthetically, some people who are now treated as patients in hospitals also have the feeling that perhaps they are not treated quite the way they would have been a few years ago.

DR. SHUBIK: Once again I must say that yesterday, having vented my spleen early in the morning and screamed that the meeting was getting off track somehow or other, it seems to have gotten on track once again, and I've never seen so many people so happy after being subjected to this torture of listening to others talk for such a long, long time. An amazing state of affairs, very remarkable, very stimulating, and excellent! I think that we should remember really that all the energy that was put into this by the program committee has really been merited. I really want to make sure that people like Dr. Mahboubi, who sits in the background and takes very little credit for much of this, should really receive our thanks for all he's done in this regard, together with Dr. Clayson.

DR. SHUBIK: The last speaker today on our program is Dr. Morris Cranmer, who also must be congratulated for taking so much trouble and helping provide so much of the assistance for the meeting; I hope he thinks he's getting his money's worth. I somehow think he is. Thank you, Morris.

21. The World-Wide Problem of Chemical Carcinogenesis: Evaluation of Risk and Extrapolation to Man

Morris Cranmer
National Center for Toxicological Research
Jefferson, Arkansas

Before I came here, and then over the last two days, I had prepared about three different talks. Everyone kept removing my slides as I went through the speeches. I have quite a stack over here, and I just want to go through them with random sort of thoughts. What I will try to do is put together some slides and a bit of opinion that might provoke some conversation, and perhaps poke a little fun at some of the things that we do and take quite seriously from time to time.

Well, my topic is "The Worldwide Problem of Chemical Carcinogenesis: Evaluation of Risk and Extrapolation to Man." We left out the "phase of the moon," but it is a rather broad topic. As I came to this conference I asked myself some questions and thought that if we tackled these questions appropriately, the comments, at least for me personally, would be well worth the while.

First question: Is it appropriate that such great attention be given to chemical carcinogenesis, and is the problem of chemical carcinogenesis worldwide or is it limited to chemically industrialized nations?

The second question: Are there methods, now available or reasonably likely to be developed, appropriate for the evaluation of relative risk to human population?

Further, can we extrapolate from high doses in man or in animals to risks at lower doses in man or animals? And, finally, can we extrapolate from animals to man, and what are the current limitations, and what are suggestions for the future?

Well, as I listened to the topics that were discussed by our numerous and excellent speakers, I asked myself first: "What sort of statements could we make about the international distribution of various forms of cancer?"

I don't know whether my chart is very clear, but it's an age-adjusted mortality rate for all malignant neoplasms in various countries. I think if you just wanted to make the point, even accepting the fact that there are many errors in terms of reporting systems and differences in the competing causes of risks, etc., there's a big difference in mortality from country to country.

How does the distribution of cancer by site vary from one country to another? I think the point was well made many different times that there is ample reason to believe a true variation exists from site to site. How do cancer mortality rates from migrants to the United States compare to rates in the countries of origin? This topic was covered very well, and I think it convinced all of us that there is ample reason to use this information.

What epidemiological inferences have been made from the differences in these cancer rates? And I think, of course, discussions of diet and many other factors have clearly hit the point.

How does cancer compare with other diseases as a cause of death in the United States? Well, these are the trends and the incidences of mortality by race and sex in the United States and I think the point has been well made when related to cigarette smoking. There is an increase in white males, and some sort of a decrease in white females, but there is an alarming increase in black males and black females.

Further, how does the occurrence of cancer vary by site? Are there certain trends or inferences that we can be made from this? The one I come away with that is most striking is that there is an urbanization correlation with cancer rates, quite aside from all the various things, whether it's air pollution, industrial chemicals, or life-styles, or drinking too much, or heavier smoking, or whatever. There's a change in the distribution across the United States.

Then the question that I would ask simply in my own mind, at least, since there are these urban-rural differences: What is the probability that a person will die from cancer? Is that changing? I think it is changing, and as our older population of the graying of America phenomenon (if I can borrow from a *Time* magazine cover), certainly is going to be changing, what relationship, for instance, does cancer hold to the other major causes of death in the country? Of course we know that cancer is the second leading cause; it seems to me as the age of the population increases that ratio will ease upward.

I did a calculation relating deaths occurring in an aging population with other types of phenomena that we're, perhaps, a little more familiar with on a personal basis, say, automobile accidents. There is about three times the loss of life in terms of man-years due to cancer as there is from automobile accidents, and although we can debate the accuracy of that statement, I think it's close enough to make the point.

What are the economic costs of cancer now, leaving out the pain and suffering and so forth? The NCI's figures it's about $2 billion if you're looking at direct costs, and maybe $20 billion a year if the loss of productivity and other types of costs are considered.

How much would the elimination of cancer as a cause of death benefit society? Well, there are many ways of looking at this. One of them is again taken from statements of the National Cancer Institute, that the average lifespan of the American people could be increased by about two years. To the individuals who may have cancer, however, the effect is considerably different, and if it happens to be certain cancers that appear early in life, it's a dramatic difference in terms of this effect.

I think the point was made by many of the speakers today and yesterday that the resources allocated to solving the problem of cancer, cancers due to chemicals, and environmental factors are certainly miniscule in comparison to allocations for other types of causes. The point was made time and time again. One thing I thought was that toxicologists have been taking a beating occasionally for alarming people as to rates and effects of some of their animal findings pertinent to the human population. For example, in *Medical News* for May 16 of this year the observation was made of what appeared to be a rather dramatic increase in cancer risk—that it had risen from 167.6 per 100,000 to 176.3. This is an increase of 5.2% in a very short period of time, and it got a lot of people upset. Statements were issued by the Office of the President as well as the federal agencies as to why this was happening. There were recriminations as to whether or not the efforts to cure cancer were correct.

Well, I think if you'll read this article it will give you the reasons for the increase; we had an influenza problem, we changed the mortality rates in certain parts of the population, and we had only 10% of the sample that we were looking at. When we got through with the data, we find, as a matter of fact, that the adjusted rate increase went down just a shade below what they had expected it to be. I wonder if we got equal newspaper coverage of that as we did the other? I somehow missed that; I didn't miss the first statement.

The third area that I think I'd like to talk about is factors associated with high and low risks of cancer: what can we predict? The case against cigarette smoking and the use of tobacco products in general worldwide, is a dead horse and doesn't need to be beaten anymore. I think it is a crying shame that more is not being done about it. I certainly hope that the new types of cigarettes do decrease the problem. It seems to me that this is the largest single thing we can do voluntarily to reduce cancer burdens, and it is a shame that it is not received with greater enthusiasm.

Relation of diet to cancer was emphasized on a number of occasions and again this is an area where we can do something voluntarily, as a society, to change the situation. The same is true of the relation of alcohol to cancer: again voluntary action can modify the effects of cancer on society. Well, I hope that low tar cigarettes decrease the rates of cancer. I think that some the activities regarding diet are going to be a matter of fact, if I may predict what is going to happen. As our fossil fuel supply decreases, as our balance of payments problem increases, and so forth, as the world's population (and a greater proportion of it) is in nutritional distress, I think we'll find it less and less likely that we'll be feeding corn or soybeans to cattle. The cost of the method of fattening beef used in this country probably will increase, and perhaps this will cause some modification of the amount of fat that we eat in the diet. It is a very real probability that economics will enter into this particular area.

Regarding the relationships of occupations to cancer: I think Dr. Selikoff and others have spoken of this and made this point very well, whether we're talking about benzidine workers or asbestos workers or asbestos and smoking. There are a number of areas where we have clear indications that we can in a way extrapolate from higher to lower exposures. We have to take into consideration the time of development of the cancers, but there is this relationship, and we are learning more and more about it.

What I don't see enough of though, is the ability to extract, from the occupationally-exposed populations, data which will be more pertinent to give us guides to broader populational studies. When I started working in the Public Health Service, the idea of utilizing those occupationally exposed to pesticides, of course, received great emphasis. We had a population we could look at. Drawing attention to a population that was discussed by Dr. Selikoff—the chemists and the increased cancer risks to chemists—and since I've spent quite a little bit of time in a laboratory making a whole series of derivatives from some nitrosoquanidine compounds, it does give one some cause for reflection. The fact that lymphomas are so markedly increased in both the ACF study done way back in the 1960s and well as in the new study indicate that this is rather interesting.

Again, though, when I see the effort to put into perspective the changes in rates, I think it's also interesting to note that of the women chemists there was not a large enough population to show the same situation that you could for men, although the women did have a considerably increased breast cancer rate. What went without notice, but I think is important, too, is that they had five times the national suicide rate. This is, of course, an occupational hazard, too! After all, five times the national suicide rate is quite a bit, and putting these things in context from time to time may have some merit as well.

Let me now consider the relation of cancer in animals and to man. Dr. Selikoff used examples and other speakers have used examples of how experimental animals can be predictive of endpoints in man. It is unfortunate that epidemiology is very good at detecting cancers which are very rare, and the animal experiments are very good at generating cancers that are not so rare. If we have angiosarcomas or mesotheliomas or benign liver tumors, these pop out because of the low background rate in the human population. It's unfortunate that we can't then do as well with those cancer types that are of the greatest human importance; that is, for example, breast cancer. The predictive techniques in epidemiology, it seems to me, can draw more on some of the animal experiments that have been done and can be done, although there are great problems. Of course, we've all discussed that.

I think meetings of this type will bring the two groups together. We can interact on how we can design some of the laboratory experiments that would be more pertinent, and then we would be able to answer some of the questions with epidemiological studies in humans.

While I'm thinking about it, let me mention that during the discussion of the birth control pill situation and the increased risk to hepatic cancer, I believe the number that came up was something like 500 excess cases in some 50 million women that were at risk. I don't know if that's exact but it's close enough, and that's an extremely low incidence rate. The power of epidemiological studies then is great in being able to pull this out.

The study on phenobarbital (I'm talking about the type of liver lesions that were observed in experimental animals), involved something like 8,000 persons. If you applied the same criteria that were used for the birth control pills, it would be impossible to detect that incidence rate in a group of this size.

What I'm also thinking about, even though it does leave a bitter aftertaste in my mouth, is that when we're talking about the situation with saccharin, there were approximately 21,000 persons in one study using diabetics and no excess of bladder cancer was found. But at any rate, the resolving power of that particular study, in terms of the way I understand it, was that the resolving power would have detected with confidence a doubling of the bladder cancer incidence. Well, that is not what in most areas would be considered an acceptable risk. I think it is certainly beneficial to demonstrate that there is not a wholesale epidemic going on, and to demonstrate the extent of risk for some individuals who consume exceptionally high quantities of saccharin. I don't think it's as clear-cut as we might like to think; perhaps I will be attacked for making that statement.

Asking the questions, can we predict from high doses in man or animals to risks at lower doses, let's ask some of the reasons why we want to do that. The reasons for risk-benefit analysis are, of course, public health, economic development, employment, and industrial development; there are a number of reasons why we might want to conduct such an analysis. Some of the questions that we might want to ask are (a) Is the agent carcinogenic in animal models? (b) How likely is it to be a human carcinogen? (c) What is the estimated impact on human health? (d) What are the alternatives to the agent? and (e) Are the alternatives carcinogenic?

Thinking back to the hycanthone story, if we're going to extrapolate we have two problems: (1) from the high doses that we use in the toxicology study to low doses in many and (2) extrapolating from our animals to man. We dis-cussed many of the problems with that, and I'm going to bore you by going back over some of them, discussing some of the mathematical sleight-of-hand that might be useful in doing some of those things. Well, going back over some of the things that Dr. Miller, Dr. Conney, and certainly others discussed: What are some of the factors that would modify our detector, our experimental animal? Of course, we have sex, age, nutrition, etc. What are some of the factors that would affect the metabolism, assuming that Dr. Conney has worked out whether it's charcoal-broiled beef or asparagus or cabbage, or whatever it was that happens to be modifying the situation? Again we all can speak about experi-ments in which each one of these factors has had a marked influence on the out-come of the experiment, depending on the drug or compound being studied. And factors influencing the nutrition: what's required? At very high doses of certain compounds you do deplete sinks of compounds that are involved in im-portant detoxification mechanisms, so that you override other types of activity. Certainly there are environmental factors that have to be dealt with; simple things like the temperature of the room can make considerable differences in a lot of studies, including those on carcinogenicity. If you're talking about certain types of endocrine-related end points, we can show that intensity of light in animal rooms changes the related tumor.

Let's take a compound such as Dr. Miller's favorite 2-acetylaminofluorene. You can look at some of the tumor sites that you get in various species, and we can argue about whether there are others, but I think the point is that there is a variety of endpoints from the compound. We know a lot about 2AAF, that the guinea pig does not have the enzymes to produce the N-hydroxy, that the rat has the sulfur transferase, that the female rat does not get liver cancer the same way the male rat does, and that mice get bladder cancer from the compound since they have very little, if any, sulfur transferase. There are these differences.

Let's see, if we want to do this process of predicting, how are we going to do our risk assessment, and what are our techniques, and models going to be, and what assumptions are we going to make? Let's say we're enamored by safety factors, and we are going to use a 10,000-times safety factor. It's exaggerated, but let's, for the point of discussion, see what kind of problem you get into very quickly. If we had zero tumors out of 200 animals, and we placed an 95% upper confidence limit on that, that would be 2.3%. If we divided that by 10,000 (if we wanted to use the compound as a food additive at 10 ppm in the diet) we would have had to test the compound in those animals and get zero tumors in 200 animals at 10% in the diet. That's just the mathematics of the situation, and it simply won't work. Many of the compounds that we want to work with are going to be needed at 10 ppm in the finished product. Then per-cent in the diet of these compounds is going to get us into very deep trouble, regarding safety.

What are some of the common models? The logistic model was spoken about a minute ago, and there's the "one-hit model" which is popular among some persons, as well as the extreme value models; the probit models; there's a whole series of these models. As far as I'm concerned, none of them has an iota of data to suggest that it is more appropriate, than that which has been generated by experimental animals. If we look at two low dose-response curves, we can see the dosage in fractions versus percent tumors. It's practically impossible to separate probits in one hit. I'm taking two extremes of it in a certain range, and that range happens to be the one in which you usually do your experiments. Until you get down to very low levels you're not going to be able to distinguish between them and up at the top, well, it's silly to talk about it anyway, because competing causes of risks of death and other things are so complex in experiments that you can't do it. Linear extrapolation is a method in which you take the upper confidence limit of some value obtained from the animal experiment and which is presumed reasonable to extrapolate from and from this you go to zero. It's easy to do, and it lends itself to the slide rule type of safety setting. It's very easy to interpret how you're going to come out on this, and there is very little ambiguity between one person's doing it and another's. Actually it's going to put us all out of business as toxicologists, because this method eliminates almost all compounds if you presume any upper confidence limit on a reasonable number of animals under test. No excess tumors measured at all on this basis is acceptable. You find that most chemicals cannot be used.

Mantel-Bryan have a model that the FDA is proposing in a sensitivity-of-method document for animal drug residues. It is based on the relationship of distribution: standard deviations to dose. What I want to point to is that, with respect to a number of the least active potent carcinogens the slopes of the curves tend to be pretty steep. Of compounds studied in our laboratory, One compound I'll talk about a little later (2-acetyl aminofluorene) has an enormously steep slope, if you're talking about a fixed point in time as opposed to a time-to-tumor relationship. A conservative approach would be to extrapolate, using a slope of one. The reason for this is that for such items as cigarette smoking, DES, and in some experiments on aflatoxin, the curves tend to have shallow slopes. So you set your risk factor and you then determine permissible uses of the compound. If we consider the probit-logistics of the one-hit model, it develops that for the area somewhere in the 2 to 50% response range (that is those that one could likely conduct in a laboratory with any kind of precision if you take the effective dose for which you're predicting that 1% of the animals will respond) and you use the probit model, then you divide you etio-1 dose by 100 and that will give you a predicted 1-in-100-million response rate. The logistics are that you divide the etio-1 by 100,000 and the one-hit by 1 million; I think the point is obvious that the models differ greatly in terms of what happens at lower doses. Again if we take the Mantel-Bryan plot and the probit analysis, and we go for a none-to-the-hundred-million risk, and I'm going to explain what I mean by that in just a second, we talk about zero out of 50. In other words, if there were no tumors in 50 animals on test, you would take $\frac{1}{1800}$ of that dose and that would be your risk factor for 10^{-8}. If you used a slope of 2 it goes down to $\frac{1}{130}$ of the dose, so you can see how important the choice of slope is. The choice is much more important than at high levels. Again, we're completely blind in being able to suggest which is appropriate. I mentioned that some of these compounds under certain conditions do have shallow slopes.

Another model which Roy Albert, head of EPA's Cancer Assessment Group, is in favor of and has done some work on, is time-tumor models. The chart I refer to now shows the relationship between time and tumor. The slope of this relationship would be derived from formula in which an index of relative carcinogenicity is equal to the dose times time raised to some power. The slope would be the power of time. In these time-to-tumor models, you have to decide whether life-shortening effects, competing risks, log normal, or wide distributions are appropriate. There are all sorts of things on which we're just now generating experimental data so that we can decide whether it's appropriate for a few compounds to be tested in inbred strains of animals, let alone be able to talk about the human population, but at least we're making some progress along those lines.

Let me explain what one in a million means in terms of Mantel-Bryan analysis. The reason I'm bringing this up is because I was having a conversation with Umberto Saffiotti one day, and he said, "My God, Cranmer, you're saying that one in a million is an acceptable risk. That means there would be 200 excess cases of cancer." I said, "No, Umberto, that's not quite what we're saying." What we're saying is that I'm 99% sure that, after I've chosen the most sensitive animal model that I have to work with, and I've placed upper confidence limits on the data that I have, and I assume that there are no other competing causes of death, and I assume that the animal will get cancer, any time during the expected, adjusted survival lifetime for the entire population, there would be no more than one cancer. That's what we're really saying. At the same time you ought to say, "It's my best estimate that nothing is ever going to happen." But the best estimate or the worst case estimate, as I call it, in this instance could really probably differ by a million, 10 million, or 100 million. On some of the stuff that we actually tried out on human data, this suggested that a one-in-a-million risk is approximately equal in the human situation to one excess cancer among all the people who have ever lived on the earth.

Another way of looking at this is to say that it is equivalent to 1-50 millionth of an impact on our cancer situation in the persons alive today. Or, another way to express it might be to say that if this risk were spread over the entire population it would be equivalent to 1 second of increased lifespan. Still another way of looking at it would be to say that if our worst case estimate is indeed true (i.e. not exceeded), and if a certain number of chemicals have an additive rather than a potentiating effect, the presence of 20 such compounds would under this model equal a one-in-a-million risk, and would not contribute as much in terms of gained human life as that of avoiding one fatal automobile accident. I am 99% confident of this. So when we say what one in a million is, it's only fair to explain what we mean by these "worst case analyses." I don't think, at least from the impact that I see of the public understanding of what we're talking about, that we're doing a very good job.

While we're on that particular thought, I wonder if everyone who wrote to the FDA commented on the sensitivity of the methodology and the use of the Mantel-Bryan model and its appropriateness for estimating the slopes and risk factors? The fact is that many people did write in, many of them suggesting that the model was not conservative enough. They said that something like one in 100 million ought to be the risk rate, or that linear extrapolation ought to be used, as well as many other suggestions.

But the point I'm trying to make is that those in this room who have been talking for the last couple of days about real human cancers (for example, what can we do to reduce certain types, what are the relative risks, what confidences can we have in some of these things, etc.) really ought to comment on some of these activities and decisions that are going to influence in a very major way those products that we are collectively going to have available to us.

If we took two approaches, (one is a bioassay approach and one is an experimental approach). What might we do (or what I would like to see us do) at NCTR, and why are we interested in getting a better understanding of the human epidemiological data and guidance from persons in that field for setting up some of our experimental work? I think it's clear that an array that's currently popular, and I think appropriate, involves microbial systems like the Ames system, mammalian cell systems, plus learning something about the metabolism of the compound. We look at various species, perhaps two species of rodents, and perhaps for certain types of compounds we may look at dogs, and for estrogens we're looking at monkeys. We have some modest tumor incidence and latent period data, if it's a positive compound, and then we start making some rough estimates of what might happen in man. Then if this is a compound which has occupational uses, we try to get some human data into the total picture. Now that is the bioassay approach.

Now if you had the experimental approach you'll start by assuming that the compound is a carcinogen, and we have some species comparisons down here including men; let's assume it is a human carcinogen and we're trying to estimate risk and that sort of thing. We can go into the relative types of metabolism and which species might be appropriate. Or, is it an absolute increase in tumors that's important or the shift in the relative risk to a certain type of tumor? For instance, if you're talking about using a tumor count, let's use the mouse liver and tumor count, you might take a very different approach to extrapolation. You would say, what is the excess risk of that mouse or rat to liver cancer that the estrogen study was done on, or what was the excess risk and is that an appropriate excess risk for humans for that same end point? If we had more knowledge about the generation of a particular lesion, rather than just adding up tumors and dividing by some factor, we would be in a better position to predict to man.

What I'm going to ask now is that the epidemiologists take some advantage of some of the studies being done at NCTR. I have put one part of a large experiment up here on the board to consider Dr. Hammond's point about how experiments can be designed in the toxicology laboratory to address some of these particular problems. This experiment had another component which involved 24,164 female mice. You can think of it as an epidemiological study where indeed we're working with animals as nearly identical as we can get. Perhaps, they're not absolutely genetically equal, but they've gone through a minimum of 23 generations of brother-sister mating, and we've done all sorts of things to keep the drift within the breeding colonies minimized: the animals are all receiving the same "feed," etc. They're certainly bred over a period of time. Of course, you don't put that many animals on the experiment in one day. They're not all in one room, obviously, so there are many other types of variables, the positions in the room, for instance, were not the same, so during development their environment was really quite different, so they are different individuals. I would rather not get into quarreling about whether or not they're genetically equal. They certainly are different individuals and we get different distributions. But, in this particular study what we did was to put significant numbers of animals on a compound and then after six months of treatment we removed the compound, keeping groups for serial sacrifices in a lifespan study. We have another group which we set aside for the first six months and then put them on the compound for six months, and then went through the serial sacrifices. Another group was reserved for 12 months; then we put them on the compound for six months and then we went through the rest of it. The point of all this is that we try to adjust some way to make some statement about the relative sensitivity with age of the ability of this compound to produce cancer. I'm not talking about whether older animals are given a compound and they run out of time because of old age so you get fewer cancers and say young animals are more sensitive. This is the type of approach we are trying to make and the experiment was done successfully. That you can get drift in your colony is very true. A study was done on our breeding colony, starting off with 8 breeding pairs. Some of them were within 95% confidence limits and the other numbers were less than that. What we have here is a family tree, and the breeding group, within a relatively short period of time of three years, begins to drift. There are differences in the population for lung lesions. The point is you can get these shifts, within a closed population.

Let me summarize my points here. I think some facts have come out during the last couple of days. Cancer is currently the second leading cause of death and it's going to probably increase as the population ages. The population *is* aging. In my opinion, the turning point is early retirement and the escalating costs of cancer treatment which will increase the societal costs of cancer, and therefore, more than ever justify the resources that are going into it. I think most environmental influences affecting the major human cancers should be voluntarily controlled,—alcohol, cigarette smoking, modifications of diet, and other types of activities, which could have tremendous impacts on our cancer burden. Efforts to reduce these exposures voluntarily, I think, are going to run into tough times just like cigarette smoking. I really believe that occupational carcinogenesis will decrease, given enough time. I think the asbestos situation is a wave that we're going to be waiting on, but the "act" in many industries is certainly being cleaned up and the worker exposures, for instance, to some of the aromatic amines that occurred not very often, hopefully will be a situation much reduced in the future. Carbonization is going to increase and if there are true risks associated with that increase, we're going to get increased cancers. Dietary influences due to excess animal fat and protein will decrease, I think, because of the lack of availability, for economic reasons. I think the impact of natural products may very well increase.

If you remember during the era of the oil embargo and the big grain sales to Russia, there was a significant increase in the amount of aflatoxins and other types of natural toxicants in the food supply; as we run out of convenient fossil fuels to dry these farm products properly, there's every reason to believe that mold growth will increase. In addition, our farming practices, which are very, very energy-dependent, may be changing considerably in the future.

The majority of chronic studies are conducted on compounds which represent little relative cancer risks to man. I'm talking about the toxicologists now. We spend most of our time testing compounds that most of us really believe are going to turn out quite negative and so our resources are not allocated toward where the problem is. Perhaps the societal reasons for doing it that way are valid and that is a fact. Epidemiology and related techniques are improving. International comparisons are improving, record linkages will remain in my opinion a major problem. I can't see it getting anything but worse in the United States with the privacy act, and the availability of trained epidemiologists is going to be rate-limited. Major gains in cancer prevention, I think, are going to really await changes in societal attitudes toward many of these issues. I would like to see an increased effort in occupational epidemiology with respect to gleaning from these high exposure groups some information that would allow us to compare with our animal models with greater accuracy.

So what are some of the future trends that I would pick up from listening to the comments over the last couple of days? Voluntary societal activity will remain the number one item that could be changed to modify cancer risks. Inhalation smoking and the use of tobacco products may go down a little bit, but probably the impact of cigarettes which are less hazardous would have a greater effect. Alcohol abuse is certainly going to continue. There's a suggestion, of course, that it's increasing. Dietary excesses, whether we're talking about excess spices or excess consumption of total calories or excess consumption of fat, or whatever, will certainly continue. Things like sunbathing, although not chemical, have to be considered. I wonder about exposure to ultraviolet light, because there is a risk associated with that; if there is also exposure to a number of other types of chemicals, I wonder whether some type of interaction wouldn't be possible. We worry about nitrosamines all the time, and there are nitrosamines in suntan lotion, with a potential for producing cancer. In terms of the second area I think, nutrition, the natural toxicants and the decomposition-condensation products of cooking our foods, preparing them, storing them, and modifying them for palatability will be the second major thing that we could do; in other words, modify our eating habits.

The third major are that I see in the future as a problem is fossil fuels. Our change from petroleum products and natural gas to coal gasification will produce all sorts of interesting products resulting from these reactions which we know very little about, but we should be extremely suspicious about them. The increased urbanization with respect to point source is going to remain a problem. It seems to me drugs will remain a problem, and one of our choices of this risk versus that risk is made for very good reason. I think environmental chemicals and the DDT or the PBB business is going to fall down below that, in terms of what the actual impact on man would be. Occupational hazards to the total population, I think, will decrease in terms of its cause of excess cancers, but will remain very high for persons who happen to be in particular occupations. And medical treatment, I think, is going to influence the cancer rates. As we decrease the risk of other types of competing diseases, we're going to increase the risk of cancer; again, I want to emphasize that we will have an aging population.

All of these points could stimulate some conversation. Whether you agree with me or not I don't know, but at least I'll be a nice sounding board to throw rocks at.

I'm discouraged personally that there is so much that we might be able to do in terms of reducing cancer that could be accomplished voluntarily, and it seems to me the proper amount of effort is not being placed on it. Also I'm discouraged as a toxicologist that we're allocating a disproportionate amount of our effort on compounds that don't count. The third thing is, and I hope this meeting will be something that will bring about a great change in that, that there is not enough interaction between toxicologists and epidemiologists to come up with real ways to estimate risk rather than using some mathematical sleight-of-hand. Thank you very much.

Day Three—Afternoon Discussion

DR. SHUBIK: Dr. Cranmer's paper is open for discussion. Dr. Conney.

DR. CONNEY: In pharmacology a lot of work has been done over the past two or three decades relating plasma levels of drugs to pharmacological activity. There's been very little of this done in terms of carcinogens in animals. For instance, what sort of plasma concentration of the parent compound and metabolites relates to the carcinogenicity of the compound? I think that there's a need for more of these kinds of studies as well as asking the same kinds of questions in epidemiology studies, that is, what kinds of plasma concentrations and metabolites are related to carcinogenic risk in the human population? There's been an attempt at these kinds of studies relating concentrations of aflatoxin in food in Africa to liver tumors in a population. By doing these kinds of studies, I think it will be possible to get an idea of the sort of risk associated with the concentration of carcinogen and metabolites, hopefully in plasma rather than in food.

I think that the relationships will be more meaningful, if one can do this in plasma or in biological fluids from the patient. I think that the methodologies now are getting sensitive enough so that one can attempt to do this. One can measure, for instance, nitrosamine concentrations in human plasma, and I think that this is an area that should be explored a great deal more. I was interested in Dr. Selikoff's presentation measuring concentrations of the PPB's, and I think that more of these kinds of studies which follow populations and put in the extra parameter of plasma concentration would be well worthwhile, both in experimental animal studies as well as in the human studies.

DR. CRANMER: Well, I guess, plasma concentrations would be a step in the right direction. I'd like to know the concentration of the true percentage at the target site, whether the compound is taken in continuously, whether there are pulse changes—and if we're talking about certain types of compounds we've been discussing in the last few days such as estrogens, for instance—the prolactin-estrogen ratios would be the important thing.

Certainly we should get the information as to how much is there and where it is. I don't think anyone would argue with you. But the ratio between the parent compound, necessarily, and what's causing the carcinogenic effect may not be too significant.

DR. CONNEY: You're absolutely right. One can't just measure the parent compound. One has to measure metabolite(s) as well and hopefully measure the metabolite as an end product of activation. One has to know, really, two things in humans as well as in animals: What the concentration of the parent compound is in the organism, the animal or the human and second, what assessment can be made regarding metabolic activation and detoxification? I think that both aspects are important. There are ways of getting at these questions that I think can be applied both in animals and in humans.

DR. KENSLER: I've been working in the cancer chemotherapeutic area as some of you know, and we've been developing a great deal of pharmacokinetic information, such as plasma levels, half-lives, and so on. For example, for chemical which was mentioned the other day as a carcinogenic agent in mice, the plasma half-life of *that* was about 30 seconds. It's very, very rapidly removed. And I would say fine, there may be some things (estrogens, and so on) where this can be useful, but I suspect in most cases it wouldn't be. What we really need to know is what you alluded to, namely, what molecular species reside in the tissues or cells where the neoplastic changes occur? If we can find this out, we'd be in a much better position than is likely to happen, just from plasma levels.

DR. UPHOLT: I feel compelled to point out that in the discussion about extrapolation that Morris gave, there is little resemblance to the way we use it in EPA, and if you can bear with me a couple of minutes I'd like to describe very briefly how we attempt to use risk extrapolation. What Morris described in terms of risk extrapolation tended to be simply a method of arriving at a negligible risk. If this is the objective, I submit that a safety factor over a no-observed-effect level probably would give you an accurate estimation of a negligible risk.

In contrast, what we're trying to do is to estimate a risk that can be weighed some way or other against a benefit. To do that you start on an entirely different approach. The first thing you have to describe is the population at risk. We are not talking about trying to get to a risk of one in a million or one in some other particular level. We are trying to describe the population that is at risk at the present time. Then we must make some sort of an estimate of what exposure is that population is receiving. If we have that much information, then we use the extrapolation in an effort to estimate what the risk is at that level of exposure. You see we have now reversed the independent and dependent variables, compared with the way Morris mentioned.

We do not take, nor are we looking for, the dosage that produces a definite risk. We are looking for the risk that is produced by an exposure that we're actually working with in the field. We do this by two or more extrapolation models, because we don't have sufficient confidence in any one model. Morris suggested, as I recall, that Roy Albert prefers, and he implied that EPA prefers, a time-to-tumor model. It is true that Roy Albert has promoted this approach; in fact, I guess he's a leader in this area and he is in fact the chairman of our Carcinogen Assessment Group. On the other hand, he has stated in testimony in a public hearing recently that he does not believe, and that we do not believe in EPA, that time-to-tumor models are anywhere near as acceptable at the present time as some other models are, so we have not yet used that particular model in EPA, even though we would hope to move that way in the future. What we have done so far is to use at least a one-hit theory, and if we can use a second model (we try to use always two models as a minimum) it is most apt to be a log probit with a slope of experimental data, if we have any reasonable estimate of slope. If not, we would use the slope of one, as Mantel and Bryan did. Having used these two or more models, and knowing the size of the population, we come up with not one, but two or more estimates of numbers of cancers that may be occurring in that population at that level.

Now the question is: How much can we reduce this through our regulatory action? Generally speaking, we do not expect to eliminate it. We can eliminate it only if we ban the manufacture of the substance. As long as any level of that substance is in the environment, there continues to be some risk, and therefore any action we take will do somewhat less than eliminate it, so that the estimate of the number of cases is the maximum that we could obtain by regulatory actions.

I can give you one example that I happen to remember although the figures may not be exactly accurate, the situation of chloroform in drinking water. By using a one-hit theory, by monitoring the water supplies across the United States, we analyzed for chloroform. It was admittedly a small sample, but it was all we could do in the situation that we were faced with. We then counted the number of people who drank water from those chlorinated supplies, and assumed that each person drank two liters a day. We had an exposure level in a given sized population, and using the one-hit theory, going through the mathematics, we came out with a figure of something like 700 or maybe up to 7,000 cancers that might occur and might be prevented assuming they did occur. We talked only about the total number of tumors in the experimental animals in the studies on carcinogenicity of chloroform. We talked about the total number of tumors based upon the experimental animals on which we based our carcinogenistic scoreboard. What we figured—in any way you look at it, even if we could eliminate all the chloroform in the drinking supplies which we knew we could not do, but even if we could—would be the maximum number of cases of cancer that we could anticipate preventing by eliminating chlorination of drinking water.

A second model was the log probit with the slope of the experimental data coming out to a fraction so small that our statistician wanted to call it zero, but I objected to that. We knew that such a model did not give you a zero figure, so that's what it was. It came out to something like one cancer in 3½ million years.

When you give those two figures, and we presented that to the administrator of EPA to show him the maximum benefit we could achieve, what the maximum reduction in risk was that we could achieve through stopping chlorination, and then also described to him the cost to society of precipitously giving up chlorination in terms of increased risks of infectious diseases, the administrator immediately realized he had no choice. There is no way in which we could eliminate chlorination at this time, and he so stated publicly the reason why. This is but one example. Now obviously we looked at alternatives, and there were alternatives, and I won't go into all the details of that. But this is one example of the way we do it.

DR. CLAYSON: I would like to speak, not at length but briefly, to Dr. Kolbye. I passed from a stage of extreme sadness to one of outstanding rage when I heard about these extrapolations. In fact, I was going to suggest to you after the session this afternoon that (a) we've been very lucky that we haven't had too many biostatisticians here to press this extrapolation; and (b) possibly in conjunction with the other regulatory agencies, you might think of passing a form of regulation on the amount we're allowed to extrapolate, from various data. I would suggest to you that this regulation should be reasonable and that those known as scientists should be allowed a 500-fold extrapolation, which is 500-fold more than I was allowed when I was a schoolboy. Regulators will be even more kind to him and allow him 5,000-fold, whereas for statisticians who don't make their livelihood out of it, we might even allow 5 million-fold.

Quite seriously, when we look at our data and, if I can just draw something on the board very quickly to show you what I mean, this is one tumor in 10^n population. This is really where we have our experimental data, going down to 1%. Dr. Cranmer will explain to you the process of going down to 1%, the break point, and the real measure is, probably, somewhere around there. All this is extrapolation.

Now we know that we haven't got complete confidence in our animal data. We put in 95% confidence curves and they all promptly appear something like that. And with the modifying factors, which we briefly discussed at this meeting, it might vary anywhere all over the place. A 1% control tumor incidence, somebody suggested might pinch the confidence limit somewhere near the edge. I think, when you're dealing with a population of 10^8, one sees that the degree of pinch would be very small indeed.

Realistically, I think it's a waste of time. Now I don't want to be purely destructive, but I think the people working on the mechanisms of carcinogenesis, in fact, give us possible clues on how we might get out of this. I would hope in the next few years it would be possible to define mechanistically the critical stage in carcinogenesis. It should then conceivably be possible, with some of them at least, to follow the effective dose on these, further down. For example, does DNA repair become progressively more efficient as the dose of the insult is reduced? Is it a chance of interaction with a critical target reduced in a linear fashion, as in one of these models, or is it reduced in a threshold fashion as the amount of the active agent is reduced? I think if we ask that sort of question later on, and it has been suggested recently for metabolic activations and toxicology in general, we might be able to come out with some rather more meaningful answers within our animal data, possibly, even when we come to extrapolate across the species boundaries from our experimental animals to man. What we're doing at the moment is politically expedient, but don't let's pretend we're doing something scientific even if the biostatisticians tell us it's wonderful.

DR. CRANMER: I'd like to comment, if I may. I agree with much of what David has said. I'd just like to repeat one thing that I mentioned in my talk. The distinction between utility and validity with respect to some of these models, I think, may have some painful utility in very limited application. Please don't interpret that I am satisfied with even those limited applications of the model. I am fighting, at least within FDA, to avoid having people like the commissioner using mathematical models to estimate risk of incurring human cancer, for example from saccharin. You know that bothers me, that blows my mind.

I'd also like to comment that I feel we too frequently get caught up in a two-dimensional analysis of the association between exposure to a substance and the response. If we're down at low levels and responses occur, something is occurring to a much greater degree with susceptibility. I don't mean to talk down to you; I'm sure you're thinking about this more than I am, but there are some ways perhaps to control cancer by modifying the modifiers and the promoters, some of which may not be labeled at all as carcinogens. If we're going to go chasing every electrophile that's probably out there naturally or artificially in our environment, we're getting nowhere.

DR. HAMMOND: I'd like to comment briefly, mainly to congratulate Dr. Cranmer on some excellent work he's doing. Listening here, it seems to me in this particular area we're working in, specifically on animal experiments, the thing we most urgently need now is the improvement of efficiency of the animal model. There's a limited number of personnel, there's a limited number of dollars, and we have to see how to get the most out of both, whether we test 1,000 agents very crudely and sloppily, or whether we test one agent thoroughly, or whatever we do. But what I'm getting at, I think, is the experiment on a very large scale that Dr. Cranmer was speaking of, together with examining epidemiologic evidence very carefully. I wish to emphasize the need for bringing in some actuaries into this, because disregarding the age at which exposure is likely to occur may cover up the total dosage anybody is apt to get. This is something that starts in utero, as it might with saccharin; that's one thing in a cumulative lifetime dosage. If you started somebody going to work as a chemist at 25 or 30, that's something quite different. Now, I would think that with the experimental model that Dr. Cranmer told us about, plus epidemiologic evidence, plus a good hard look at our age distribution in the population as it is now and it's likely to be, then we can make much better use of the facilities and personnel we have in this field than we can at the present time. I think this is quite urgent.

I believe, Dr. Cranmer, you told me they were giving very high priority to this certain theme, did I misquote you on that? I think this should go down as one of the most important things in this meeting.

DR. SHUBIK: I would just like to add that Dr. Wynder's stress on metabolic epidemiology, I think, is extremely important, and I think we need a much better understanding of what the metabolic epidemiology is in humans and then start looking for more appropriate approaches in the experimental animal.

DR. COULSTON: You know, I appreciate very much what Dr. Upholt has told us, and it's an honest effort by both him and his colleagues at EPA to do something about a very difficult subject. How do you set a limit? The fact that with chlorination, they came up with the conclusion they did (which I think they had to come up with, socioeconomically) shows that at least they can make a decision based on whatever mathematics they use. This I think is important, and in this case I think we all agree they came up with the right answer: not to go to charcoal filtration, which would cost $100 billion in this country. I don't think we have $100 billion to spend on this. We can go to it gradually.

The other point I want to make: one of the great fallacies in this calculation is that they are assuming that the mouse or the rat or the hamster predicts for man, and we have no basis for this prediction, especially in these cases. So it's again a half-baked guess at what could be a good solution.

The second and most terrible thing to me goes now with what David Clayson said, and I couldn't agree with him more: that sloppy line that he talked about is even more sloppy, and probably not even existent, for all the reasons that we talked about, repair mechanisms, and so on. But even worse than that, since we put it on a log-dose basis, you can never get to zero because zero is one. You can never extrapolate down to zero and say, "Well, there is a dose which is absolutely safe." Dr. Henry Wills, who is here, and I once put together a paper on radiation in which we clearly showed that this is the wrong way to do it, other techniques such as log probits or whatever you want should be used, but there is a way to get away from the horrible dilemma of never getting back to zero, no matter how you extrapolate.

DR. KENSLER: I think there's another problem here; it's the high dose levels where metabolic pathways may yield molecules which you do not get at low levels. It might not even be testing the right thing. For example, we had Perry Gehring's ethylene glycol metabolism stuff mentioned earlier. Whereas at low levels it all goes to CO_2, at the higher dose levels you start to pile up oxalate. Now we're again, with industry's support, attempting a definitive study on the pharmacokinetics and metabolic pathways of methylene chloride, so that as you go down in the dose, in the ratio of CO to CO_2, some of the intermediates change. Hopefully, when this experiment is tested it won't be tested in this routine screen, which then becomes definitive for saying something's a carcinogen or not. But, we will have appropriate dose levels and appropriate metabolic information so that we may make some reasonable judgments as to the levels of risk.

DR. SELIKOFF: In this orgy of iconoclasm in this last hour I thought the apex was delivered by Fred (Coulston), and I don't hear any contradiction. Does the animal model have any relevance to human disease? If not, we're wasting a lot of time, a lot of money, a lot of good scientists, and a lot of good space at NIH.

DR. KENSLER: Well, I think Fred was so much on his own in that regard that it didn't seem to me worthwhile commenting on it. Frankly, I think that if you were to take a vote, you wouldn't find that he had a terribly large amount of backing in saying that mice, rats, and hamsters have no relevance to human disease. Can we have a vote on that? That's what you said.

DR. SELIKOFF: He really implied that they were not always relevant.

DR. COULSTON: Let me make it clear again. You know in the old days, Dr. Selikoff, you remember very well, as all of us do, that man was the test animal. We studied chemicals in man. Even as recently as 1940 the FDA never required more than a 30-day rat study and a couple of dogs to be tested to see if the dogs got sick or died. The key point is, we've become so highly sophisticated now, Dr. Selikoff, that we do not accept such a simple thing as a 30-day rat test and experience in man any longer. How do you think Demerol was discovered? How do you think neosynephrine or neoarsphenamine was discovered? A few rats, a few dogs, and the scientists went right to man. I'm not saying that was correct, but they discovered a lot of fine drugs which still exist today.

The point is we've become so sophisticated now that we are not sure of ourselves any longer; we don't want to try out things directly on man. Yet, you know I could study chemicals in man, 999 times out of 1,000 and get away with it. If I just started in man with low doses and gradually built them up, I wouldn't hurt anyone. But, I'd probably kill one in a thousand, and that's why this shouldn't be done.

The fact is, we've become so highly sophisticated with rats, mice, dogs, hamsters, monkeys, and chimpanzees in the studies on radiation and radioactive materials. We have come to genetics and mutagenicity, and we haven't stopped yet. There are going to be many, many more things down the road that we're going to use in order to prove safety. It's tough enough to prove efficacy, let alone proving safety. What I'm trying to say is, that we should resolve the problem by asking ourselves, "Is the rodent or the hamster predicting something to man?" and then spend our time trying to find that out. Now if it isn't, let's use a monkey or a dog.

Let's do the metabolism studies which tell us whether these animals are truly handling the chemical like man. We've heard no discussion of that in this meeting, by the way. But that's what happens when toxicologists get together. I'm simply trying to say that this is all guess, and as David Clayson said, we shouldn't put too much faith in it; yet I don't know how to do it better.

DR. SELIKOFF: I think we have to agree with you.

DR. CLEMMESEN: The only point I'd like to make is that I see very few epidemiological studies that can deal with more than, say, two competing factors, and that's going to be the shock in epidemiology. Do we go any further, and we are very often amiss?

DR. WYNDER: You know those of us in preventive medicine have a disadvantage in that it takes a long time for the psyche to know whether we've been right or wrong. And this is one advantage that our colleagues in therapy have; they know quite often whether they are right or wrong right away; unfortunately, mostly wrong.

I reflect that I've been in cancer research 30 years. I heard similar discussion 30 years ago, and during these 30 years lung cancer has continued to increase, so we have not been very effective. Although we have known the major causes sometimes, stomach cancer has gone down, and we have not really willingly or knowingly contributed to that. Breast cancer has gone up in incidence, and so has colon cancer. The fact is, we have related to life-style variables which we have discussed very little. I certainly agree with Dr. Kolbye that modifying factors are very important. I would like to end up on this point of caution: If nothing else, economics will force us to assign priorities. At the current time 8.6% of our GNP goes for disease care. Health care cost $40 billion in 1976, and it is estimated it will be 10% of our GNP by 1980, or $200 billion. So you say, what does it mean to us? What it means to us is that there is only so much money available for health care activities, and I can assure you that if we don't watch out, more and more will go into therapy; we already know this at the National Cancer Institute, because much of the money goes into therapy and therefore less money is available for fundamental and preventive research. Therefore, if for no other reason, we'd better very carefully select our priorities, those that are likely to have the highest payoff, and as I mentioned in my talk, the highest payoff is certainly related to the major cancers of which we already know the major causes. I think we ought to concentrate on those.

A final point. There are only so many good scientists and cancer research workers available in this country. Too many scientists work in areas that are too erudite and not really related to the major public interest; sufficient scientists are not available for the major causes. I believe that we as scientists should have not only in mind our own curiosity but should really relate our efforts to those cancers that do in the most of us.

DR. SHUBIK(?): Dr. Upholt is going to address us for approximately a minute or less.

DR. UPHOLT: I think I can keep it to less than a minute. I completely agree with Dr. Clayson that extrapolation is unscientific. I would suggest that much of the other extrapolation we've been talking about this week is unscientific as well. I would agree with Dr. Coulston that there is little alternative for the regulatory agencies except to go beyond science. Unfortunately, scientists do not give us a zero level or a no-risk level; therefore, I hope that as scientists you will continue to provide us some dosage-response information, and some basis upon which we can move toward a quantification of risk so that instead of making our decisions purely on the basis of what the attorneys interpret or what the public demands, we can begin to give a little bit of quantification to both risk and benefit. Thank you.

DR. COULSTON: Hear, hear!

DR. KERST: I don't know how you worked that out. I am Fred Kerst from Velsicol Chemical Corporation, and I'm not going to make some comments I would like to make. I want to ask one question, and possibly somebody could have some of this information tomorrow. Both Drs. Wynder and Cranmer have reflected and indicated the allocation of resources toward the problems associated with the incidence of cancer. I would assume that somebody in this group, or somebody in this nation at least, has the information that would indicate or suggest the resources available to allocate for the various problems. I could predict with some knowledge, where I think the bulk of it's being put, but I would like to avoid doing that. Possibly some can by tomorrow morning quantify some of this. But if no one can, I'd like to pick up and make a few comments then on how we're misappropriating our resources and why, and I'll do it on a qualitative basis if someone can't quantify it. So I'll stop there.

22. Overall View of the Conference

Frederick Coulston

DR. CLAYSON: I think it's time that we should start our wrap-up session. I know that some of you want to go out and see the very exciting primate colony, some 6 miles away on the military base. We would like, if we can, to finish this meeting by 10 o'clock this morning.

What I'm hoping we'll be able to do is that Dr. Coulston will give an overview, Dr. Clemmesen will speak about the epidemiology, and then we'll open this meeting for comments from the floor. I will try to make a brief summary of some of the things which impressed me during the last three days. So I'd like to ask Dr. Coulston if he would state his feelings about what we have achieved and what we've omitted during the last three days.

DR. COULSTON: Thank you.

This part of the meeting is the best part really, where we can all voice our opinions and more or less say what we think about what we've accomplished in the past two or three days. Certainly, I feel it's been a successful meeting; we have accomplished something which according to Dr. Hammond, Dr. Wynder, and Dr. Selikoff has never been done before, and I'm quoting them. Epidemiologists have met and discussed safety evaluation of problems together with toxicologists, biochemists and pathologists. Dr. Hammond told us yesterday that there's nothing new about this meeting: he tried it 25 years ago, but it accomplished nothing. The toxicologists tried to impress everybody that they knew all the answers, and the epidemiologists did the same thing, and they got nowhere. This meeting, I think, has accomplished something very remarkable in the sense that some of us have seen more clearly what we can do in toxicology along the lines of what the epidemiologist does.

This to me is a breakthrough. I think that in the future some of us will perform more meaningful chronic toxicity studies, and the question is whether we can convince the scientists and the regulatory agencies that that is the correct way to go.

It means to me that the epidemiologist will give more of his time to the problems of the animal experimentalists vis à vis the setting up of experiments. They will contribute more than just say, "Oh, you don't have enough monkeys in this group to be statistically significant, two years from now," or "You ought to add 25 rats per group, males and females." The real help we need is to try to understand what we're doing, particularly with "hindsight" chemicals, old chemicals, relating our animal experimentation to the human experience. The toxicologist is limited, he's very limited, in the interpretation of animal data to man. As many of you know, there are centers where we have carried animal studies of chemicals to man. It's a tribute to the FDA that, as long ago as 1964, they requested from our Institute that we not only study compounds in animals, but that we take these compounds to man (methoxychlor, parathion, cyclamate and many others, just to use a few examples).

The first real attempt to relate animal toxicology to man was sponsored by the Food and Drug Administration. Some of these chemicals were pesticides and a few were food additives.

The fact is that these animal and human studies can be done and are still going on. There is no reason why chemicals should not also be tested in man, if great masses of the population are to be exposed to these chemicals, just as we do with drugs. I certainly think a food additive, before it is allowed on the market, should have some testing in man. In general, we go from dogs and rats and put the additive out in the general population and just hope for the best. It is a dreadful mistake to do this, and I've always thought this way. There are procedures to evaluate the safety of compounds, even chlorinated hydrocarbons and cholinesterase inhibitors, in a limited number of people to make sure that the chemical is generally safe, even if the specific details of toxicity to man are unknown. At least you're not going to cause a toxicological calamity, and it's essential, I think, that somehow we get some information in man. Now you can get to safety evaluation in man in many ways, and we discussed these in this meeting. We can study the factory environment where the chemicals are being made. We can study the vicinity where the smokestack of the factory pours out chemical substances into the community. We can get to man by epidemiological studies. Unfortunately, you can only do that with compounds that have been around for a while, and where large numbers of people have been exposed. The epidemiologist needs to figure out ways to do his studies on small populations as well as on large ones. Peter Greenwald would have said, "I must have 100,000 people (cases) or I won't touch it." But, it seems to me, studies can also be done on 600 people or less, if that's all they can find exposed to a chemical. The epidemiologist must work out methods to do this. The average epidemiologist wants large numbers of people in order to validate statistically small changes that may occur. But, perhaps, we should worry about the qualitative rather than the quantitative changes, at least that could establish some degree of safety. Dr. Shubik spoke about the statement of the problem and put it just about as well as anyone. We can do so much in animals, but we need to learn how to interpret what goes on when we extrapolate to man.

Dr. Conney presented his own wonderful work and that of his colleagues, and he delineated the kind of changes that can occur with carcinogenic and non-carcinogenic agents, the relationship of various subcellular biochemical actions, as well as subcellular organelles, to the formation of cancer. He pointed out very clearly that there was hope in the future to develop some sort of chemical system that might be antidotal to set into equilibrium and normalize a carcinogenic activity. To me that's a dream, but a very important dream, and we wish him well in the future.

Dr. Herman Kraybill actually said some things which I think are very startling. Of course, the statement that sticks in my mind the most is that there was actually an experiment using the maximum tolerated dose and half that dose, which utilized in one rat study the total animal production of that chemical in the United States. I think this points out the ridiculousness of a-priori setting doses in a cookbook fashion. Herman did a magnificent job of pointing out this fallacy. Of course, he said many other things and I could paraphrase almost everything he said, but it is sufficient to point out his key and cardinal rule: Select the dose for the animal study based upon the intended use of that chemical in our society, which is usually known by scientists. Extrapolate from that dose a safety factor suitable for that chemical. For example, if you were simply going to add an antioxidant to a food material, obviously you'd have to have a safety factor that's very high, maybe even a hundred times, based upon the intended and correct use dose of that chemical. But if I were going to work with an alkylating agent such as an anticancer drug, if I took even a 10 times safety factor, I'd kill every animal; with some of the agents even twice the use dose would kill every animal. You cannot set a guideline, you have to interpret every chemical and every chemical group for the purposes of your test. That to me was one of the highlights of the meeting. Dr. Kraybill and others talked about changes in the current carcinogenic testing along these lines.

Dr. Klein, presenting Dr. Korte's paper, raised some very pertinent issues which Dr. Miller discussed later; namely, he made the statement that it's very difficult for them to convince themselves that covalent binding exists, and that in their case they could find only one real reference to a covalent binding situation that seemed chemically real enough. Now this, of course, is exceedingly important. If what they say is correct, and I assure you this is open to much question, then one of the basic tenets of how carcinogenesis occurs has to be re-examined. These men are good organic chemists, some of the best in the world. We should listen to them.

Dr. Gingell discussed in great detail the metabolism of DDT and some other compounds in different animal species. He made some very important points, particularly that, depending on the animal species, there were differences in metabolism, and how you relate this to man is, of course, the issue.

Dr. Mohr, an outstanding pathologist, with a worldwide reputation, told us about his work and his interesting new techniques of putting chemicals in the trachea, as well as by inhalation and by oral administration. The point that he was making is that depending on the way that the chemical was administered, he could find lung lesions or he could not find lung lesions. This was a very important contribution in a very difficult area, namely, inhalation toxicology. One of his key points was the nature of the lesion as developed, based upon the route of administration. He clearly showed that many compounds if given orally produced no effect, and if even given by inhalation produced little or no effect, but if they were actually put down the trachea, they would produce effects.

Dr. Jim Miller gave an outstanding presentation. He certainly paved the way for the understanding of relationships between animal and man. His discussion of electrophiles and their counterparts—what did you call them, nucleophiles?—is an important consideration, and leads again to the hope that someday we can do something about not just chemical carcinogens but perhaps the cause of all cancers. Dr. Miller discussed at great length the paper of Dr. Klein and Dr. Korte and made it clear that he believes in covalent binding, but he also presented some data from some other people where another method not involving covalent binding led to carcinogenesis; I think that's important. I don't like all-or-none theories; usually, you find an exception to them, and it's the exception that usually leads to the truth. You try to find out why this is the exception, and perhaps this can lead to another paramater and a new theory.

Dr. Conney then talked about polycyclic hydrocarbons in carcinogenesis and the role of metabolism and presented evidence that these compounds are handled differently in different species. He made again the contribution that it is important to understand the underlying basic principles of how the chemical is handled, bound, excreted, secreted, and stored in the body of a mammal. Further, he made some predictions relating to how these same reactions would occur in man.

Dr. Clayson talked about animal studies and gave us the kind of background that he does so well and admirably. Dr. Clayson showed us many ways in which carcinogens can be studied, and he pointed out very clearly the various parameters of human cancer and how these can be studied. We owe him a great debt of gratitude.

I guess one would say that Dr. Mays's program was the hit of the show, because of his kodachromes, showing not just the beauty of the model before surgery, but also the beauty of the scar after surgery. All surgeons are proud of how they can perform their surgery and end up with a good scar that's not too objectionable.

Dr. Mays's paper to me was very important for toxicologists. I knew about this story, I'd heard about it from many people, particularly Phil Shubik, but to see the actual presentation of the effect of certain estrogens and the gory kodachromes, if you will, was indeed a shocker. For one thing the lesions that he described, if common in the population, should have led the FDA to ban all contraceptive pills by now. But there are mitigating factors. Most of these liver lesions, as he pointed out, occurred with one kind of drug, in other words, the estrogen-progestin combination effect appears to be related to its content of a certain type of chemical. This does not paint with a bad brush all of these drugs and combinations. Second, the incidence of these lesions in women makes one wonder why they were not found more nationwide or worldwide and why so many were picked up in his area to begin with, although they are occurring in other areas, I hasten to add. But there were many questions that were raised. The fact is that this is an unusual lesion to find, and certainly much thought has to be given to its relationship to animal carcinogenic-type studies and toxicologic studies, in general.

Dr. Shellenberger showed very well the role of estrogens and animal cancer and went into great detail presenting the data; it's clear that for many chemicals, the animal—the rat particularly—is a good species to work with, and another as we know, is the nonhuman primate. The dog seems to be a very bad choice for estrogenic studies. He gave a very thorough discussion of this.

Dr. Peter Greenwald showed very clearly certain relationships between estrogens and human cancer. Some of his work was questioned by various epidemiologists in the room, but basically they agreed with his findings. This is an example, again, particularly in the case of estrogens and the offspring of mothers that had received stilbestrol. In looking at his data, I was not as convinced that stilbestrol caused these changes in the vagina of the daughters of women which had received stillbestrol. I've said this belongs publicly, and I say it again. There are actually very few cases that really prove the point, less than 100, but the brush is painted broadly and people talk about thousands of cases. It's not so. The question of whether there are changes in the reproductive system of men is even more open to question, in my view. Based upon the data that I have seen and examined there seems to be some causal relationship, but it's not as serious as one might expect. The fact that you can prove even 10 cases related epidemiologically this way is an important discovery of a principle, but I don't like to see it blown up out of proportion so that every woman in American is now wondering: "Did the doctor give me stilbestrol?" The odds are he did in those days. You know it's a paradox; these children now are grown up and maybe have vaginal carcinoma due to the treatment of their mothers, but you can look at it the other way. Maybe they wouldn't be here at all if it weren't for the treatment with stilbestrol, and it's a half of one and a half of another whether should you not be born at all or be born and have a carcinoma which can be treated and cured. The cure rate is high. I wish Dr. Robert Furman was here to discuss this. It's an interesting question, but the paper was good and presented very clearly.

The paper by Dr. Clemmesen on phenobarbital and its epidemiology is a classic. He updated his work and responded very well to the questions of the other epidemiologists and people in the audience. He pointed out once again that he could not find any causal relationship between a known inducer in animals (phenobarbital) and human experience based on some 35 to 40 years of coverage in thousands of people. This work of Dr. Clemmesen is classic in the sense that it's one of the few times we have had the data that he has accumulated, and is continuing to accumulate, to show us the way chemicals may differ between animals and man. The presentation by Dr. Wynder clearly demonstrates that a causal relationship exists between cigarette smoke and lung cancer. It's why we have it on the program. But there is no animal evidence of any single (or even multiple) chemical that shows what there is in cigarette smoke, that causes cancer.

This is an example, the reverse of which is, let's say, DDT. It has been beautifully shown by many people including Tomatis and others in my own laboratory, that a high dose of DDT produces hepatic nodules, some of which break down and produce a cancer, perhaps not related to the chemical at all, but as secondary changes that have occurred in the cells and tissues. But when you go to man there is absolutely no evidence that DDT ever caused a cancer. With smoking you've got just the reverse. Human experience has proven cancer occurs, but animal data is still lacking. This is the kind of thing that this meeting was supposed to bring out, and I think it has. Nothing happens in the rat or monkeys with DDT. The only species in which anything happens is the mouse, and certain strains of mice produce these hepatic nodules. In the study done by the Cancer Institute in Lyon, rats produced nothing, and other strains of mice produced nothing, it's only the strain that Tomatis used that produced the nodules. The Moscow group found nothing, the Milano group found nothing, but the Lyon group found in mice a dose-response and some cancer in the higher dose group.[1]

The issue is smoking causes cancer in man and not animals, while with DDT or dieldrin the animal data is positive in terms of dose-relationships and lesions but there is no human counterpart of the data.

This is the issue of the day in my view. Why should we believe the data from the mouse alone? Why should a regulatory agency believe the mouse which has a different metabolism of the chemical in almost every case from that of the rat, monkey, or man. And yet we base everything on the fact that a lesion was produced.

Dr. Wynder presented much interesting data and made a great plea that what should now be created in his country are environmental carcinogenesis

---

[1]Recently, the National Cancer Institute has stated that DDT is not a carcinogen in mice or rats.

centers. And who can deny that he's right? The question is how do you do it, and how do you implement it? He made the case very strongly.

Carcinogens in food as discussed by Dr. Kolbye was one of the outstanding and provocative speeches of the day. In fact, it led the audience to cheer him when he finished. What he did was simply to point out the myths, the fallacies, and the problems of a regulator who is also a scientist and a lawyer. I think his forthright presentation will be read by many, many people for years to come. He concluded very simply that we need more information. We need more data related to man, and how to get that is the issue of the day.

Dr. Selikoff, in his usual fashion, presented an extremely informative and delightful paper. He waved his flag just as I would wave my flag, and his interest is in better working conditions, better factory controls, and better protection of the population. No one can deny that he is an outstanding proponent of this type of philosophy. He presented some of the old ways that epidemiologists studied things and the new ways, and it turned out that they're not that far apart; some of the old methods still persist.

Dr. Lyon talked about alcohol, and obviously he was a very conservative man. He did not attempt to scare anybody by saying that alcohol as such produced or caused cancer. It may, but the point was in conjunction with other things that the evidence, based on epidemiology such as that applied to smoking, seemed to indicate that if you're an alcoholic and a heavy smoker, this would produce something in addition to what either alone might do. It was a provocative paper and certainly anyone who has worked with alcohol over the years knows that it's a potent drug, and I call it a drug deliberately. It has great and profound metabolic effects on the tissue. Why shouldn't it? It's a dehydrating fluid of the first order, used by chemists and pathologists for years!

Then we had the classic paper by Dr. Kensler. Charlie told me that this was the first time in ten years he had talked so much at a meeting. He commented, "It must have been a great meeting, because I felt relaxed and could talk freely among friends." And from Charlie Kensler, I think that's a compliment to all of us. He showed the remarkable work that's been done over the years to try and find the key factor in cigarette smoke that causes cancer, and of course he couldn't do it any more than anybody else. Whether it's benzo(a)-pyrene or not, nobody really knows. More work has been done on benzo(a)-pyrene to prove it to be the causative agent in cigarette smoking than I think on any other chemical for any disease that I know of. And yet the point is, you can't prove it. His presentation was more than just an animal model for tobacco safety. It showed how one could systematically go about trying to find the needle in the haystack, the true causal agent of a disease. I think he did it very well, and we were very pleased to have him present it.

Dr. Hammond talked in the afternoon about tobacco epidemiology, and let us say he is a master. He is one of the real founding fathers of modern epidemiology, and some of the things he said were very provocative and indicated how people in the animal field could perhaps benefit by making their experimental approach more like the approach of the epidemiologist. I think this can be done, and I think it's a very exciting way to do it. It will certainly lead to much discussion. He said to me after the meeting, and I hope he'll forgive me if I repeat it, "You know, there's nothing new in the meeting you had; I did this 25 years ago. But my meeting was a complete failure." He said, "The toxicologists talked to themselves and tried to convince the epidemiologists how good they were, and the epidemiologists did the same back to the toxicologists." He continued, "Your meeting was outstanding because we talked to one another, we didn't get angry, and maybe we all profited by it." It was a nice remark from a grand person.

Dr. Cranmer summed up the basic problems. He showed some of the issues worldwide, what the problems were, and how cancer was increasing in certain countries and in certain areas of some countries and that certain kinds of cancer seemed prevalent in certain areas, even in some counties in the United States. This is a big puzzle, and it almost leads one to believe that there is a question of chemical carcinogenesis in an area.

Dr. Peter Greenwald has done a lot of work in New York State on the distribution in the various counties of cancer. And it's easy to say, "Oh boy, it's chemicals that are doing it," but it isn't that easy. There are all kinds of genetic factors, families marrying within family groups, the genetic background groups, or people from Europe who congregated in one township, so that genetic factors are involved as well as chemical factors. And too glibly people are apt to say, "Well, if this area produced a lot of leukemias, therefore it's a chemical that caused it." This is still to be proven to my satisfaction. There's no doubt chemicals play a role, but there are other factors; this is the point. And I think this came out very clearly in Dr. Cranmer's paper. He went on to show the kinds of studies that can be done to evaluate the pros and cons of extrapolation to man, and I think his paper in its entirety presented the facts to us so that we could understand them.

I hope in the next half-hour we can make some further statements concerning today's remarks.

Final Discussion

DR. CLAYSON: Thank you very much, Dr. Coulston. Dr. Clemmesen, would you like to make your remarks at this stage please?

DR. CLEMMESEN: I must apologize if some of my remarks, in trying to propose some positive things that can be done, may give an impression of a negative attitude. It may be advantageous to consider some the things that really could be done and are in reach.

Some years ago, 40 years ago, I think, Mellanby had some funds to examine the effects of diet on cancer. He had to use mice, because rats didn't respond to carcinogens, and since he was a practical man and wanted to do something useful with what money there might be left, he took 120 mice and subdivided them into groups fed on brains, spleen, kidney, liver, etc. To his unpleasant surprise he discovered that those which were fed on liver had more cancer of the skin than the others. These were the days of the antipernicious anemia factor in the liver and this looked interesting. But some bright fellow on his staff found out that perhpas it was the fat in the liver that did the trick. So the dietary factor disappeared. And what was more, when they smeared the skin of rats in which, as we all know, the epidermis is more like that of man than mouse cells, then they could also produce cancer in rats.

So what was this? Is fat now a cocarcinogen? It is a modifying factor, but it may be useful to define such statements, perhaps, in a more uniform language, so that we know where we are. This might also do away with some of the differences which we are prone to ascribe to dietary factors, and others to species differences.

We are in the position in which numerous active chemicals are thrown on the market, and the reason why so many are carcinogenic is that factories prefer very reactive compounds. That leaves us not only with large numbers of compounds, but also with the fact that we are testing them on animals and on man. We can deal with their metabolites, and that gives a wide range of questions.

We have, whether we like it or not, three possible ways of proceeding. We have cell and tissue studies, we can study animals, and we can study man. And the cells have, after all, some advantages. They show things rapidly and there is no difficulty with numbers. We may even use human cells, and it is in that field I think that too little has been done; and too little has also been done on tissue cultures, not only cell cultures but tissue cultures. Since, according to modern philosophies, changes in the nuclei of the cells are a common factor in cancer, it may be a very important thing whether we like it or not. We prefer, of course, to use animals, and here it is gratifying to know that the demands for large numbers are not as bad as they are sometimes believed to be. But when we speak about rodents we have to do with a set of metabolites which may not be identical to those in man; this is a most important thing to bear in mind.

I think it might be more logical to subdivide into rodents, women, and man, according to what was presented yesterday. There's such a wide knowledge of the effect of hormones that it should really be possible to compare directly the differences in hormonal behavior of mammary cancer in women and in mice. As you all know, mammary cancer is more frequent among mice who have bred, whereas in women it is more frequent among those who have not had children.

This is one of the factors. Another most important factor is that both the cells and the animals give us results at once, whereas experience from epidemiology refers to things that happened 25 years ago. And what is more, it is extremely difficult to study more than two factors at a time, and we do know that we are living in a "sea of carcinogens." So this is a most serious limitation to epidemiology, and there are others which are inherently problems; the true latent period is very difficult to define in man, also because of cocarcinogens and environmental factors. To that come things that could be eliminated at once. Now the legal difficulties: we have legal difficulties coming up in your and in various countries. The computer scare is producing difficulties in obtaining information from civil records, which are just as important as the records of cancer patients. This is not always realized, and as Dr. Wynder pointed out, there are even more difficulties coming up with people, that you have to request through various authorities before you can start at all. There, I think, physicians could be of considerable help.

It is really too bad, as I can see in my own hospital, that cancer patients are admitted without any mention in the case record of their smoking habits. That ought to be obligatory in any case record. Of course we have, furthermore, the difficulties involved in having death certificates which are thought to refer only to the patients that were not cured.

All these things could, and should, be taken up with lawyers and perhaps politicians. I have proposed that it should be within the authority of medical authorities or clinicians of chemical works to impose upon the factory or laboratory the duty to keep medical records for all the cases. Such an obvious measure has been sidetracked, but this could be done just as the situation is now.

I think that this meeting has been very, very useful in laying down the difficulties with which we are confronted. Thank you.

DR. CLAYSON: I would now like to ask for comments from the floor. If you have any gripes or anything to praise about this meeting, I think that's one type of comment. The other type is if you would like to see any positive statement come out of this meeting. Now is the last chance to state it. I'll take you first, Dr. Mofidi.

DR. MOFIDI: I was struck by what Dr. Coulston said about Dr. Mays' paper, which, of course, made a very deep impression on all of us. Dr. Coulston said it looked a little strange that there should be so many cases of hepatoma in Dr. Mays' area. I think this is a very good question and of great practical value.

I, as a clinician, cannot accept the fact that in so many other areas and countries with good hospitals so many hepatomas would have been missed; therefore, it may well be that there is a cluster. If this is so, we ought to find out why because we might be able to do something about it.

There might well be a cofactor; otherwise this would be difficult to explain. I believe that it would not be too difficult to find out in many other places what the incidence of hepatomas really is; I believe that this is very good area to work in for both the epidemiologist and the experimentalist, because they could try to find in their animals what is what. Thank you very much.

DR. CLAYSON: Thank you very much indeed. I don't know whether Dr. Mahboubi is still here. I think not, but his problem in trying to persuade the commissions to tell him when these cases arise, and remember they don't automatically go to any registry, would indicate to me that these cases probably exist in other parts of the country, but because nobody has shown an interest in them at all they just haven't surfaced. I think our total number of hepatoma cases, before the American College of Surgeons started looking into it, was about 100;

this number has nearly quadrupled and I don't think I would necessarily presume there was a cofactor. There may be a susceptible population. But this is still very much a matter of debate and a very worthwhile point to look into.

DR. BLAIR: I would like to speak in the position of an industrial scientist and as an administrator. I believe this conference has been extremely worthwhile, and there are a few comments I would like to make because while you see the world in a certain way, many of us who represent your scientific colleagues working in chemical concerns see it somewhat differently.

Many of us are subjected to legal action. I myself have been subpoenaed. I have been forced into kangaroo courts dealing with carcinogenicity. Today we are in a society which is as caught up in cancer as we were caught up in Communism 20 years ago. Your subject is the subject of all this activity. Either you will use your knowledge and lead, or the lawyers and the political arena will take over and you will no longer be in control.

Action such as that of the Consumer Protection Agency is banning the tris (2,3-dibromopropyl) phosphate, in effect, essentially certified the Ames test. I can assure you that probably every agency now will be asking for more and more data of this type.

It has been reported that OSHA's action on the *14 carcinogens* was such that the University of Minnesota administration has now banned all 14 carcinogens in its laboratories. There is an attempt in New Jersey to ban all 14 carcinogens from that state. Of course, these actions bring about terribly difficult problems.

I was forced into a kangaroo court by politicians over a product which the Dow Company said had no activity at all, and that was a polybrominated biphenyl. The only purpose of bringing me there under a subpoena was to pound to death the company involved, on the following day. So this is the type of world that really we're living in and I am truly greatly concerned about it, because I'm fearful that many of us in the scientific arena, when confronted with political pressures and legal action, will also find ourselves in a difficult situation. Three weeks ago I was the only scientist attending a meeting of 150 lawyers. Their subject was: How do we deal with the toxic substances control act? I would like to know how many in this room have ever read that document. Would you hold your hands up? Very good. I think maybe a third of you have, but I can assure you that that document will have a profound effect upon how you practice chemistry in your laboratory.

Enough for the comments, as far as this meeting is concerned. I am particularly interested in epidemiology because I believe there is much information available within our organization, and we could get to it if we knew how to utilize it. These are very, very difficult problems. When I listen to you talk about the problems of hospitals I think of another problem. Just imagine now that under EEO we'll be forced to *allow* women of childbearing age to work in a carcinogen plant within American industry.

You talk about the effect of birth control pills. What about this new dimension? I'm concerned that as in many sciences we get so involved in the details of the past and in mechanistic studies—and I used to do a lot of this in the organophosphate field where I find it very stimulating and exciting—but decisions are being made which will have a profound impact in the future such as those I have mentioned: women in the work place. Just a few minutes ago it was said we were living in a "sea of carcinogens." That very type of statement absolutely polarizes the situation regarding insurance rates, delayed retirement effects, or exposures. Do they go on for two hours at a time, what's the level, etc.?

These are the problems that we're facing today. I think that we have got to come to grips with the world of today, and while it's interesting to speculate on the world of the past, if we continue to concentrate only on that we'll be like anthropologists. We will not be dealing with what we must actually deal with, and that is the multitude of chemicals that we have and the multitudes of laws that have been swept in on us, and while I would think that this should promote the need for more toxicologists, I can assure you it's promoting the need for more lawyers.

Our hiring of legal talent is proceeding at a more rapid rate than the hiring of scientists. However, on the positive side, I can assure you that I think the industry will respond very positively. I believe it has done a fairly good job in most of the areas it has attempted to deal with; it will move more rapidly than most universities and others in molding together multidisciplinary task forces to deal with these kinds of problems. This has been its strength, and I'm sure there are many industries represented here today which are putting together toxicological groups, epidemiological groups, medical groups, and analytical groups as teams. This has been a great strength of the chemical industry. They can report back, hopefully at future meetings, more than they have at this meeting. We need new and more rapid means of analysis and new methodologies. Dr. Coulston talked about this as did others—how to get data more rapidly and utilize it.

We must find ways to come to grips with some of our colleagues who polarize the situation by their use of information. There's a great tendency for many to play to the presses, and even just the statement that 80% of all carcinogens are environmentally induced has cost millions and millions of dollars in this country.

Much of our resources is directed now into defensive, legalistic trial types of activities. I think this is a loss of our talents today in our company, and we're still pouring in millions of dollars yearly to defend a low volume herbicide because it was used in Vietnam.

I do want to thank all, especially Dr. Coulston, who saw to it that a few of us in the industry were invited and also thank those of you who put together this program. I certainly would like to see it repeated and expanded to include a current problem that really we're living with, such as I just mentioned. Thank you.

DR. MILLER: In relation to what Dr. Blair has just said, there are things I thought about quite a bit and which I would really like to ask some of the epidemiologists. We so often hear this remark that we're "living in a sea of carcinogens," but cancer really isn't a new disease, is it? I believe that mummies have been discovered who had cancer.

Can the epidemiologists tell us how much cancer there was around about 1800, 1750, or 1776? That's an important date in American history. How much cancer really is caused by the new chemicals introduced into the environment? I believe absolutely that the majority of cancer is caused by chemicals but I'm reminded of a well-known statement that Eric Boyland, the English cancerologist made, that I always show on my slides. I haven't got them with me. He said that 80% to 90% of cancer is caused by chemicals, some of which are exogenous and some of which are endogenous. We don't know how much of each. So what I'm really asking the epidemiologist is, just how much more cancer is there, since we had a chemical industry, than there was before?

DR. HAMMOND: That can be answered, not with any exactness, but as for data, there is plenty. The best set of records I have seen is in a hospital in a small town south of Toledo (Spain). All of the hospital's records from about 1450 on have been kept. Part is written in Arabic, and if somebody knows how to read it I'd like him to translate the records sometime; the rest is in Latin. The extraordinary part is the part that's in Latin. Almost the same terminology was used that we are use today, and there was a large number of cases that were beautifully described. They didn't have the histology, of course. They didn't have our modern methods, but in reading those case histories you have no real doubt at all what it was. There was plenty of cancer.

DR. MAGEE: May I make the comment on the "80 or 90% environmental cancer rate?" That 100% is environmental? It is. One hundred percent is also genetic. It is. Everything that happens to any living organism results from an interaction between hereditary factors and environmental factors; all of it is environmental. Now there is considerable evidence that for most cancers, whether the person gets them or not, are much more caused by environment than they are by heredity. But what does the word environment mean? The only meaningful environment in terms of cancer is environment at the cellular level, not just what you eat or what gets to certain tissues. We're dealing with clones of cells. And a very large part of that environmental factor is endogenous in terms of hormones, in terms of metabolic reactions, and what not. When I have talked about environment I meant all that: I was talking about environment at the cellular level. I didn't mean the environment that we are sitting in in this room. And this has been very, very badly misunderstood. I have told the press this time and time again, and I repeated it at the Science Writers' Meeting. But that doesn't make a very good story.

DR. MILLER: Well, I was going to make this comment before Dr. Blair and Dr. Magee made their comments, and I think I'll still go ahead and do it. Dr. Clemmesen raised some interesting points, and I agree with him on many things. However, I think he made one very unfortunate statement, that is, that "we live in a sea of carcinogens." That's one of those half-truths. It's a catchy phrase, and it's easy to make hay on it in the public media. And it's one of those phrases that you have to expand to make it resemble the real situation. True, we *do* live in a very dilute sea of compounds, some of which, with sufficient dosage, in time would induce cancer in experimental animals and in man.

We have no choice. And, of course, that kind of thing is not going to get quoted in the media. As Dr. Magee pointed out, tumors have been seen in fossils of prehistoric animals and in mummies. Dr. Hammond just pointed out how prevalent cancer has been in the past industrialization. We've got to get across to the public somehow the idea that not *every* chemical is carcinogenic and that dose-response is an important aspect of carcinogenesis. I think it's very unfortunate to repeat this phrase that "we live in a sea of carcinogens."

DR. COULSTON: You know, I'm quoting Dr. Tomatis (WHO) when I say there are approximately 1,600 known chemical carcinogens for mice and rodents in general. But there are only approximately 15 known to ever cause cancer in man, such as the β-naphthylamines and the estrogens, and so on. Most of us could name most of the compounds involved—alkylating agents, and so on. Now this is an astonishing thing. If regulatory agencies were to do their job and ban these 1,600 compounds, then, I think, we would be in great trouble both scientifically as well as economically. The fact is there are only 15 known carcinogens in man. Where does this magical figure that 80% of cancer is due to environmental chemicals come from? I wish Herman Kraybill was here because he gives a remarkable story on that, and I'll try to get him to write it up for the proceedings.

I heard on the platform of the Society of Toxicology meeting one time a very eminent man from the National Cancer Institute who started his talk by saying 60% of all cancers was due to chemicals. Before he ended the talk a half hour later, it was up to 90%. He went from 60 to 90% in the same talk. And the truth is there are no data to say 80% or 60% or 90%. It's simply based on a statement that came from England that then was amplified, and everybody uses this statement; there is no validation of this statement. Thank you, Mr. Chairman.

DR. CLAYSON: Thank you, Dr. Coulston. I think if we were to use the term "environmental factor" concerning carcinogenesis, one would have very little difficulty in getting somewhere in that range between 60 and 90%. I've tried this exercise on the British male population pursuing immigrant data which suggested environmental factors, to determine certain types of human cancer and I was, like you, amazed when without working for more than half an hour on the problem, I came up with a figure of 50% to 60% of cancer dependent on environmental factors of one sort or another.

This includes about 80% of lung cancer-related tumors, things like the colon where we have environmental factors, and other tissues. But I think we must make it absolutely clear at every stage that cancer is not due to specific industrial chemicals as far as we can tell at this stage, or specific anything else.

DR. MAGEE: I'm going to sound, Dr. Miller, as if I'm violently disagreeing with you, but in a moment you'll see that I'm not. We do live in a sea of chemicals—of carcinogens—in the sense of promoters. We're all exposed to cosmic rays and we're all exposed to background radiation. As long as there's been fire on earth there's been benzo(a)pyrene, and German chemists tell me that benzo(a)pyrene is necessary for cell growth in plants. To get rid of benzo(a)-pyrene, we have to get rid of plants, and we also have to get rid of our food supply, which would not be exactly beneficial. My own very strong feeling at the present time is that exposure to large amounts of individual promoters has almost nothing to do with cancer in the general human population at all, except in a very few instances, and these are mostly industrial workers.

I do not believe for one moment that the key to the cancer problem will be found in a search for promoters. I have a totally different theory of carcinogenicity from the one generally held. At the next meeting of this group I think I'll present you with some data and some computer models of what's going on.

DR. ZAPP: The problem that Dr. Miller has referred to, and that we've just been discussing, and I say this is a problem not a conclusion, was stated very clearly, I think, in some words uttered by Ralph Nader. He made three statements which went as follows: It is now generally agreed among experts that 60% to 90% of all cancer is caused by environmental factors. Second statement: Industries are introducing thousands of new and untested chemicals into our environment every year. And this is not true. Third statement: We should stop calling it environmental cancer and call it corporate cancer. Now I think that leads us from the fact to the absurd, but it's the *absurd* that's causing us the problem.

DR. CLAYSON: Thank you. I'm told by Dr. Coulston that we've got to finish very quickly. Dr. Mrak.

DR. MRAK: Thank you very much. I felt this meeting was terrific, and all the way along I've been wondering, how do you get this information to the decision-makers? I'm a little bit involved in the $5 million study that the National Research Council made with respect to the decision-making process and EPA. There are 7 volumes, and I think I've read 3 of them so far. You might want to get them. I don't think they've helped me a bit. I think if we hold another meeting or two, we ought to get some of the people who are heavily involved in the decision-making process to listen in and if you do that, have those people who get so complicated that they go over the heads of many people summarize with a simple statement that even a lawyer will understand. Thank you.

Concluding Statement: David B. Clayson

Thank you, Dr. Mrak. I'm going to take the chairman's privilege now and make a few comments of my own. I'll not allow anybody to answer them. I must confess, Dr. Coulston, that on the first day of this meeting I had the feeling of disappointment, and to some extent, despair, that we weren't really going to get off the ground. This feeling completely evaporated during the past 2 days, and I think the meeting has been highly successful.

The purposes of the conference were to: (1) bring together epidemiologists, toxicologists and those interested in mechanisms to discuss progress in their own areas; (2) to discuss possible ways in which joint endeavors concerned with the definition and solution of public health problems may be forwarded and (3) to define the nature of the more important public health problems in the cancer area.

Each discipline has its own contribution to make. Epidemiologists are concerned primarily with disease in man and what causes it. Their major limitation is that they cannot perform until there has been effective human exposure and they can count the bodies. Toxicologists have two areas of interest—both requiring the use of surrogate species—first, the confirmation of the results of present exposures, usually and most effectively, those already demonstrated epidemiologically in man; and, second, the prediction of what may be carcinogenically effective in man if allowed to enter the environment. Those concerned with mechanisms have in the past been a relatively exclusive club of playboys, mainly concerned with pursuing their own academic interests. Their great strides in recent years will, I am sure, elevate them to the forefront of the battle, because it is through their efforts that ultimately we may be able to consider classes of chemicals rather than having to battle with a never-ending and overwhelming succession of single materials whose individual properties must be painstakingly evaluated one by one.

In support of this main phalanx of talent are several other cohorts. The most vital is the "astute clinician" whose inquiring mind associates the appearance of a series of tumors with a possible causative factor. We had an excellent talk from Dr. Mays on oral contraceptives and benign liver tumors as an example of what the astute clinician can do. Then there are the regulators whose function is to translate the results of the field and laboratory workers into action to protect the public. Despite many fears that regulators are merely rather dull officers of government, interpreting laws mechanically in an attempt to deprive the general public of its pleasures, and industry of its profits, I think Dr. Kolbye clearly defined their dilemma, perched as they are between a paranoid public and publicity-prone politicians. The final support group yet to come into position are the psychologists and/or publicity men whose task will be to persuade the public that they enjoy being deprived of potentially dangerous, but pleasurable, items or activities, such as cigarette smoking, a harmful diet, saccharin, or red dye No. 2, to name but a few.

Organizationally, this multidisciplinary force is disjointed. Dr. Wynder suggested that environmental cancer centers be organized to bring together the various disciplines needed to make a real impact on environmental carcinogenesis. I think we all realize the benefits of such an approach at the national or international level, although I personally have some reservations about bringing any but the most carefully selected clinician into a chemical group, and I do not

409

know where the necessary new expertise would come from. We have at this meeting, I think, experienced some difficulty in appreciating the significance of each others' efforts, despite the very limited range of expertise represented here.

Dr. Wynder also emphasized the importance of studying the etiology of common human tumors such as those of the colon, in which he used the work of his own Institute as an example, as well as studies on the breast and the prostate. He introduced the concept of metabolic epidemiology as the way to approach these difficult problems and as a way to identify high risk groups. High-risk groups would make feasible the economic introduction of cancer detection and control programs.

Two other points have also come from this meeting: (1) a rapid cancer prevention information service is needed, which perhaps could derive from the NCI/ SRI CIDAC program; and (2) should NCI and other federal staff be subject to similar peer review, as are their scientific colleagues outside the government, as far as intramural research is concerned? All these ideas derived some support and some reservations from the meeting as a whole.

What else should I say without repeating every single word uttered during this meeting? Dr. Shubik, in opening, drew attention to many shady areas in single-compound environmental carcinogenesis, ranging from the necessary balance between the scientific credibility of decisions which have a vast economic impact on the community, to the desirability (or otherwise) of a safer cigarette. Dr. Hammond's brilliant exposition of the mortality consequences of even a safer cigarette excited me. However, while we may attempt to estimate the health benefits in billions of dollars/decade of less harmful cigarettes, I have on several occasions noted a complete failure to consider the increased costs of maintaining an aging population, advancing in years and senile. A complete and comfortable retirement at 60 or 65 is likely to be an early casualty. Dr. Shubik also mentioned two points which hid beneath the surface for most of the meeting: the question of carcinogenesis modification and the problem of dose-relatedness of carcinogens. The first of these, if we go beyond the often quoted phorbol ester, is sufficient for several more meetings. The second, dose-relatedness and extrapolation, can produce more heat than light, as I think became briefly evident yesterday.

Dr. Kraybill in a talk of great wisdom, drew attention to the varied problems of "maximum tolerated dose" and the occurrence of thresholds, both needing frank and full discussion at this time. There were, of course, areas of frank disagreement, as with chemically-induced cancer immunology, where Drs. Zapp and Magee appeared to be at odds.

I was sorry that our discussions on chlorinated pesticides were not more incisive. We heard interesting papers on recent metabolic work in this area, but failed to come to any conclusion about the consequences of this information. I suspect it is their persistence rather than their carcinogenicity which is the real environmental problem.

I can only congratulate Drs. Miller and Conney for the satisfaction and intellectual stimulation given by their three papers on mechanisms of action of carcinogens. We always expect something good, and were not disappointed. However, as we have several times stressed in the course of this meeting, there is a need to explain to the layman (whether a scientist of another discipline or a reasonably educated member of the public) what this means, and I would ask them both to consider this additional chore as an important extra task vitally necessary to the maintenance of the impetus they have given to the intellectual satisfaction of the study of carcinogenesis.

Our discussions on problems related to drugs were to me particularly satisfying. Some implications, for example, of Dr. Greenwald's paper were worrying. Drugs, especially estrogens, could approach cigarette smoking as causes of human cancer. The regulatory authorities clearly recognize that risks have to be taken with drugs, but I think they are still unsure of the level of risk the public will tolerate in this area. The temptation not to take even apparently reasonable risks, when you have the feeling that your families' economic standard of living may depend on it, must be exceedingly great.

Dr. Wynder yesterday gave us the background to his suggestion that the largest problems need most urgent attention. The worst must be first. Nevertheless, however admirable this sentiment is, scientists, too, must make a living in a rapidly hardening world. A balance has to be struck between the possible (i.e., the achievable) and the desirable. Even Dr. Wynder stated that it was a good day if he had prolonged a single human life by persuading someone to stop smoking. Perhaps scientists may be permitted some satisfaction with progress on smaller, but real, problems and, as for example, with cancer related to alcoholic beverages which may be due to a carcinogenesis modifying factor or to real carcinogens present in liquor.

I'm not trying to say that we should not work on colon cancer, prostate and breast cancer, but really to make progress I think we must all admit we need ideas as well as just experiments.

I think Dr. Selikoff introduced us to a very difficult area: the modes of action for different carcinogens. He illustrated this with his own work with cigarette smoking and asbestos. He mentioned uranium and asbestos, and there must be thousands of other examples in the environment, which if we only knew something about them, might make the tasks of the regulators a lot easier.

I indicated yesterday afternoon my own unhappiness with the present efforts to extrapolate from high doses of carcinogens and low doses of carcinogens. I quite realize that the regulatory agencies have a terribly difficult problem here. They feel that they must make their decisions appear scientific if they are only really pseudoscientific.

My own feeling for the approach to this problem now, rather than sometime in the distant future when we know better science, is that we might think about the economic and health aspects of some of these problems and lookfor the best technologically achievable levels of some of the carcinogens we cannot dispense with, rather than the setting of artificial levels.

You must remember that technology hopefully will continue to improve in the same way that it has in the past 50 years. And that the technologically best level at this stage does not mean that we are stuck with it forever, but merely that we have something which can be worked on, which can be improved on if we find, or we believe, that it is necessary, and one in which we could probably convert some of our worst problems to lesser problems without causing the great economic disruptions which some decisions appear to be doing at the moment.

This is a personal view. I don't know whether or not it's the right view, but I think we do need in this area not only good science, not only good law, but just one tremendous amount of common sense.

The one question which we did not discuss was what to do about carcinogens which for one reason or another we need in, or cannot remove from, the environment. In some cases, such as aflatoxin, we are for practical reasons forced to set levels too near those biologically effective in rodents. With others, we may be able to set socially acceptable limits, especially if we help to inform the public about the meaning of the risks we are all taking.

Dr. Upholt explained one way of setting such levels which I feel, although convenient, is so scientifically unsound that it can only lead to future trouble. I much prefer the concept of the use of the best available technology consistent with economic resources to reduce the levels of unavoidable carcinogens to a pragmatic minimum and the use of such pragmatically set levels as present but revisable standards. This was the approach taken with radiation, and if I am correct, I think the health record of the atomic energy industry (excluding uranium mining and processing), which worked under this principle has been more acceptable than some would have us believe.

We will close now. I would like to thank Drs. Coulston and Cranmer, Dr. Mahboubi, the speakers, Mrs. Ruth Magee and her staff, Mrs. Rose Houle, the hotel staff for all they have done for us. Particularly, I wish to thank Dr. Coulston, for all of us, for conceiving the idea of this meeting and for being such a wonderful host while we were at this meeting. I hope this will not be the last time we shall meet to discuss this important interface between disciplines.

Index

*For individual chemical compounds and groups thereof, *see* also under the headings Chemical carcinogens, Mutagenicity, and Xenobiotic metabolism.

Carcinogenicity testing *(cont.)*
  dosages of chemical pesticides
    appropriate for, 39
  dose-response relationships in, 22, 40-48
  extreme value models in, 381
  linear extrapolation in, 43, 381, 383,
    391, 393, 411
  nutritional factors in, 24-27, 380
  pharmacohinetics in, 40, 45, 105, 307,
    387
  probit models in, 381
  statistical evaluation of results of, 21,
    32-33, 43, 46-47, 256, 261, 311-
    12, 316, 334, 362-64, 372-73,
    380
Case histories, proper recording of, 129-30
Center for Disease Control, 232
Charcoal-broiled beef, effects on drug
    metabolism, 60-63, 380
Chemical carcinogens, suspected or
    demonstrated
  2-acetylaminofluorene (AA7), 126, 129,
    136, 139-41, 253, 267, 380
  2-AAF-N-Sulfate, 139-40
  N-acetoxy-AA7, 141
    O-glucuronide of, 141
  1'-acetoxysafrole, 146
  actinomycin D, 137
  adriamycin, 137
  aflatoxims, 12, 27, 105, 136, 139, 147,
    276, 315, 385, 387
  antilipidemic agents, 272
  arsenic compounds, 35-36, 53
  asbestos, 14, 124, 231, 334-37, 378,
    385, 411
  azo dyes, 56, 77, 122, 133
  benzene, 335
  benzidine, 378
  benzo(a) anthrocene, 57, 172
  benzo(a) pyrene, and metabolites thereof,
    8, 108-15, 123, 136, 161-72,
    266, 332-33
  beryllium, 228
  β-blocking agents, 272
  cadmium, 228
  carbozole, 9
  carbon tetrachloride, 43, 47, 103
  chlondecone (Kepone), 231
  chlormadinone, 272
  chlornaphazin, 186-87, 329, 331
  chloroform, 34, 43, 47, 388
  chromates, 228

Chemical carcinogens *(cont.)*
  chrysene, 175
  cobalt, 228
  croton oil, 122
  cycasin, 136
  cyclamate, 31, 54, 75, 396
  DDD, 101
  DDT, 11, 31, 41, 44-45, 53, 100-4,
    125, 127, 131, 315, 386, 400,
    410
  dibenzo(a,h)anthracene, 57, 175
  dibenzo(c,g)carbazole, 9
  dieldrin, 43, 92, 400
  diethylstilbestrol (DES) 29, 31, 130,
    188-89, 193, 209-10, 213-20,
    233-37, 268-71, 276, 381, 399
  dimethylaminoazobenzene, 25
  7, 12-dimethyl benzanthracene, and
    derivatives thereof, 174-75
  dioxane, 32
  dioxins, 26
  drugs, 129-30, 185-94
  17β-estradiol, 214, 220-22
  estrogens, 189, 199-201, 212, 226-27,
    267-68, 275-76, 279, 399, 407,
    411
  estrone, 133
  ethinyl estradiol, 201, 212
  ethionine, 136
  ethyl alcohol, 293, 319-24
  2, 7-FAA, 41
  flurocarbon compounds, 79, 82
  griseofulvin, 11, 136, 277-78, 338
  hair dyes, 131
  hexachlorobenzene, 118
  hycanthone, 192, 379
  hydrozines, 9
  N-hydroxy-AA7, 139
  1'-hydroxysafrole, 93, 146-47
  in automobile exhausts, 107-13
  in birth control pills, 11-12, 190, 197-
    201, 207, 268
  in charcoal-broiled beef, 60
  in cigarette smoke, 9-10, 57-59, 115-16,
    119, 126, 231, 287, 401
  in coal tar, 7-9, 57, 107, 115, 333, 341
  in foods, 12, 60, 120-21, 311-16, 401
  inorganic, 35-36, 134, 227-28
  in petroleum fractions, 9, 107-13
  in tobacco tar, 9
  isoniazid, 10-11, 193
  lindane, 41